Respiratory Medicine
Lecture Notes

Respiratory Medicine
Lecture Notes

Stephen J. Bourke

Consultant Physician
Royal Victoria Infirmary
Newcastle upon Tyne;
Honorary Senior Lecturer
Newcastle University

Graham P. Burns

Consultant Physician
Royal Victoria Infirmary
Newcastle upon Tyne;
Honorary Senior Lecturer
Newcastle University

Ninth Edition

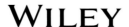

WILEY

This edition first published 2015 © 2015 by John Wiley & Sons, Ltd.

Registered office: John Wiley & Sons, Ltd, The Atrium, Southern Gate, Chichester, West Sussex, PO19 8SQ, UK

Editorial offices: 9600 Garsington Road, Oxford, OX4 2DQ, UK

The Atrium, Southern Gate, Chichester, West Sussex, PO19 8SQ, UK

111 River Street, Hoboken, NJ 07030-5774, USA

For details of our global editorial offices, for customer services and for information about how to apply for permission to reuse the copyright material in this book please see our website at www.wiley.com/wiley-blackwell

Library of Congress Cataloging-in-Publication Data

Bourke, S. J., author.

Lecture notes. Respiratory medicine / Stephen J. Bourke, Graham P. Burns. – Ninth edition.

p. ; cm.

Respiratory medicine

Includes bibliographical references and index.

ISBN 978-1-118-65232-9 (pbk. : alk. paper)

I. Burns, Graham P., author. II. Title. III. Title: Respiratory medicine.

[DNLM: 1. Respiratory Tract Diseases. WF 140]

RC731

616.2 – dc23

2015006394

A catalogue record for this book is available from the British Library.

Wiley also publishes its books in a variety of electronic formats. Some content that appears in print may not be available in electronic books.

Cover image: iStockphoto © sankalpmaya

Set in 8.5/11pt, UtopiaStd by Laserwords Private Limited, Chennai, India
Printed and bound in Malaysia by Vivar Printing Sdn Bhd

1   2015

To Dr R.A.L. Brewis

Contents

Preface

It is now 40 years since the first edition of *Lecture Notes: Respiratory Medicine* was written by our predecessor and colleague, Dr Alistair Brewis.

Alistair Brewis, who sadly died in 2014, was inspirational to generations of students and doctors. He was something of a polymath. As consultant in the Royal Victoria Infirmary, Newcastle, he was a very highly regarded physician. With a natural ability to communicate, his calm, friendly chats with patients were remarkably insightful, putting them at ease as he pieced together the clinical jigsaw. As a teacher, he had the ability to make almost any topic seem surprisingly understandable. Over the years, he inspired many to take up careers in respiratory medicine. Alistair was also an accomplished artist. He illustrated the first edition of *Lecture Notes* with sketches and diagrams that both amused and genuinely facilitated understanding; many have been retained in this ninth edition. As a mentor, he was a reliable source of sage advice, a wise man who understood the human condition.

From its first edition, *Lectures Notes: Respiratory Medicine* was a classic textbook, opening the eyes of generations of students to the special fascinations of the subject. Subsequent editions map the developments in this very broad-ranging specialty, dealing with diseases from cystic fibrosis to lung cancer, COPD to pneumonia, asthma to tuberculosis, sleep disorders to occupational lung diseases.

In the ninth edition, the text has been revised and expanded to provide a concise up-to-date summary of respiratory medicine for undergraduate students and junior doctors preparing for postgraduate examinations. A particular feature of respiratory medicine in recent years has been multidisciplinary team work, utilising the skills from a variety of disciplines to provide the best care for patients with respiratory diseases. This book should be useful to colleagues such as physiotherapists, lung-function physiologists and respiratory nurse specialists. The emphasis of *Lecture Notes: Respiratory Medicine* has always been on information that is useful and relevant to everyday clinical medicine, and the ninth edition remains a patient-based book to be read before and after visits to the wards and clinics where clinical medicine is learnt and practised. As *Lecture Notes: Respiratory Medicine* develops over time, we remain grateful to our teachers and their teachers, and we pass on our evolving knowledge of respiratory medicine to our students and their students.

S.J. Bourke
G.P. Burns

About the Companion Website

This book is accompanied by a companion website:

www.lecturenoteseries.com/Respiratory

The website includes:

- Interactive multiple choice questions
- PDFs of figures from the book
- PDFs of key points from the book
- PDFs of web links from the book

Part 1

Structure and function

Anatomy and physiology of the lungs

The anatomy and physiology of the respiratory system are designed in such a way as to bring air from the atmosphere and blood from the circulation into close proximity across the alveolar capillary membrane. This facilitates the exchange of oxygen and carbon dioxide between the blood and the outside world.

A brief revision of clinically relevant anatomy

Bronchial tree and alveoli

The **trachea** has cartilaginous horseshoe-shaped 'rings' supporting its anterior and lateral walls. The posterior wall is flaccid and bulges forward during coughing. This results in narrowing of the lumen, which increases the shearing force from the moving air on the mucus lying on the tracheal walls.

The trachea divides into the right and left main bronchi at the level of the sternal angle (angle of Louis). The **left main bronchus** is longer than the right and leaves the trachea at a more abrupt angle. The **right main bronchus** is more directly in line with the trachea, so that inhaled material tends to enter the right lung more readily than the left.

The main bronchi divide into **lobar bronchi** (upper, middle and lower on the right; upper and lower on the left) and then **segmental bronchi**, as shown in Fig. 1.1. The position of the lungs in relation to external landmarks is shown in Fig. 1.2. **Bronchi** are airways with cartilage in their walls, and there are about 10 divisions of bronchi beyond the tracheal bifurcation. Smaller airways without cartilage in their walls are referred to as **bronchioles**. **Respiratory bronchioles** are peripheral bronchioles with alveoli in their walls. Bronchioles immediately proximal to alveoli are known as **terminal bronchioles**. In the bronchi, smooth muscle is arranged in a spiral fashion internal to the cartilaginous plates. The muscle coat becomes more complete distally as the cartilaginous plates become more fragmentary.

The epithelial lining is ciliated and includes goblet cells. The cilia beat with a whip-like action, and waves of contraction pass in an organised fashion from cell to cell so that material trapped in the sticky mucus layer above the cilia is moved upwards and out of the lung. This mucociliary escalator is an important part of the lung's defences. Larger bronchi also have acinar mucus-secreting glands in the submucosa, which are hypertrophied in chronic bronchitis.

Alveoli are about 0.1–0.2 mm in diameter and are lined by a thin layer of cells, of which there are two types: type I pneumocytes have flattened processes that extend to cover most of the internal surface of the alveoli; type II pneumocytes are less numerous and contain lamellated structures, which are concerned with the production of surfactant (Fig. 1.3). There is a potential space between the alveolar cells and the capillary basement membrane, which is only apparent in disease states, when it may contain fluid, fibrous tissue or a cellular infiltrate.

Lung perfusion

The lungs receive a blood supply from both the pulmonary and the systemic circulations.

The **pulmonary artery** arises from the right ventricle and divides into left and right pulmonary arteries, which further divide into branches accompanying the bronchial tree. The pulmonary capillary network

Respiratory Medicine Lecture Notes, Ninth Edition. Stephen J. Bourke and Graham P. Burns.
© 2015 John Wiley & Sons, Ltd. Published 2015 by John Wiley & Sons, Ltd.
Companion Website: www.lecturenoteseries.com/Respiratory

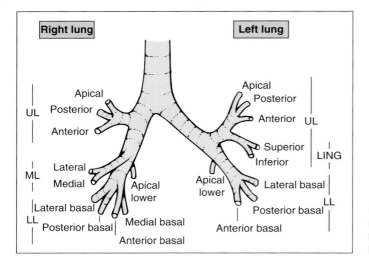

Figure 1.1 Diagram of bronchopulmonary segments. LING, lingula; LL, lower lobe; ML, middle lobe; UL, upper lobe.

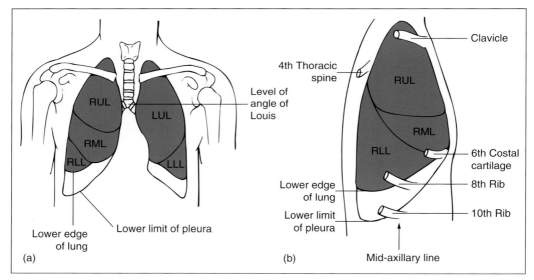

Figure 1.2 Surface anatomy. (a) Anterior view of the lungs. (b) Lateral view of the right side of the chest at resting end-expiratory position. LLL, left lower lobe; LUL, left upper lobe; RLL, right lower lobe; RML, right middle lobe; RUL, right upper lobe.

in the alveolar walls is very dense and provides a very large surface area for gas exchange. The pulmonary venules drain laterally to the periphery of lung lobules and then pass centrally into the interlobular and intersegmental septa, ultimately joining together to form the four main pulmonary veins, which empty into the left atrium.

Several small **bronchial arteries** usually arise from the descending aorta and travel in the outer layers of the bronchi and bronchioles, supplying the tissues of the airways down to the level of the respiratory bronchiole. Most of the blood drains into radicles of the pulmonary vein, contributing a small amount of desaturated blood, which accounts for part of the 'physiological shunt' (blood passing through the lungs without being oxygenated) observed in normal individuals. The bronchial arteries may undergo hypertrophy when there is chronic pulmonary inflammation, and major haemoptysis in diseases such as bronchiectasis or aspergilloma usually arises

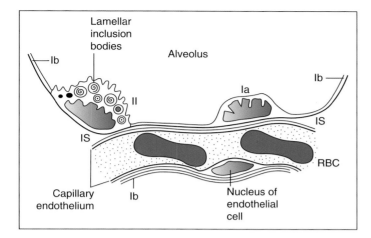

Figure 1.3 Structure of the alveolar wall as revealed by electron microscopy. Ia, type I pneumocyte; Ib, flattened extension of type I pneumocyte covering most of the internal surface of the alveolus; II, type II pneumocyte with lamellar inclusion bodies, which are probably the site of surfactant formation; IS, interstitial space; RBC, red blood corpuscle. Pneumocytes and endothelial cells rest upon thin continuous basement membranes, which are not shown.

from the bronchial rather than the pulmonary arteries and may be treated by therapeutic bronchial artery embolisation. The pulmonary circulation normally offers a much lower resistance and operates at a lower perfusion pressure than the systemic circulation. The pulmonary capillaries may be compressed as they pass through the alveolar walls if alveolar pressure rises above capillary pressure.

Physiology

The core business of the lungs is to bring oxygen into the body and to take carbon dioxide out.

This is brought about by a process best considered in two steps:

1 **Ventilation.** The movement of air in and out of the lungs (between the outside world and the alveoli).
2 **Gas exchange.** The exchange of oxygen and carbon dioxide between the airspace of the alveoli and the blood.

This process continues throughout life, largely unconsciously, coordinated by a centre in the brain stem. The factors that regulate the process, 'the control of breathing', will also be considered here.

Ventilation

To understand this process, we need to consider the muscles that 'drive the pump' and the resistive forces they have to overcome. These forces include the inherent elastic property of the lungs and the resistance to airflow through the bronchi (airway resistance).

The muscles that drive the pump

Inspiration requires muscular work. The diaphragm is the principal muscle of inspiration. At the end of an expiration, the diaphragm sits in a high, domed position in the thorax (Fig. 1.4). To inspire, the strong muscular sheet contracts, stiffens and tends to push

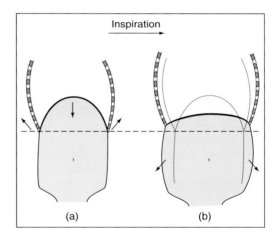

Figure 1.4 Effect of diaphragmatic contraction. Diagram of the ribcage, abdominal cavity and diaphragm showing the position at the end of resting expiration (a). As the diaphragm contracts, it pushes the abdominal contents down (the abdominal wall moves outwards) and reduces pressure within the thorax, which 'sucks' air in through the mouth (inspiration). (b) As the diaphragm shortens and descends, it also stiffens. The diaphragm meets a variable degree of resistance to downward discursion, which forces the lower ribs to move up and outward to accommodate its new position.

the abdominal contents down. There is variable resistance to this downward pressure by the abdomen, which means that in order to accommodate the new shape of the diaphragm, the lower ribs (to which it is attached) also move upwards and outwards. (When airway resistance is present, as in asthma or chronic obstructive pulmonary disease (COPD), the situation is very different; see Chapter 11.) The degree of resistance the abdomen presents can be voluntarily increased by contracting the abdominal muscles; inspiration then leads to a visible expansion of the thorax, rather than a distension of the abdomen (try it). The resistance may also be increased by abdominal obesity. In such circumstances, there is an involuntary limitation to the downward excursion of the diaphragm and, as the potential for upward movement of the ribs is limited, the capacity for full inspiration is diminished. This inability to fully inflate the lungs is an example of a **restrictive ventilatory defect** (see Chapter 3).

Other muscles are also involved in inspiration. The scalene muscles elevate the upper ribs and sternum. These were once considered, along with the sternocleidomastoids, to be '**accessory muscles of respiration**', only brought into play during the exaggerated ventilatory effort of acute respiratory distress. Electromyographic studies, however, have demonstrated that these muscles are active even in quiet breathing, although less obviously so.

The intercostal muscles bind the ribs to ensure the integrity of the chest wall. They therefore transfer the effects of actions on the upper or lower ribs to the whole rib cage. They also brace the chest wall, resisting the bulging or in-drawing effect of changes in pleural pressure during breathing. This bracing effect can be overcome to some extent by the exaggerated pressure changes seen during periods of more extreme respiratory effort, and in slim individuals **intercostal recession** may be observed as a sign of respiratory distress.

Whilst inspiration is the result of active muscular effort, quiet expiration is a more passive process. The inspiratory muscles steadily release their contraction and the elastic recoil of the lungs brings the tidal breathing cycle back to its start point. Forced expiration, however – either volitional or as in coughing, for example – requires muscular effort. The abdominal musculature is the principal agent in this.

The inherent elastic property of the lungs

Lung tissue has a natural elasticity. Left to its own devices, a lung would tend to shrink to little more than the size of a tennis ball. This can sometimes be observed radiographically in the context of a complete **pneumothorax** (see Chapter 16). The lung's tendency to contract is counteracted by the semi-rigid chest wall, which has a tendency to spring outward from its usual position. At the end of a normal tidal expiration, the two opposing forces are nicely balanced and no muscular effort is required to hold this 'neutral' position. Breathing at close to this lung volume (normal tidal breathing) is therefore relatively efficient and minimises work. It is rather like gently stretching and relaxing a spring from its neutral, tension-free position. Unfortunately, in some diseases (asthma or COPD), tidal ventilation is obliged to occur at higher lung volumes (see Chapter 3). Breathing then is rather like stretching and relaxing a spring that is already under a considerable degree of tension. The **work of breathing** is therefore increased, a factor that contributes to the sensation of breathlessness. Test this yourself: take a good breath in and try to breathe normally at this high lung volume for a minute.

The natural tendencies for the chest wall to spring outwards and the lung to contract down present opposing forces, which generate a negative pressure within the pleural space. This negative pressure ('vacuum') maintains the lung in its stretched state. Clearly, at higher lung volumes, the lung is at greater stretch and a more negative pleural pressure is required to hold it in position. The relationship between pleural pressure (the force on the lung) and lung volume can be plotted graphically (Fig. 1.5). The lung does not behave as a perfect spring, however. You may recall that the length of a spring is proportional to the force applied to it (Hooke's law). In the case of the lung, as its volume increases, greater and greater force is needed to achieve the same additional increase in volume; that is, the lung becomes less 'compliant' as its volume increases. **Lung compliance** is defined as 'the change in lung volume brought about by a unit change in transpulmonary (intrapleural) pressure'.

Airway resistance

In addition to overcoming the elastic properties of the lungs and the chest wall, during active breathing the muscles of respiration also have to overcome the frictional forces opposing flow up and down the airways.

Site of maximal resistance

It is generally understood that resistance to flow in a tube increases sharply as luminal radius (r) decreases (with laminar flow, resistance is inversely proportional to r^4). It seems rather contradictory,

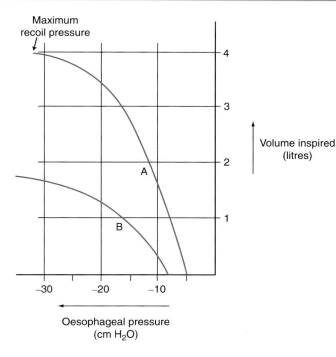

Figure 1.5 Graph of (static) lung volume against oesophageal pressure (a surrogate for intrapleural pressure). In both subjects A and B, we see that *lung compliance* – the change in lung volume per unit change in intrapleural pressure (or slope of the curve) is reduced at higher lung volumes. A: normal individual. B: individual with reduced lung compliance, such as lung fibrosis.

therefore, to learn that in a healthy individual, the greater part of total airway resistance is situated in the large airways (larynx, trachea and main bronchi) rather than in the small airways. This is in part due to the fact that the flow velocity is greatest and flow most turbulent in the central airways, but also due to the much greater *total* cross-sectional area in the later generations of airway (Fig. 1.6). Remember, we only have one trachea, but by the 10th division we have very many small airways, which effectively function in parallel.

Conditions may be different in disease states. Asthma and COPD – diseases that affect airway calibre – tend to have a greater proportionate effect on smaller generations of airway. The reduced calibre of the smaller airways then becomes overwhelmingly important and the site of principal resistance moves distally.

Consider the model of the lung represented in Fig. 1.7. Here, the tube represents a route through generations of airways from the alveoli to the mouth. The smaller generations, without cartilaginous support, are represented by the 'floppy' segment (B). Airways are embedded within the lung and are attached externally to lung tissue whose elastic recoil and ultimate connection to the chest wall supports the floppy segments. This recoil force is represented by the springs.

During expiration, a positive pressure is generated in the alveolar space (A). Air flows from A along the

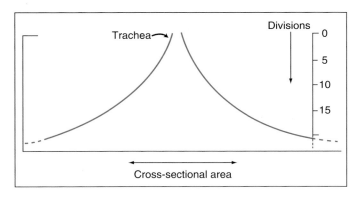

Figure 1.6 Diagrammatic representation of the increase in total cross-sectional area of the airways at successive divisions.

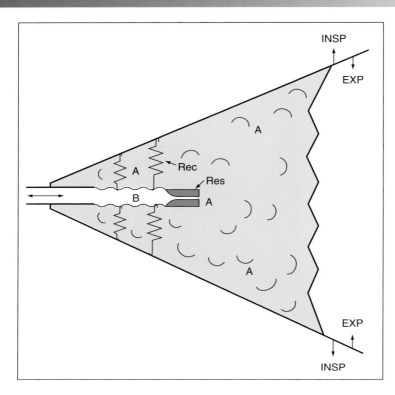

airway, past B, where the pressure is lower (it must be, otherwise the air would not have flowed in this direction), and on to the mouth, where the pressure is nominally 'zero'.

The pressure difference across the walls of the floppy segment (A minus B) would tend to cause this part of the airway to collapse. It is prevented from doing so by the retractile force of lung recoil (tension within the springs).

The flow-limiting mechanism

During expiration, the extent of the pressure drop between A and B is proportional to the flow rate. Clearly, with increased effort, flow rate will be increased … up to a point. Eventually, a critical flow rate will be reached, where the pressure gradient between A and B is sufficient to overcome the retractile force of the lung, the airway wall collapses and airflow ceases. Once there is no flow, the pressure inside the airway at point B quickly equilibrates with that at A. With no pressure difference forcing the airway wall to collapse, the retractile force of the lung reopens the airway and flow recommences. This brings us back to where we started and the cycle begins again. It will be apparent that this mechanism determines a maximum flow rate along the airway. Any attempt to increase flow rate (associated with a

greater pressure difference A to B) will simply result in airway closure. As each route out of the lung will similarly have a maximal possible flow rate, the expiratory flow from the lung as a whole will have an absolute limit. It can be seen that this limit is set by the internal mechanics of the lung, not by muscular effort (above a certain level of effort). That is perhaps fortunate: if it were not the case then lung function tests such as **peak expiratory flow rate** (PEFR) would not be tests of lung function at all, but of muscular strength.

The effects of disease on maximum flow rate

In asthma (see Chapter 10), airway narrowing occurs, leading to a greater resistance between point A (the alveolus) and point B. The pressure drop, A to B, for any given flow rate will therefore be greater than in the healthy lung, and the critical (maximal) flow rate (when the pressure difference between A and B is just enough to overcome the retractile force of the lung) will be lower. You may have known for some time that peak expiratory flow is reduced in asthma, but now you understand why.

In COPD (see Chapter 11), the loss of alveolar walls (emphysema) reduces the elastic recoil of the lung. There is therefore less protective retractile force on the airway wall and the critical pressure drop along the airway required to cause airway collapse will occur at a lower flow rate. Thus, maximum expiratory flow is also reduced in COPD.

Airway resistance and lung volume

It can easily be seen in the model that, as lung volume decreases, lung elastic recoil (tension within the springs) diminishes, providing less and less support for the floppy airway. It is clear, therefore, that the maximum flow rate achievable is dependent on lung volume and is reduced as lung volume is reduced. For any given lung volume, there will be a maximum expiratory flow that cannot be exceeded, no matter what the effort. You can confirm this by inspecting the shape of a flow loop, which is effectively a graph of the maximal flow rate achievable at each lung volume (see Chapter 3). A true PEFR can only be achieved by beginning forced expiration from a position of full inspiration. I would suggest you've been aware of this fact for longer than you realise. Immediately prior to blowing out the candles on your second-birthday cake, you probably took a big breath in. At the age of two, you had an intuitive understanding of the volume dependence of maximal expiratory flow rate.

Lung volume and site of maximal airway resistance

As we have already discussed, the greater part of airway resistance resides in the central airways. These airways are well supported by cartilage and so generally maintain their calibre even at low lung volumes. The calibre of the small airways, without cartilaginous support, is heavily dependent on lung volume. At lower lung volumes, their calibre is reduced, and resistance is increased. During expiration, therefore, as lung volume declines, the site of principal resistance moves from the large central airways to the small peripheral airways. The PEFR (see Chapter 3) tests expiratory flow at high lung volume and is therefore determined largely by the central airways. The **forced expiratory volume in 1 second** (FEV_1; see Chapter 3) is also heavily influenced by the central airway, though not as much as PEFR. Specialised lung-function tests that measure expiratory flow at lower lung volumes (e.g. FEF_{25-75} and $\dot{V}_{max50}$; see Chapter 3) are believed to provide more information about the smaller airways.

Gas exchange

The lung is ventilated by air and perfused by blood. For gas exchange, to occur these two elements must come into intimate contact.

Where does the air go?

An inspired breath brings air into the lung. That air does not distribute itself evenly, however. Some parts of the lung are more compliant than others, and are therefore more accommodating. This variability in compliance occurs on a gross scale across the lungs (upper zones verses lower zones) and also on a very small scale in a more random pattern. At the gross level, the lungs can be imagined as 'hanging' inside the thorax; the effect of gravity means that the upper parts of the lungs are under considerable stretch, whilst the bases sit relatively compressed on the diaphragm. During inspiration, as the upper parts of the lung are already stretched, it is difficult for them to accommodate more air; the bases, on the other hand, are ripe for inflation. Therefore, far more of each inspired breath ends up in the lower zones than the upper zones.

On a small scale, adjacent lobules or even alveoli may not have the same compliance. Airway anatomy is not precisely uniform either, and airway resistance between individual lung units will vary. It can therefore be seen that ventilation will vary in an apparently random fashion on a small scale throughout the lung. This phenomenon may be rather modest in health, but is likely to be exaggerated in many lung diseases in which airway resistance or lung compliance is affected.

Where does the blood go?

The pulmonary circulation operates under much lower pressure than the systemic circulation. At rest, the driving pressure is only on the order of 15 mmHg. In the upright posture, therefore, there is barely enough pressure to fill the upper parts of the system and the apices of the lung receive very little perfusion at all from the pulmonary circulation. The relative overperfusion of the bases mirrors the pattern seen with ventilation (which is fortunate, if our aim is to bring blood and air into contact), but the disparity is even greater in the case of perfusion. Thus, at the bases of the lungs, perfusion exceeds ventilation, while, at the apices, ventilation exceeds perfusion.

The distribution of perfusion is also heavily influenced by another factor: hypoxia. By a mechanism we do not fully understand, low oxygen levels in a region of the lung have a direct vasoconstrictor effect on the pulmonary artery supplying that region. This has the beneficial effect of diverting blood away from the areas of lung that are poorly ventilated towards the well-ventilated areas. This 'automatic' **ventilation/perfusion (V/Q) matching system** aims to maximise the contact between air and blood and is critically important to gas exchange.

Relationship between the partial pressures of O_2 and CO_2

During steady-state conditions, the relationship between the amount of carbon dioxide produced by the body and the amount of oxygen absorbed depends upon the metabolic activity of the body. This is referred to as the 'respiratory quotient' (RQ).

$$RQ = \frac{CO_2 \text{ produced}}{O_2 \text{ absorbed}}$$

The actual value varies from 0.7 during pure fat metabolism to 1.0 during pure carbohydrate metabolism. The RQ is usually about 0.8, and it is assumed to be such for everyday clinical calculations.

Carbon dioxide

If carbon dioxide is being produced by the body at a constant rate then the partial pressure of CO_2 (Pco_2) of alveolar air (written P_Aco_2) depends only upon the amount of outside air with which the carbon dioxide is mixed in the alveoli; that is, it depends only upon alveolar ventilation. If alveolar ventilation increases, P_Aco_2 will fall; if alveolar ventilation decreases, P_Aco_2 will rise. P_Aco_2 (as well as arterial Pco_2, P_aco_2) is a sensitive index of alveolar ventilation.

Oxygen

The partial pressure of alveolar O_2 (P_Ao_2) also varies with alveolar ventilation. If alveolar ventilation increases greatly then P_Ao_2 will rise and begin to approach the Po_2 of the inspired air. If alveolar ventilation is reduced, P_Ao_2 will also be reduced. Whilst arterial Po_2 (P_ao_2) also varies with alveolar ventilation (in the same direction as alveolar Po_2), it is not a reliable index of alveolar ventilation, as it is also profoundly affected by regional changes in ventilation/perfusion (V/Q) matching (see later in this chapter).

The possible combinations of Pco_2 and Po_2 in alveolar gas are shown in Fig. 1.8. Moist atmospheric air at 37 °C has a Po_2 is between 20 and 21 kPa. In this model, oxygen can be exchanged with carbon dioxide in the alveoli to produce any combination of P_Ao_2 and P_Aco_2 described by the oblique line which joins P_Ao_2 20 kPa and P_Aco_2 20 kPa. The position of the cross on this line represents the composition of a hypothetical sample of alveolar air. A fall in alveolar ventilation will result in an upward movement of this point along the line; conversely, an increase in alveolar ventilation will result in a downward movement of the point.

In practice, RQ is not 1.0 but closer to 0.8. In other words:

$$\text{alveolar } Po_2 + \left(\frac{\text{alveolar } Pco_2}{0.8} \right) = 20 \text{ KPa}$$

This is represented by the dotted line in Fig. 1.8.

Point (a) represents the Pco_2 and Po_2 of **arterial blood** (it lies a little to the left of the RQ 0.8 line because of the small normal alveolar–arterial oxygen tension difference). Point (b) represents the arterial gas tension following a period of underventilation. If the P_aco_2 and P_ao_2 were those represented by point

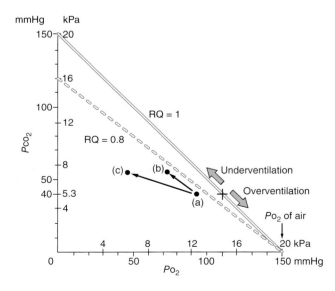

Figure 1.8 Oxygen–carbon dioxide diagram. The continuous and interrupted lines describe the possible combinations of Pco_2 and Po_2 in alveolar air when the RQ is 1 versus 0.8. (a) A hypothetical sample of arterial blood. (b) Progressive underventilation. (c) Po_2 lower than can be accounted for by underventilation alone.

(c), this would imply that the fall in P_aO_2 was more than could be accounted for by reduced alveolar ventilation alone.

The carriage of CO_2 and O_2 by blood

Blood will carry different quantities of a gas when it is at different partial pressures, as described by a dissociation curve. The dissociation curves for oxygen and carbon dioxide are very different (they are shown together on the same scale in Fig. 1.9). The amount of carbon dioxide carried by the blood is roughly proportional to the P_aCO_2 over the whole range normally encountered, whereas the quantity of oxygen carried is only proportional to the P_aO_2 over a very limited range of about 3–7 kPa (22–52 mmHg). Above 13.3 kPa (100 mmHg), the haemoglobin is fully saturated. Further increases in partial pressure result in hardly any additional oxygen being carried.

Effect of local differences in V/Q

In the normal lung, the vast majority of alveoli receive ventilation and perfusion in about the correct proportion (Fig. 1.10a). In diffuse disease of the lung, however, it is usual for ventilation and perfusion to be

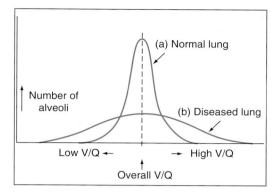

Figure 1.10 Distribution of ventilation/perfusion (V/Q) relationships within the lungs. Although the overall V/Q ratio is the same in the two examples shown, the increased spread of V/Q ratios within the diseased lung (b) will result in a lower arterial oxygen tension and content than in the normal lung (a). Arterial Pco₂ will be similar in both cases.

irregularly distributed, so that a greater scatter of V/Q ratios is encountered (Fig. 1.10b). Even if the overall V/Q remains normal, there is wide local variation in V/Q. Looking at Fig. 1.10, it is tempting to suppose the effects of the alveoli with low V/Q might be nicely balanced by the alveoli with high V/Q. In fact, this is not the case: the increased range of V/Q within the lung affects the transport of CO_2 and O_2 differently.

Fig. 1.11b and c show regions of low and high V/Q, respectively, while Fig. 1.11d shows the result of mixing blood from these two regions. Fig. 1.11a shows normal V/Q, for contrast.

Effect on arterial CO_2 content

Blood with a high CO_2 content returning from low-V/Q areas mixes with blood with a low CO_2 content returning from high-V/Q areas. The net CO_2 content of arterial blood may be near normal, as the two balance out.

Effect on arterial O_2 content

Here the situation is different. Blood returning from low-V/Q areas has a low Po_2 and low O_2 content, but there is a limit to how far this deficit can be made good by mixture with blood returning from high-V/Q areas. Blood returning from a high-V/Q area will have a high Po_2 but is unable to carry more than the 'normal' quantity of oxygen, as the haemoglobin will already be saturated.

- Areas of low V/Q result in a rise in arterial CO_2 and a fall in arterial O_2 content.

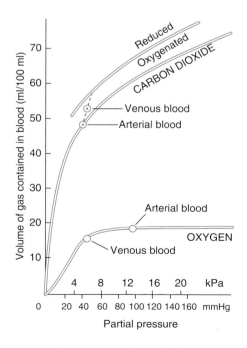

Figure 1.9 Blood oxygen and carbon dioxide dissociation curves drawn to the same scale.

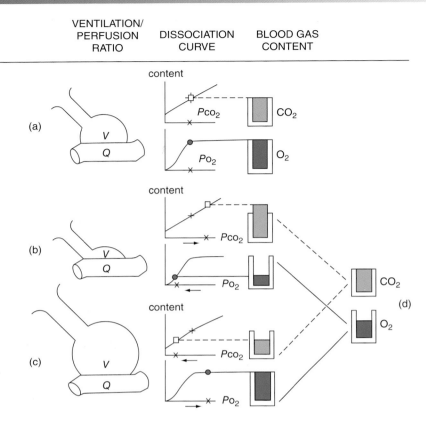

Figure 1.11 Effect of ventilation/perfusion (V/Q) imbalance. (a) Appropriate V/Q. The V/Q ratio is shown diagrammatically on the left. When ventilation is appropriately matched to perfusion in an alveolus or in the lung as a whole, the Pco_2 is about 5.3 kPa (40 mmHg) and the Po_2 is about 12.6 kPa (95 mmHg). The dissociation curves shown in the centre of the diagram describe the relationship between the blood gas tension and the amount of gas carried by the blood. The normal blood gas contents are represented very diagrammatically on the right. (b) Low V/Q. Reduced ventilation relative to blood flow results in a rise in arterial Pco_2 and a fall in Po_2. Reference to the dissociation curves shows that this produces a rise in arterial CO_2 content and a fall in O_2 content. (c) High V/Q. Increased ventilation relative to blood flow results in a fall in Pco_2 and a rise in Po_2. Reference to the dissociation curves shows that this results in a fall in CO_2 content below the normal level but no increase in O_2 content. In health, the vast majority of alveoli have an appropriate balance of ventilation and perfusion and the arterial blood has a normal CO_2 and O_2 content, as shown in (a). In many disease states, the V/Q ratio varies widely between areas. Such variation always results in a disturbance of blood gas content. The effects of areas of low V/Q are not corrected by areas of high V/Q. The result of mixing blood from areas of low and high V/Q is shown diagrammatically on the extreme right (d). It can be seen that, with respect to CO_2 content, the high content of blood from underventilated areas is balanced by the low content from overventilated areas. However, in the case of O_2, the low content of blood from underventilated areas cannot be compensated for by an equivalent increase in the O_2 content of blood from overventilated areas. *Arterial hypoxaemia is inevitable if there are areas of low V/Q (relative underventilation or overperfusion).*

- Increased ventilation in areas of high V/Q may balance the effect on CO_2 content but will only partially correct the reduction in O_2 content; a degree of hypoxaemia is inevitable.
- It follows that, where arterial oxygen levels are lower than would be expected from consideration

of P_aco_2 (overall ventilation) alone, there must be a disturbance to the normal V/Q matching system in the lung; that is, there is likely to be an intrinsic problem with the lung or its vasculature.

When interpreting arterial blood gas results, it is often important to know whether an observed low

P_ao_2 can be explained by underventilation alone or whether a problem with the lung or pulmonary vasculature is present. The tool we use for this task is the **alveolar gas equation**.

The alveolar gas equation

An understanding of the relationship between P_aco_2 and P_ao_2 is critical to the interpretation of blood gases (see Chapter 3). The relationship can be summarised in an equation known as the alveolar gas equation.

- Pure underventilation leads to an increase in P_aco_2 and a 'proportionate' fall in P_ao_2. This is known as **type 2 respiratory failure**.
- A disturbance in V/Q matching leads to a fall in P_ao_2 but no change in P_aco_2. This is known as a **type 1 respiratory failure.**
- Because these two problems can occur simultaneously, the alveolar gas equation is needed to determine whether an observed fall in P_ao_2 can be accounted for by underventilation alone or whether there is also an intrinsic problem with the lungs.

Rather than merely memorise the alveolar gas equation, spend just a moment here understanding its derivation (this is *not* a rigorous mathematical derivation, merely an attempt to impart some insight into its meaning).

Imagine a lung, disconnected from the circulation, being ventilated. Clearly, in a short space of time, P_Ao_2 will come to equal the partial pressure of oxygen in the inspired air (P_Io_2):

$$P_Ao_2 = P_Io_2$$

In real life, the pulmonary circulation is in intimate contact with the lungs and is continuously removing O_2 from the alveoli. The alveolar partial pressure of O_2 is therefore equal to the partial pressure in the inspired air minus the amount removed.

If the exchange of oxygen for carbon dioxide were a 1 : 1 swap then the amount of O_2 removed would equal the amount of CO_2 added to the alveoli and the equation would become:

$$P_Ao_2 = P_Io_2 - P_Aco_2$$

The $CO_2 : O_2$ exchange, as already discussed, is, however, not usually 1 : 1. The RQ is usually taken to be 0.8. Thus:

$$P_Ao_2 = P_Io_2 - (P_Aco_2/0.8)$$

As CO_2 is a very soluble gas, P_Aco_2 is virtually the same as P_aco_2. P_aco_2 (available from the blood gas measurement) can therefore be used in the equation in place of P_Aco_2:

$$P_Ao_2 = P_Io_2 - (P_aco_2/0.8)$$

This is (the simplified version of) the alveolar gas equation. If P_Io_2 is known then P_Ao_2 can be calculated.

But, so what? What do we do with the P_Ao_2?

Unlike in the case of CO_2, there is normally a difference between alveolar and arterial Po_2 (which should be the greater?). The difference $P_Ao_2 - P_ao_2$ is often written $P_{A-a}o_2$ and is known as the **alveolar–arterial (A–a) gradient**. In healthy young adults, breathing air, this gradient is small; it would be expected to be comfortably less than 2 kPa. If the gradient is greater than this then the abnormality in the blood gas result cannot be accounted for by a change in ventilation alone; there must be an abnormality intrinsic to the lung or its vasculature causing a disturbance of V/Q matching. For examples, see the multiple choice questions at the end of the chapter.

The control of breathing

To understand this, we first have to remember why we breathe. Whilst oxygen is an essential requirement for life, we do not need the high level of oxygenation usually seen in health for mere survival. We operate with a substantial margin of safety. This safety margin allows us to vary our ventilation (sometimes at the expense of a normal oxygen level) in order to precisely regulate the CO_2 content of the blood. CO_2 is intimately linked with pH. Whilst it is possible to live for years with lower than normal oxygen levels, we cannot survive long at all with pH outside of the normal range. Keeping pH in the normal range is therefore the priority, and CO_2 rather than O_2 is the principal driver of ventilation.

In health, Pco_2 is maintained at very close to 5.3 kPa (40 mmHg). Any increase above this level provokes hyperventilation; any dip leads to hypoventilation. In practice, Pco_2 is so tightly regulated that such fluctuations are not observable. Even when substantial demands are placed on the respiratory system, such as hard physical exercise (with its dramatic increase in O_2 utilisation and CO_2 production), the arterial Pco_2 will barely budge.

Like any finely tuned sensor, however, if the respiratory system is exposed to concentrations it's not designed to deal with for long periods, it will tend to break. In some patients with chronic lung disease (commonly COPD), the CO_2 sensor begins to fail. Underventilation then occurs, and, over time, Pco_2

drifts upward (and P_{O_2} downward). Despite the fall in P_{O_2}, initially at least, nothing much happens. Although there is a separate sensor monitoring levels of hypoxia, it remains blissfully unconcerned by modest reductions in P_{O_2} (because of the margin of safety just discussed). Only when P_{O_2} reaches a levels that could have an impact on bodily function (around 8 kPa; 60 mmHg), does the hypoxic sensor wake up and decide to take action. Happy to tolerate a certain degree of hypoxia, it won't allow the P_{O_2} to fall below this important threshold, which is marginal to the sustainability of life.

When this occurs, hypoxia then takes up the reins as the driver to ventilation and prevents what would have been a progressive decline to death. Once an individual is dependent on this '**hypoxic drive**', a degree of hypoxia is (obviously) necessary to drive ventilation. This is not always appreciated. At times, a 'high-flow' oxygen mask may be applied to a patient by a well-meaning doctor in an attempt to raise the P_{O_2} to a more normal level. But no hypoxia means no drive to breathe. The result can be catastrophic underventilation, which, if not dealt with properly, can be fatal. When treating hypoxic patients who may have chronic lung disease, until their ventilatory drive is known (from arterial blood gas analysis), oxygen should be judiciously controlled to achieve an oxygen saturation (based on pulse oxymetry) between 88 and 92%. In this 'Goldilocks' zone, the patient will not die of hypoxia and ventilation is unlikely to be depressed to any significant degree.

 KEY POINTS

- The essential function of the lungs is the exchange of oxygen and carbon dioxide between the blood and the atmosphere.
- Ventilation is the process of moving air in and out of the lungs, and it depends on the tidal volume, respiratory rate, resistance of the airways and compliance of the lungs. A fall in ventilation leads to a rise in P_{CO_2} and a fall in P_{O_2}: type 2 respiratory failure.
- Derangement in the matching of ventilation and perfusion in the lungs (which may be caused by any disease intrinsic to the lung or its vasculature) leads to a fall in P_{O_2}: type 1 respiratory failure.
- The respiratory centre in the brain stem is responsible for the control of breathing. pH and P_{CO_2} are the primary stimuli to ventilation. Hypoxia only acts as a stimulant when $P_{O_2} <$ about 8 kPa.

 FURTHER READING

Brewis RAL, White FE. Anatomy of the thorax. In: Gibson GJ, Geddes DM, Costabel U, Sterk PJ, Corrin B, eds. *Respiratory Medicine*. Edinburgh: Elsevier Science, 2003: 3–33.

Cotes JE. *Lung Function: Assessment and Application in Medicine*. Oxford: Blackwell Science, 1993.

Gibson GJ. *Clinical Tests of Respiratory Function*. Oxford: Chapman and Hall, 2009.

West JB. *Pulmonary Pathophysiology – The Essentials*. Baltimore, MD: Williams and Wilkins, 1987.

Multiple choice questions

1.1 The principal muscle(s) involved in forced expirations is (are):
A the diaphragm
B rectus abdominus
C the scalene muscles
D sternocleidomastoids
E the intercostals

1.2 Lung compliance:
A increases as lung volume increases
B is reduced in emphysema
C is reduced in lung fibrosis
D is the change in pleural pressure per unit change in lung volume
E is the principal factor determining forced expiratory flow

1.3 In relation to airway resistance:
A overall airway resistance increases as lung volume increases
B in health, at high lung volume, the greater part of airway resistance is situated in the small airways
C airway resistance is reduced in emphysema due to diminished retractile force on the airway
D airway resistance is proportional to the cubed power of the radius of the airway (r^3)
E in asthma, the greater part of airway resistance is situated in the small airways

1.4 In relation to ventilation (V) and perfusion (Q):
A the upper zones of the lungs are ventilated more than the lower zones
B the upper zones of the lungs receive more perfusion than the lower zones
C V/Q is greater in the lower zones
D VQ matching is unaffected in asthma
E reduced overall ventilation leads to a fall in Po_2

1.5 In a patient breathing room air at sea level, the arterial blood gases were: pH 7.36, Pco_2 4.0, Po_2 10.5, $aHCO_3^-$ 19, base excess −5. The alveolar–arterial gradient is:
A 2.5 kPa
B 5.0 kPa
C 5.5 kPa
D 6.5 kPa
E 10.0 kPa

1.6 During inspiration, the diaphragm:
A rises
B relaxes
C shortens
D is inactive
E causes a rise in intrathoracic pressure

1.7 An increase in ventilation leads to:
A a rise in pCO_2 and pO_2
B a fall in pCO_2 and pO_2
C a rise in pCO_2 and a fall in pO_2
D a fall in pCO_2 and a rise in pO_2
E a rise in pCO_2 and no change in pO_2

1.8 VQ mismatching leads to:
A a rise in pCO_2 and pO_2
B a fall in pCO_2 and pO_2
C a rise in pCO_2 and a fall in pO_2
D a fall in pCO_2 and a rise in pO_2
E no change in pCO_2 and a fall in pO_2

1.9 In relation to the control of breathing:
A hypoxia is irrelevant
B a rise of 0.2 kPa in pCO_2 is required before ventilation is driven to increase
C a metabolic alkalosis can reduce ventilation and therefore pO_2
D a rise in blood pH will tend to reduce ventilation
E a fall in pH implies there has been a reduction in ventilation

1.10 In relation to airway resistance:
A resistance increases as lung volume is reduced
B the site of principal resistance moves to the larger airways as lung volume is reduced
C maximum forced expiratory flow can be achieved at mid lung volume
D FEF_{25-75} provides accurate information on the calibre of the large airways
E FEF_{25-75} provides accurate information on the calibre of the small airways

Multiple choice answers

1.1 B

The diaphragm is the main muscle of inspiration; quiet expiration is a rather passive process. Forced expiration requires positive pressure to be quickly generated in the thorax. To achieve this, the abdominal musculature contracts quickly, which increases the intra-abdominal pressure, forcing the diaphragm up into the thorax.

1.2 C

Lung compliance is the change in lung volume brought about by a unit change in transpulmonary (intrapleural) pressure. The fibrotic lung is less compliant.

1.3 E

Airway resistance in health resides principally in the central (large) airways at high lung volume. As lung volume decreases, it moves peripherally to the smaller airways. It is increased in emphysema and is proportional to r^4.

1.4 E

Most of the ventilation goes to the bases, but an even greater proportion of the perfusion goes to the bases. Poor V/Q leads to a fall in Po_2 but does not affect Pco_2. Reduced overall ventilation causes a rise in Pco_2 and a fall in Po_2.

1.5 C

$$P_{AO_2} = P_{IO_2} - \frac{P_{aCO_2}}{0.8}$$

$$P_{AO_2} = 21 - \frac{4.0}{0.8} = 16$$

$$P_{AO_2} - P_{aO_2} = 16 - 10.5 = 5.5 \text{ kPa}$$

This is elevated, implying a problem with VQ matching within the lung.

1.6 C

During inspiration, the diaphragm contracts and stiffens, pushing the abdominal contents down and reducing pressure in the thorax, which 'sucks' air in.

1.7 D

Increasing ventilation 'blows off' more CO_2 (leading to a fall in pCO_2) and replenishes the alveolar oxygen, leading to an increase in alveolar O_2 and therefore arterial pO_2, although the O_2 saturation of the blood may alter very little.

1.8 E

See Figure 1.11.

1.9 C

The sensitivity to changes in pH and pCO_2 is so exquisite that adjustments are made before any measurable change can occur.

Hypoxia does matter, but only has significant impact on the drive to breathe when pO_2 falls significantly (approx 8 kPa). A low pH can be caused by either reduced ventilation or a metabolic disturbance (in which case, it would lead to a rise in ventilation).

1.10 A

As lung volume is reduced, the small airways narrow and the site of principal resistance moves peripherally. Resistance is lowest (and therefore max forced flow rate is achieved) when the lungs are full. FEF_{25-75} provides information on the calibre of the small airways, but it can be a rather noisy signal.

Part 2

History taking, examination and investigations

2

History taking and examination

History taking

History taking is of paramount importance in the assessment of a patient with respiratory disease. Difficult diagnostic problems are more often solved by a carefully taken history than by laboratory tests. It is also during history taking that the doctor gets to know the patient and their fears and concerns. The relationship of trust thus established forms the basis of the therapeutic partnership. The doctor should start by asking the patient to describe their symptoms in their own words. Listening to the patient's account of the symptoms is an active process, in which the doctor is seeking clues to underlying processes, judging which items require further exploration and noting the patient's attitude and anxieties. By carefully posing questions, the skilled clinician directs the patient to focus on pertinent points, to clarify crucial details and to explore areas of possible importance. History-taking skills develop with experience and with a greater knowledge of respiratory disease.

It is important to appreciate the differences between **symptoms**, which are a patient's subjective description of a change in the body or its functions that might indicate disease; **signs**, which are abnormal features noted by the doctor on examination; and **tests**, which are objective measurements undertaken at the bedside or in the diagnostic laboratory. Thus, for example, a patient might complain of pain on breathing, the doctor might elicit tenderness on pressing on the chest and an X-ray might show a fractured rib.

Symptoms

Table 2.1 lists the main respiratory symptoms that might be encountered in history taking.

Dyspnoea

Dyspnoea (breathlessness) is something everyone understands but no one can satisfactorily define. It is a **subjective** sensation and thus as much about the mind's interpretation of the signals it receives from the body as about what's going on in the lungs. Dyspnoea is an **unpleasant sensation**, an **awareness of breathing** that seems **inappropriately difficult** for the demands that have been placed upon the body. It is *not* tachypnoea (increased respiratory rate), which is a sign noted by the doctor. For example, an athlete at the end of a modest training run will be tachypnoeic but is unlikely to complain of breathlessness.

In history taking, when attempting to determine the cause of dyspnoea, careful assessment includes taking note of the speed of onset, progression, periodicity and precipitating/relieving factors. The severity of dyspnoea is graded according to the patient's exercise tolerance (e.g. dyspnoeic on climbing a flight of stairs or at rest). Onset may be sudden, as in the case of a pneumothorax, or gradual and progressive, as in chronic obstructive pulmonary disease (COPD). An episodic dyspnoea pattern is characteristic of asthma, with symptoms typically being precipitated by cold air or exercise and often displaying **diurnal variability** (varying with the

Respiratory Medicine Lecture Notes, Ninth Edition. Stephen J. Bourke and Graham P. Burns.
© 2015 John Wiley & Sons, Ltd. Published 2015 by John Wiley & Sons, Ltd.
Companion Website: www.lecturenoteseries.com/Respiratory

Table 2.1 **Main respiratory symptoms**
• Dyspnoea • Wheeze • Cough • Sputum • Haemoptysis • Chest pain

time of day). **Orthopnoea** is dyspnoea that occurs when lying flat and is relieved by sitting upright. It is a characteristic feature of pulmonary oedema or diaphragm paralysis but can be found in most respiratory diseases if very severe. **Paroxysmal nocturnal dyspnoea** (PND) is the phenomenon of waking up breathless at night. Most medical students assume this implies pulmonary oedema, but it is also a cardinal feature of asthma. An exploration of other features of these two conditions is needed before a conclusion about cause can be drawn. It is important to note what words the patient uses to describe the symptoms: 'tightness in the chest' may indicate breathlessness or angina. Dyspnoea is not a symptom that is specific to respiratory disease and it may be associated with various cardiac diseases, anxiety, anaemia and metabolic states such as ketoacidosis.

Wheeze

This is a whistling or sighing noise that is characteristic of air passing through a narrow tube. The sound of wheeze can be mimicked by breathing out almost to residual volume and then giving a further sharp, forced expiration. Wheeze is a characteristic feature of airway obstruction caused by asthma or COPD but can also occur in pulmonary oedema when airway walls are swollen with fluid. In asthma, wheeze is characteristically worse on waking in the morning and may be precipitated by exercise or cold air. Wheeze that improves at weekends or on holidays away from work and deteriorates on return to the work environment is suggestive of occupational asthma. Wheeze occurs in expiration. 'Wheeze' on inspiration is not wheeze, it is **stridor** – indicating obstruction of the central airways (e.g. obstruction of the trachea by a carcinoma): an important distinction not to miss.

When wheeze is present, airway obstruction is present. Wheeze, however, is not a reliable indicator of obstruction. It is often absent in COPD. Severe, life-threatening asthma may be associated with a '**silent chest**'.

Cough and sputum

Cough begins with closure of the vocal cords; this allows the forced contraction of the abdominal muscles and bracing by the intercostal muscles to generate a large positive pressure within the thorax. Sudden opening of the vocal cords then results in a forceful expiratory blast. The expiratory flow rate produced is much greater than that during voluntary forced expiration; the resultant shearing forces are particularly effective at removing secretions or inhaled solid material. When the vocal cords cannot be opposed, cough is much less effective and its character is quite different (see discussion of **bovine cough** later in this chapter).

Cough is a protective reflex provoked by physical or chemical stimulation of irritant receptors in the larynx, trachea or bronchial tree. It may be dry or associated with sputum production. The duration and nature of a cough should be assessed, and precipitating and relieving factors should be explored. It is important to examine any **sputum** produced, noting whether it is mucoid, purulent or bloodstained, for example. Cough occurring on exercise or disturbing sleep at night is a feature of asthma. A transient cough productive of purulent sputum is very common in respiratory tract infections. A weak, ineffective cough that fails to clear secretions from the airways is a feature of bulbar palsy or expiratory muscle weakness, and predisposes the patient to aspiration pneumonia. Cough is often triggered by the accumulation of sputum in the respiratory tract. Chronic bronchitis is defined as cough productive of sputum on most days for at least 3 months of 2 consecutive years. Bronchiectasis is characterised by the production of copious amounts of purulent sputum. A chronic cough may also be caused by gastro-oesophageal reflux (with or without aspiration), sinusitis with post-nasal drip and, occasionally, drugs (e.g. ACE inhibitors). Violent coughing can generate sufficient force to produce a '**cough fracture**' of a rib or to impede venous return and cerebral perfusion, causing '**cough syncope**'. Patients with **in situ pulmonary adenocarcinoma** (bronchoalveolar cell carcinoma) sometimes produce very large volumes of watery sputum: **bronchorrhoea**.

Haemoptysis

Haemoptysis is the **coughing up of blood**. It is a very important symptom that requires investigation. In particular, it may be the first clue to the presence of bronchial carcinoma. All patients with haemoptysis should have a chest X-ray performed, and further

Table 2.2 Major causes of haemoptysis

Tumours

- Bronchial carcinoma
- Laryngeal carcinoma

Infections

- Tuberculosis
- Pneumonia
- Bronchiectasis
- Infective bronchitis

Infarction

- Pulmonary embolism

Pulmonary oedema (sputum usually pink and frothy)

- Left ventricular failure
- Mitral stenosis

Pulmonary vasculitis

- Goodpasture's syndrome
- granulomatosis with polyangiitis (GPA)

investigations such as bronchoscopy, computed tomography (CT), sputum cytology and microbiology may be indicated, depending on the circumstances. The most important causes of haemoptysis are bronchial carcinoma, lung infections (pneumonia, bronchiectasis, tuberculosis), chronic bronchitis, pulmonary infarction, pulmonary vasculitis and pulmonary oedema (pink frothy sputum) (Table 2.2). In some cases, no cause is found, and the origin of the blood may have been in the upper airway (e.g. nose (epistaxis), pharynx or gums).

Chest pain

Pain that is aggravated by inspiration or coughing is described as **pleuritic pain**, and the patient can often be seen to wince when breathing in, as the pain 'catches'. Irritation of the pleura may result from inflammation (pleurisy), infection (pneumonia), infarction of underlying lung (pulmonary embolism) or tumour (malignant pleural effusion). Chest wall pain resulting from injury to the intercostal muscles or fractured ribs, for example, is also aggravated by inspiration or coughing and is associated with tenderness at the point of injury.

Associated symptoms

In addition to these major respiratory symptoms, it is important to consider other associated symptoms.

For example, **anorexia** and **weight loss** are features of malignancy or chronic lung infections (e.g. lung abscess). **Pyrexia** and **sweating** are features of acute (e.g. pneumonia) and chronic (e.g. tuberculosis) infections. **Lethargy**, malaise and confusion may be features of hypoxaemia. **Headaches**, particularly on awakening in the morning, may be a symptom of hypercapnia. **Oedema** may indicate cor pulmonale. **Snoring** and daytime **somnolence** may indicate obstructive sleep apnoea syndrome. **Hoarseness** of the voice may indicate damage to the recurrent laryngeal nerve by a tumour.

Many respiratory diseases have their roots in previous **childhood lung disease** or in the **patient's environment**, so that it is crucial to make specific enquiries concerning these points during history taking.

History

Past medical history

Did the patient suffer any major illness in childhood? Did the patient have frequent absences from school? Was the patient able to play games at school? Did any abnormalities declare themselves at a pre-employment medical examination or on chest X-ray? Has the patient ever been admitted to hospital with chest disease? A long history of childhood 'bronchitis' may in fact indicate asthma. Severe whooping cough or measles in childhood may cause bronchiectasis. Tuberculosis acquired early in life may reactivate many years later.

General medical history

Has the patient any systemic illness that may involve the lungs (e.g. rheumatoid arthritis)? Is the patient taking any medications that might affect the lungs (e.g. amiodarone or nitrofurantoin), which can cause interstitial lung disease, or β-blockers (e.g. atenolol), which may provoke bronchospasm? What effect will the patient's lung disease have on other illnesses (e.g. fitness for surgery?).

Family history

Is there any history of lung disease in the family? An increased prevalence of lung disease in a family may result from 'shared genes' (inherited traits such as cystic fibrosis, α_1-anti-trypsin deficiency or asthmatic tendency) or 'shared environment' (e.g. tuberculosis).

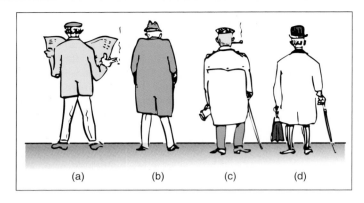

Figure 2.1 Which man has airway obstruction? (Answer at foot of this page.)

(a)   (b)   (c)   (d)

Social history

Does the patient smoke, or have they ever smoked? Is the patient exposed to passive smoking at home? It is important to obtain a clear account of total smoking exposure over the years so as to assess the patient's risk for diseases such as lung cancer or COPD. Pack-year history should be calculated: smoking one pack (20 cigarettes) per day for 1 year equates to 1 pack-year. Does the patient keep any pets or participate in any sports (e.g. diving) or hobbies (e.g. pigeon racing) that might be important in assessing the lung disease?

Occupational history

What occupations has the patient had over the years, what tasks were performed and what materials were used? Do symptoms show a direct relationship to the work environment, as in the case of occupational asthma improving away from work and deteriorating on return to work? Has the patient been exposed to substances that might give rise to disease many years later, as in the case of mesothelioma arising from exposure to asbestos 20–40 years previously (see Chapter14)?

Examination

Some physical signs in medicine are difficult to assess, and examination skills may take years to refine (e.g. identifying the nature of a heart murmur). By contrast, most of the signs in respiratory disease are easy to elicit and interpret. Despite this, evidence of respiratory disease is often entirely overlooked.

Answer to question in Fig. 2.1: (b) has airway obstruction – note the high position of the shoulders.

The expertise in respiratory examination lies in knowing what to look for. Read the following and you will become expert. You will discover the insightful experience that is respiratory examination; ordinary doctors will be in awe of your deductive abilities.

General examination

Be alert to clues to respiratory disease that may be evident from the moment the patient is first seen (Fig. 2.1) or that become apparent during history taking. These include the rate and **character of breathing**, signs of respiratory distress such as **use of accessory muscles** of respiration (e.g. sternocleidomastoids), the **shape of the chest**, spine and shoulders and the character of any **cough**. **Hoarseness** of the voice may be a clue to recurrent laryngeal nerve damage by a carcinoma. **Wheeze** may be audible. **Stridor** is most commonly picked up during history taking, rather than examination.

Avoid proceeding directly to examination of the chest; first pause and ask the patient to cough.

Cough

A voluntarily produced cough is an extremely useful but much neglected sign in respiratory examination. It is probably wise to start with it, lest it be missed. The clues it provides to later examination findings are so useful it can almost feel like cheating.

From the explanation of cough given earlier, it can be seen that when the vocal cords are not opposed, cough will no longer have its normal distinct, crisp start. Such a cough is known as **bovine cough** (cows don't have vocal cords). It is a sign not to be missed, as it may result from tumour in the left side of the chest, causing recurrent laryngeal nerve palsy. The **hoarse voice** that accompanies this abnormality may be missed, particularly if the doctor and patient are meeting for the first time.

If airway obstruction is present, the cough will have a **wheezy quality** (listen out for it). As described already, the expiratory flow rate during a cough is greater than that generated in a normal forced expiration. Therefore, if airway obstruction is mild, it may be that wheeze is only heard during a cough.

When reporting a cough, a patient is usually asked if they produce sputum. The answer 'no' normally results in the doctor documenting that the cough is 'dry'. Beware: an inability to 'bring up' sputum doesn't imply it isn't there. Consciously listening to the quality of a cough will avoid such a mistake.

Knowing whether a cough is **wet or dry** can be invaluable when it comes to determining the nature of the crackles heard later in the examination. Whilst in theory the 'coarse' crackles of bronchiectasis are different to the 'fine' crackles of fibrosis, in practice – on sound quality alone – it can be a difficult call. If you've already listened to the quality of the cough by the time of auscultation, your ability to distinguish fine from course will be uncannily good.

A loud, booming cough heard from one end of the ward to the other is a sign of craved attention.

Next, start with the hands and look for signs en route to the chest.

Hands

Look for **clubbing**, **tar staining** or **features of rheumatoid arthritis**. Signs of CO_2 retention include peripheral **vasodilatation** and **asterixis**: a flapping tremor detected by asking the patient to spread their fingers, cock their wrists back and close their eyes. CO_2 retention dulls proprioception and the hands tend to drift forward, particularly when the eyes are closed. Eventually, an awareness that the hands are no longer in position leads to a sudden corrective movement. In understanding the underlying mechanism of this sign, it should be clear why a doctor holding the patient's hands in place (as many do) will always miss it. Count the **pulse rate** and note any abnormalities in rhythm (e.g. atrial fibrillation) or character (e.g. a bounding pulse of carbon dioxide retention). Count the **respiratory rate** over a period of at least **30 seconds**. The respiratory rate is best counted surreptitiously, perhaps whilst feeling the pulse, as patients tend to breathe faster if they are aware that a doctor is focusing on their breathing. The respiratory rate is an incredibly easy observation to make and is a highly sensitive index of physiological derangement (as such, it is an integral part of all early-warning systems in hospital), yet it is all too frequently missed. Do it. Do it properly.

Clubbing

Clubbing is increased curvature of the nail, with loss of the angle between the nail and the nail bed (Fig. 2.2). It is a very important sign that is associated with a number of diseases (Table 2.3), most notably bronchial carcinoma, bronchiectasis and fibrotic lung disease, such as idiopathic pulmonary fibrosis. Clubbing also occurs in asbestosis, although usually only in more advanced disease. Advanced clubbing is sometimes associated with hypertrophic pulmonary osteoarthropathy, in which there is new bone formation in the subperiosteal region of the long bones of the arms and legs, which is detectable on X-ray and is associated with pain and tenderness.

Next examine the head and neck. Check for elevation of **jugular venous pressure** or **lymph node enlargement**. In the face, seek signs of **cyanosis** and **anaemia** (pallor of conjunctiva). Be alert for uncommon signs such as **Horner's syndrome** (ptosis, meiosis, enophthalmos, anhydrosis), which indicates damage to the sympathetic nerves by a tumour situated at the lung apex (see Chapter 4).

Jugular veins

The jugular veins are examined with the patient in a semi-reclining position, with the trunk at an angle of about 45° from the horizontal. The head is turned slightly to the opposite side and fully supported so that the sternocleidomastoid muscles are relaxed. The jugular venous pulse is seen as a diffuse superficial pulsation of multiple waveform that is distinct from the carotid arterial pulse. The height of the pulse wave is measured as the **vertical height** of the top of the oscillating column of blood above the sternal angle. The jugular venous pressure normally falls during inspiration. It is elevated in right-heart failure, which may occur as a result of pulmonary embolism or cor pulmonale in COPD, for example. Other signs of right-heart failure, such as hepatomegaly and peripheral oedema, may also be present.

Cyanosis

This is a bluish discolouration of the skin and mucous membranes that results from an excessive amount of reduced (deoxygenated) haemoglobin (usually >5 g/dl). It follows, therefore, that it will be more readily observed in those with polycythaemia than anaemia. **Central cyanosis** is best seen on the tip of the tongue and is the cardinal sign of hypoxaemia, although it is not a sensitive sign because it is not usually detectable until the oxygen saturation has

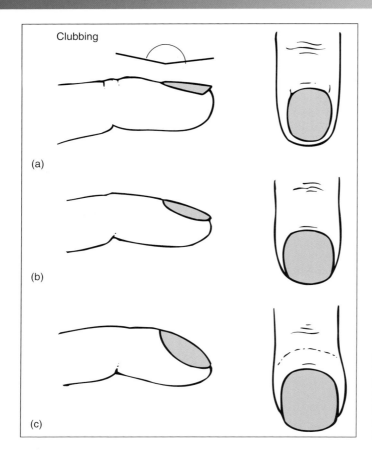

Clubbing

(a)

(b)

(c)

Figure 2.2 Clubbing. (a) Normal: the 'angle' is shown. (b) Early: the angle is absent. (c) Advanced: the nail shows increased curvature in all directions, the angle is absent, the base of the nail is raised up by spongy tissue and the end of the digit is expanded.

fallen to well below 85%, corresponding to a P_{O_2} of <8 kPa (60 mmHg). Cyanosis is more difficult to detect if the patient has dark-coloured skin. Because of the poor sensitivity of cyanosis, it is essential to measure oxygenation by oximetry or arterial blood gas sampling in patients at risk for hypoxaemia. **Peripheral cyanosis** will be present if there is central cyanosis, but it may also be caused by local circulatory slowing in the peripheries, resulting in more complete extraction of oxygen from the blood (e.g. blue hands and ears in cold weather).

Chest

Ask the patient to undress to the waist and examine the chest in a methodical way: **inspection, palpation, percussion and auscultation**.

Tip: in isolation, a particular finding (e.g. percussion note or breath sound) is often difficult to call as normal or abnormal. ***Difference*** *is much easier to detect. Remember: the only*

reason we have two lungs is to allow doctors to compare one side with the other. Make full use of that fact on examination of the chest.

Inspection

When airway obstruction is present, tidal breathing occurs at a higher lung volume; in part, this is an unconscious attempt to hold the airways open. This **hyperinflation** can be even more pronounced if the obstruction is due to emphysema, when the loss of lung elastic recoil allows the chest wall to find its neutral rest position with the lung at a more expanded volume (see Chapter 1). Many of the physical signs of airway obstruction are actually signs of hyperinflation.

Look at the chest from the front, back and sides, noting the overall **shape** and any **asymmetry**, **scars** or **skeletal abnormality**. The normal chest is flattened anteroposteriorly, whereas the hyperinflated chest of COPD is barrel-shaped, with an increased anteroposterior diameter. In airway obstruction, patients tend to

Table 2.3 **Causes of clubbing**

Respiratory

- Neoplastic
  - Bronchial carcinoma
  - Mesothelioma
- Infections
  - Bronchiectasis
  - Cystic fibrosis
  - Chronic empyema
  - Lung abscess
- Fibrosis
  - Idiopathic pulmonary fibrosis
  - Asbestosis

Cardiac

- Bacterial endocarditis
- Cyanotic congenital heart disease
- Atrial myxoma

Gastrointestinal

- Hepatic cirrhosis
- Crohn's disease
- Coeliac disease

Congenital

- Idiopathic familial clubbing

adopt a **high shoulder position** (assisting the lungs in holding a more inflated volume).

Watch the pattern of breathing. In health, a breath in takes about as long as a breath out. In airway obstruction, careful observation will reveal the **prolonged expiratory phase** to respiration. **Pursed lips** during expiration maintain a positive back pressure, holding small airways open longer, reducing gas trapping and allowing patients with airway obstruction to achieve better tidal ventilation at a more comfortable lung volume.

Watch the **movement** of the chest carefully as the patient breathes in and out. The ribs move in a way akin to the handle on a bucket. At low lung volume, the movement is predominately outward; at high lung volume, it is predominantly upward. If, on observation, the front of the chest is seen to move upward on inspiration, hyperinflation (airway obstruction) is present. Diminished movement of one side of the chest is a clue to disease *on that side*. Overall movement is reduced if the lungs have reduced compliance (e.g. fibrosis).

In health, the whole rib cage expands during inspiration, the lower costal margins moving upwards and outwards as the chest expands. This is due to the downward discursion and stiffening of the diaphragm (see Chapter 1). In a chest that is already severely overinflated (e.g. in COPD), inspiration begins with the diaphragm already in a low, flat position. The contraction it undergoes during inspiration therefore tends to pull in the lower costal margin (to which it is attached). This inward movement of the lower costal margin during inspiration appears paradoxical. **Costal margin paradox** (Fig. 2.3) is the single most reliable sign of airway obstruction. It is both sensitive and specific. It is far more reliable than wheeze. All doctors remember to listen for wheeze; few remember to look for lower costal margin paradox.

The abdominal wall normally moves outwards on inspiration, as the diaphragm descends. **Abdominal paradox**, in which the abdominal wall moves inwards during inspiration when the patient is supine, is a sign of diaphragm weakness.

Palpation

Every medical student knows to go through the motions of examining **chest expansion**; few bother to note the findings with much care. That may be because they are unsure of the interpretation or because they are in a hurry to get to auscultation, where they assume they'll find out what's actually going on. Symmetry of chest expansion is extraordinarily useful if examined properly. Examine it properly. Interpretation of the finding isn't difficult: *whatever the abnormality* (consolidation, collapse, effusion, pneumothorax etc.), remember this (you may wish to write it down and spend time trying to memorise it): *the abnormal side moves less*. Of course, that won't tell you what the abnormality is, but knowing which side the abnormality is on is very useful. Imagine that, on auscultation, the breath sounds on the left are quieter than those on the right. It can be a difficult call to decide whether you're listening to bronchial breathing on the right or diminished breath sounds on the left. Knowing before you get to auscultation that the left is the abnormal side makes interpretation strangely easy. Chest movements during respiration are best appreciated by placing the hands exactly symmetrically on either side of the chest, with the thumbs parallel with each other in the midline. The relative movement of the two hands and the separation of the thumbs reflect the overall movement of the chest and any asymmetry between the two sides.

The position of the mediastinum is assessed by locating the **tracheal position** and the cardiac **apex beat**. To locate the position of the trachea, first, don't

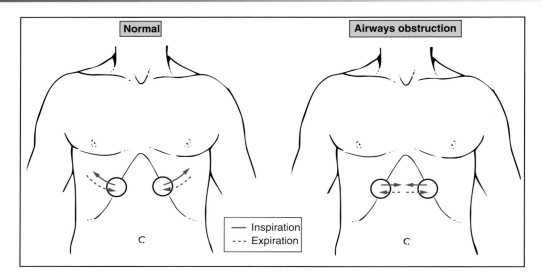

Figure 2.3 Movement of the costal margin. The arrows indicate the direction of movement in normal individuals and in those with airway obstruction (see text). The sign is most easily detected by placing the first and second fingers of each hand in the positions shown (*on* the costal margin in the positions approximating to the line of the lateral border of rectus abdominus).

touch the trachea (not until 'centre' has been established). Place the middle finger in the sternal notch (which is, by definition, 'central') and, keeping it in the notch, gently slide it back towards the trachea. The position at which the trachea is first felt on the tip of the finger immediately informs you whether the trachea is central or deviated. This technique avoids the uncomfortable poking around that usually accompanies palpation of the trachea. Note the distance between the cricoid cartilage and the sternal notch (normally the width of three fingers). Reduction in the **crico-sternal distance** is a sign of a hyperinflated chest. It is not usually necessary to actually poke three fingers into this space to determine that the distance is less than three finger breadths. The apex beat is the most inferior and lateral point at which the cardiac impulse can be felt. The intercostal space in which the apex beat is felt should be counted down from the second intercostal space, which is just below the sternal angle, and its location should also be related to landmarks such as the mid-clavicular or anterior axillary lines. It is normally located in the fifth left intercostal space in the mid-clavicular line. The mediastinum may be deviated towards or away from the side of disease. For example, lobar collapse may *pull* the trachea to that side, whereas a large pleural effusion or tension pneumothorax may *push* the trachea and apex beat away from it.

Percussion

Percussion over normal air-filled lung produces a **resonant note**, whereas percussion over solid organs, such as the liver or heart, produces a **dull note**. The percussion note over an area of consolidation is dull; over an effusion, the note is particularly dull ('**stony dull**'). **Hyper-resonance** may be present in emphysema or over the area of a pneumothorax, although it is rarely a reliable sign. Percussion technique is important and requires practice. The resting finger should be placed flat against the chest wall in an intercostal space (tip: focus on getting the middle phalanx, rather than the whole finger, flat against the chest). The percussing finger should strike the dorsal surface of the middle phalanx and should be lifted clear after each percussion stroke. All areas should be percussed. The order should allow immediate comparison of one area with the equivalent area on the opposite side. To recognize a particular note as hyper-resonant takes years of practice and a well-tuned ear. To pick up a difference between one side and the other is significantly easier. Remember why we have two lungs! When percussing the back of the chest, it is helpful to ask the patient to cross their arms over in front of them, such that one elbow is placed on top of the other. This brings the scapulae forward and out of the way.

Auscultation

Listen with the stethoscope to the **intensity** and **character** of the **breath sounds**, comparing both sides symmetrically, and note any **added sounds** (e.g. wheeze, crackles, pleural rub).

Breath sounds

The source of breath sounds in the lungs is turbulent airflow in the larynx and central airways. The quality of the breath sound (as well as the sound of the voice) heard at the chest wall will vary depending on the medium it has to travel through (Fig. 2.4). A normally aerated lung will conduct low-pitched sounds modestly but high-pitched sounds very poorly. Normal breath sounds are therefore rather low-pitched and faint, and are slightly longer in inspiration than expiration. The rate of airflow at the periphery of the lung is so slow it generates no audible sound at all. Therefore, terms such as 'good air entry' and 'vesicular breath sounds' are clearly wrong and should be avoided. Normal breath sounds should be called **normal breath sounds** – it's that easy.

A solid medium (consolidated lung) conducts sound better, particularly high-pitched sound. Breath sounds heard over a consolidated lung are therefore similar to those heard with the stethoscope held over the larynx and are referred to as **bronchial breathing**. The sound is louder and harsher, has a higher frequency 'hiss' and tends to be similar in inspiration and expiration.

Vocal resonance is assessed by listening over the chest with the stethoscope as the patient says 'ninety-nine'. Normal aerated lung transmits the 'booming' low-pitched components of speech and attenuates the high frequencies. Consolidated lung, however, transmits the higher frequencies better, so that speech takes on a bleating quality known as **aegophony**. Whispering 'ninety-nine' produces only high-pitched sounds. This can barely be heard over normally aerated lung but is transmitted surprising well over consolidated lung and is referred to as **whispering pectoriloquy**.

A reduction in the intensity of breath sounds (**diminished breath sounds**) over an area of lung may indicate obstruction of a large bronchus and collapse of a lobe of the lung. A pleural effusion produces an air–fluid interface, which sound just bounces off. Breath and voice sounds are usually **absent over an effusion**.

Added sounds

In normal individuals, at auscultation, the **inspiratory phase** of respiration seems longer than the **expiratory phase**. Prolongation of the expiratory

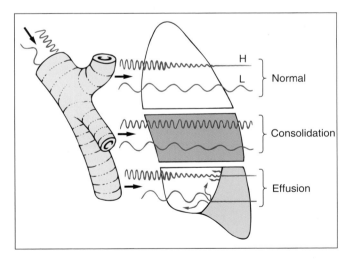

Figure 2.4 Summary of sound transmission in the lung. Sound is generated either by turbulence in the larynx and large airways or by the voice. Both sources are a mixture of high (H) and low (L)-pitched components. Normal aerated lung filters off the high-pitched component but transmits the low-pitched component quite well. This results in soft, low-pitched breath sounds and low-pitched vocal resonance. *Consolidated lung* transmits high-pitched sound particularly well. This results in loud, high-pitched breath sounds (bronchial breathing), high-pitched bleating vocal resonance (aegophony) and easy transmission of whispered (high-pitched) speech (whispering pectoriloquy). *Pleural effusion* causes reduction in the transmission of all sound, probably because of reflection of sound waves at the air–fluid interface. Breath sounds are absent and vocal resonance is much reduced or absent.

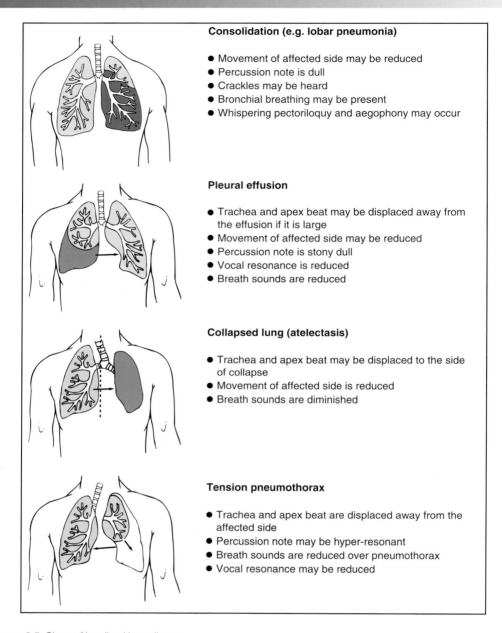

Consolidation (e.g. lobar pneumonia)

- Movement of affected side may be reduced
- Percussion note is dull
- Crackles may be heard
- Bronchial breathing may be present
- Whispering pectoriloquy and aegophony may occur

Pleural effusion

- Trachea and apex beat may be displaced away from the effusion if it is large
- Movement of affected side may be reduced
- Percussion note is stony dull
- Vocal resonance is reduced
- Breath sounds are reduced

Collapsed lung (atelectasis)

- Trachea and apex beat may be displaced to the side of collapse
- Movement of affected side is reduced
- Breath sounds are diminished

Tension pneumothorax

- Trachea and apex beat are displaced away from the affected side
- Percussion note may be hyper-resonant
- Breath sounds are reduced over pneumothorax
- Vocal resonance may be reduced

Figure 2.5 Signs of localised lung disease.

phase is a feature of airway obstruction and is often accompanied by **wheeze** ('rhonchi' is redundant and should be avoided): a high-pitched whistling or sighing sound. Diffuse wheeze is a feature of asthma. This can also be heard in COPD, but diminished breath sounds are more common.

Wheeze localised to one side, or one area of the lung, suggests obstruction of a bronchus by a carcinoma or foreign body (e.g. an inhaled peanut). Remember, inspiratory wheeze is not wheeze, it's stridor. Stridor indicates the site of obstruction as being in the trachea or main bronchi.

Avoid the term 'crepitations' when describing **crackles**: the existence of two terms only causes confusion. (Most people have a clear idea of what the difference in meaning between the two terms is.

Unfortunately, everyone's idea is different.) Language is to facilitate communication, so keep it simple: if the crackles are coarse, they should be described as **coarse crackles**; if they are fine, they should be called **fine crackles**. It is thought that crackles are produced by the opening of previously closed bronchioles. **Early inspiratory crackles** are sometimes heard in patients with a little excess airway mucus (e.g. COPD), but these may diminish or even disappear when the patient is asked to cough. **Late inspiratory crackles** can sometimes be heard at the lung bases in obese individuals as the poorly ventilated areas open at the end of a deep breath. **Pan-inspiratory crackles** can be fine (like **Velcro**), representing lung fibrosis or pulmonary oedema. Coarse pan-inspiratory crackles usually imply excess purulent airway secretions, as seen in bronchiectasis. Remember: distinguishing coarse from fine is much easier if you remembered to ask the patient to cough at the start of the examination.

Pleural rubs are 'creaking' sounds. They are often quite localised and indicate roughening of the normally slippery pleural surfaces. They are heard in the context of pleural inflammation due to either infection or infarction (pulmonary embolism).

Signs

See Fig. 2.5 for signs of localised lung disease. It is important to realise that major disease of the lungs may be present without any detectable physical signs, and it is therefore essential to obtain a chest X-ray when there is good reason to suspect localised lung disease.

 KEY POINTS

- The main respiratory symptoms are breathlessness, wheeze, cough, sputum, haemoptysis and chest pain.
- Haemoptysis is an important symptom that requires investigation, as it may indicate lung cancer, laryngeal cancer, bronchitis, tuberculosis etc.
- Diminished movement of one side of the chest on inspiration is a clue to disease on that side.
- Major disease of the chest may be present without detectable signs, and tests (e.g. chest X-ray) are required where there is suspicion of lung disease.

 FURTHER READING

Alverti A, Quaranta M, Chakrabarti B, et al. Paradoxical movement of the lower rib cage at rest and during exercise in COPD patients. *Eur Respir J* 2009; **33**: 49–60.

Douglas G, Nicol F, Robertson C. *Macleod's Clinical Examination.* London: Churchill Livingston Elsevier, 2009.

Morice AH, McGarvey L, Pavord I, British Thoracic Society Guideline Group. Recommendations for the management of cough in adults. *Thorax* 2006; **61** (Suppl. 1): 1–24.

Spiteri M, Cook D, Clarke S. Reliability of eliciting physical signs in examination of the chest. *Lancet* 1988; **1**: 873–5.

Vyshedsky A, Alhashem RM, Paciej R, et al. Mechanism of inspiratory and expiratory crackles. *Chest* 2009; **135**: 156–64.

Multiple choice questions

2.1 A 72-year-old man presents with breathlessness, clubbing and prominent fine bibasal crackles on auscultation of his chest. The most likely diagnosis is:
- A pulmonary oedema
- B idiopathic pulmonary fibrosis
- C bronchiectasis
- D emphysema
- E lung cancer

2.2 A 76-year-old man presents with breathlessness. On examination, there is diminished expansion of the left hemithorax, dullness to percussion and decreased breath sounds at the left base posteriorly. These features suggest:
- A a pleural effusion
- B pneumonic consolidation
- C a pneumothorax
- D atelectasis
- E bronchiectasis

2.3 A 45-year-old woman is admitted to hospital with a 3-day history of cough, breathlessness and right pleuritic pain. She has smoked 20 cigarettes/day for 25 years. On examination, chest expansion is diminished on the right. There is dullness over the right lung base with bronchial breathing and crackles. These features suggest:
- A atelectasis due to a bronchial carcinoma
- B pneumonic consolidation
- C pneumothorax
- D emphysema
- E a pleural effusion

2.4 A 25-year-old man presents with a sudden onset of right pleuritic pain while playing rugby. He has smoked 10 cigarettes/day for 8 years. On examination, there are decreased breath sounds over the right hemithorax with hyper-resonance on percussion. The trachea is central, jugular venous pressure is normal, heart sounds are normal and there is no tenderness on palpation of the chest. These features suggest:
- A a pulmonary embolism
- B pleurisy with a pleural effusion
- C a traumatic rib fracture
- D pneumonic consolidation with pleurisy
- E a pneumothorax

2.5 An 80-year-old man presents with progressive breathlessness. He stopped smoking 10 years ago, having previously smoked 20 cigarettes/day for 50 years. He had worked as a coalminer for 30 years. On examination, he is not clubbed. Respiratory rate is 22/min. He is cyanosed. His chest is hyperinflated with decreased cricosternal distance. The lower costal margin moves inwards during inspiration. The chest is hyper-resonant to percussion on both sides. There are diminished breath sounds but no crackles. These features suggest a diagnosis of:
- A chronic obstructive pulmonary disease
- B asthma
- C coalminer's pneumoconiosis
- D pneumothorax
- E pulmonary oedema

2.6 A bovine cough is characteristic of:
- A pharyngitis
- B pertusis
- C farmer's lung
- D cancer in the left lung
- E asthma

2.7 Signs of airways obstruction include:
- A tracheal tug
- B reduced expansion
- C lower costal margin paradox
- D prolonged expiratory phase to respiration
- E pursed lip breath

2.8 Causes of clubbing include:
- A lung cancer
- B COPD
- C pulmonary fibrosis
- D atrial septal defect
- E bronchiectasis

2.9 Diminished chest expansion on the SAME side can be caused by:
- A consolidation
- B lobar collapse
- C pleural effusion
- D pneumothorax

2.10 A tension pneumothorax on the LEFT would cause:
- A trachea deviated to the left
- B dull percussion note on the left
- C diminished breath sound on the left
- D diminished expansion on the left (compared to the right)
- E diminished vocal resonance on the left

Multiple choice answers

2.1 B

Bilateral crackles and clubbing are characteristic features of pulmonary fibrosis.

2.2 A

Dullness to percussion suggests a pleural effusion, pleural thickening or pneumonic consolidation. In consolidation, tactile vocal fremitus is often increased, whereas in a pleural effusion it is characteristically reduced.

2.3 B

Pneumonic consolidation is characterised by dullness to percussion, increased tactile vocal fremitus, bronchial breathing and crackles. Pneumonia is sometimes associated with inflammation of the overlying pleura, causing pleuritic pain.

2.4 E

Pneumothorax typically causes acute pleuritic pain and is characterised by reduced breath sounds and hyper-resonance on the side of the pneumothorax.

2.5 A

He has been a smoker and shows features of airways obstruction with paradoxical inward movement of the costal margins on inspiration (in a normal person they move outwards), with a hyperinflated chest (reduced cricosternal distance) and wheeze. The presence of cyanosis indicates hypoxia and respiratory failure.

2.6 D

Suggesting involvement of the recurrent laryngeal nerve.

2.7 All true except B

2.8 A,C,E

2.9 All true

Whatever the abnormality, the abnormal side moves less.

2.10 C,D,E

3

Pulmonary function tests

Despite the bewildering array of sophisticated tests and investigations now available, a few, fairly basic tests of lung function remain central to clinical practice. Together with a good history, clinical examination and a chest X-ray, these tests provide most of the information needed for diagnosis, quantification of severity and monitoring of disease.

This chapter covers all you will probably ever need to know about lung function. The tests are not difficult to understand, yet despite their simplicity, they are all too often misinterpreted or even misunderstood. Master the next few pages and you may find you acquire the status of 'expert' in whatever medical circle you move in.

Normal values

Ventilatory performance varies greatly with patient height, age and sex. Tables and prediction equations are available to help determine a patient's 'predicted normal value'. The patient's test result may be compared with the mean reference value and the standard deviation of results obtained in the healthy population or (more commonly, though less usefully) may be expressed as a percentage of the population's mean reference value. For example: the standard deviation for vital capacity is about 500 ml. If a medium-sized adult has a vital capacity 750 ml below the predicted value, this may be the result of respiratory disease; on the other hand, being only 1.5 standard deviations from the mean, many normal individuals (of the same age and size) with no apparent lung disease will have values lower than this. The same result could be expressed as 75% of the predicted mean, but an injudicious interpretation of this might lead to the mistaken assumption that there is a 25% 'disability'.

Pulmonary function tests should not be interpreted in isolation and should be considered in the context of all additional information concerning the patient.

In this chapter, we will look at:

- simple tests of ventilatory function;
- transfer factor; and
- arterial blood gases.

Simple tests of ventilatory function

Ventilation refers to the process of moving air in and out of the lungs.

Lung volumes

Fig. 3.1 shows an overview of lung capacity and its subdivisions. The **tidal volume** is the volume of air that enters and leaves the lungs during normal breathing. The volume of gas within the lungs at the end of a normal expiration is the **functional residual capacity**. The volume of gas in the lungs after a full inspiration is the **total lung capacity** (TLC). After a full expiration, there will still be some gas remaining in the lungs: the **residual volume**. **Vital capacity** (VC) is the volume of air expelled by a full expiration from a position of full inspiration. VC and its subdivisions can be measured directly by spirometry, whereas measurements of residual volume and TLC require the use of gas dilution or plethysmography methods.

Spirometry

Spirometry is the most commonly used test of pulmonary function. It is a measurement of the amount (volume) and/or speed (flow) of air that

Respiratory Medicine Lecture Notes, Ninth Edition. Stephen J. Bourke and Graham P. Burns.
© 2015 John Wiley & Sons, Ltd. Published 2015 by John Wiley & Sons, Ltd.
Companion Website: www.lecturenoteseries.com/Respiratory

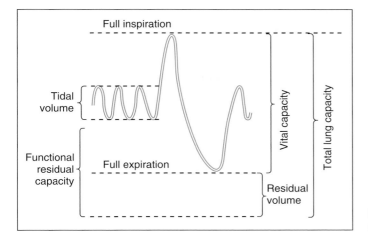

Figure 3.1 Total lung capacity and its subdivisions.

can be exhaled. Traditionally, the result of this test is represented graphically as a plot of the volume of air exhaled against time during a forced expiratory manoeuvre: the **forced expiratory spirogram** (Fig. 3.2).

Vital capacity

VC is the **volume of air expelled by a full expiration from a position of full inspiration**. The patient is usually encouraged to exhale with maximum effort, referred to as **forced vital capacity** (FVC). VC may also be measured by a slow exhalation, sometimes referred to as **'slow' VC**. In normal individuals, slow VC and FVC are very similar, but in patients with airway obstruction, air trapping occurs during forced expiration, so that the FVC may be significantly smaller than the slow VC. VC may be reduced by any condition that limits the lung's ability to achieve a 'full' inspiration, such as:

- reduced lung compliance (e.g. lung fibrosis, loss of lung volume);
- chest deformity (e.g. kyphoscoliosis, ankylosing spondylitis); or
- muscle weakness (e.g. myopathy, myasthenia gravis).

It may also be reduced in chronic obstructive pulmonary disease (COPD), when air trapping causes increased residual volume.

Forced expiratory volume in 1 second and FEV$_1$: FVC ratio

The forced expiratory volume in 1 second (FEV$_1$) is the volume of air expelled in the first second of a maximal forced expiration from a position of full inspiration. It is reduced in any condition that reduces VC, but is particularly reduced when there is diffuse airway obstruction. Normally, during a forced expiratory manoeuvre, at least 70% of the air is expelled in the first second. In diffuse airway obstruction, the FEV$_1$ is affected to a greater extent than the FVC, and the ratio **FEV$_1$: FVC** is reduced to <0.70. This pattern is referred to as an **obstructive defect** and is most commonly seen in asthma and COPD. When lung volume is restricted (by e.g. reduced lung compliance chest deformity or muscle weakness), the VC and the FEV$_1$ are reduced roughly in proportion, so that the FEV$_1$: FVC ratio is essentially normal. This pattern of ventilatory impairment is referred to as a **restrictive defect**.

Maximal mid-expiratory flow

In addition to FEV$_1$ and FVC, a number of other indices may be calculated from a forced expiratory spirogram. The forced expiratory flow measured over the middle half of expiration (**FEF$_{25-75\%}$**) reflects changes in the **smaller peripheral airways**, whereas peak expiratory flow (PEF) and FEV$_1$ are predominantly influenced by diffuse changes in the medium-sized and larger central airways, at least in health (see Chapter 1).

Peak expiratory flow

PEF is the maximum rate of airflow that can be achieved during a sudden forced expiration from a position of full inspiration. The best of three attempts is usually accepted as the peak flow rate. It is somewhat dependent on effort, but is mainly determined

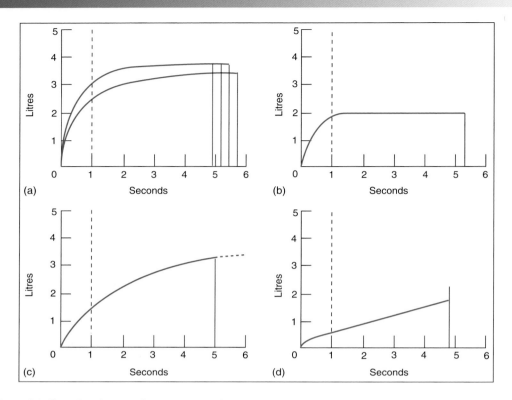

Figure 3.2 Forced expiratory spirogram tracing obtained with a spirometer. (a) *Normal*. Four expirations have been made. Three of these are true maximal forced expirations, as indicated by their *reproducibility*. The FEV$_1$ is 3.2 l and the FVC is 3.8 l. The forced expiratory ratio (FEV$_1$: FVC) is 84%. (b) *Restrictive ventilatory defect*. Patient with pulmonary fibrosis. The FVC in this case is 2 l less than the predicted value for the subject. The FEV$_1$ is also reduced below the predicted value, but it represents a large part of the FVC. The forced expiratory ratio is >90%. (c) *Obstructive ventilatory defect*. The FEV$_1$ is much reduced. The rate of airflow is severely reduced, as indicated by the reduced slope of the curve. Note that the forced expiratory time is increased: the patient is still blowing out at 5 seconds. The VC has not been adequately recorded in this case, because the patient did not continue the expiration after 5 seconds; he or she could have expired further. (This is a common technical error). (d) *Severe airway obstruction*. The FEV$_1$ is about 0.5 l. The FVC is also reduced, but not so strikingly as FEV$_1$. Forced expiratory ratio is 23%. Very low expiratory flow rate. This pattern of a very brief initial rapid phase followed by a straight line indicating little change in maximal flow rate with change in lung volume is sometimes thought to be indicative of severe emphysema, although identical results can be observed in severe asthma. (e) *Airway obstruction and bronchial hyperreactivity*. Five expirations have been made. FEV$_1$ and FVC become lower with each expiration. Patient with asthma. These features suggest poor control of asthma and liability to severe attacks. (f) *A non-maximal expiration*. Compare with (a). In a true forced expiration, the steepest part of the curve always occurs at the beginning of expiration, which is not the case here. A falsely low FEV$_1$ and forced expiratory ratio are obtained. Usually, the patient has not understood what is required or is unable to coordinate his or her actions. Some patients wish to appear worse than they really are. This pattern is unlikely to be mistaken for a true forced expiration because of its shape and because it cannot be reproduced repeatedly. (g) *Escape of air* from the nose or lips during expiration. (h) *Inability to perform the manoeuvre*. Five attempts have been made. In some, the patient has breathed in and out. Other attempts are either not maximal forced expirations or are unfinished. Bizarre patterns such as this are often seen in patients with psychogenic breathlessness or in the elderly. Even with poor cooperation, it is often possible to obtain useful information. In the example shown, significant airway obstruction can be excluded because of the steep slope of at least two of the expirations, which follow an identical course and show appropriate curvature (dotted line), and the FVC can be estimated as not less than 3.2 l. The pattern seen in large airway obstruction is shown in Figs. 3.5 and 3.6.

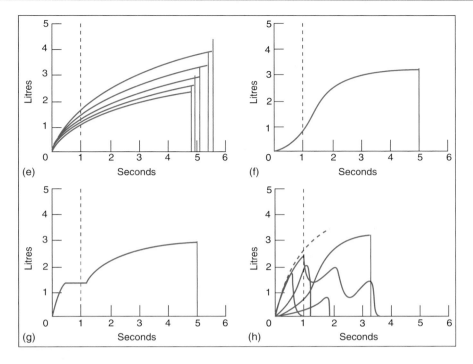

Figure 3.2 *(Continued)*

by the calibre of the airways, and is therefore an index of diffuse airway obstruction. Its principal advantage is derived from its portability and low cost (Fig. 3.3). This allows multiple measurements to be performed independently by patients at different times and in different environments. Variability can thus be observed, which makes it useful in the diagnosis and monitoring of asthma (see Chapter 10).

Flow/volume loop

The familiar spirogram plots volume against time (Fig. 3.2). Forced expiratory manoeuvres may also be displayed by plotting flow against volume. Although the result may be less familiar, it is worth remembering that it contains precisely the same information. When an inspiratory manoeuvre is also included, the trace returns to its starting point and a flow/volume loop is formed. A normal flow/volume loop is shown in Fig. 3.4.

By convention, the starting point of full inspiration (TLC) is to the left, expiratory flow appears above the horizontal and inspiratory flow is shown below it. At TLC, the airways are at their most stretched (dilated) and airway resistance is minimised, so the

maximum (peak) expiratory flow is reached quickly after the start of forced expiration (see Chapter 1). As expiration continues, lung volume progressively diminishes, airway resistance increases and the maximum flow achievable (for the given lung volume) declines. In health, this declining portion of the expiratory limb is surprisingly straight. When no further air can be exhaled, flow is zero and the loop reaches the horizontal axis. The inspiratory manoeuvre can then begin. This tends to be more effort-dependent and therefore less reproducible. Even when perfectly performed, the inspiratory limb is *not* a mirror image of the expiratory limb. Whilst airway calibre would again favour faster flow nearer TLC, mechanical advantage for the muscles of inspiration means more inspiratory force can be applied nearer residual volume. The coexistence of these two factors produces a more symmetrical inspiratory portion to the loop, with maximum inspiratory flow being at the midpoint of inspiration. Note, too, that maximum inspiratory flow is less than maximum expiratory flow.

The flow/volume loop really comes into its own when assessing localised narrowing of the central airways, as illustrated in Figs 3.5 and 3.6. Although the traditional spirogram has a characteristic appearance

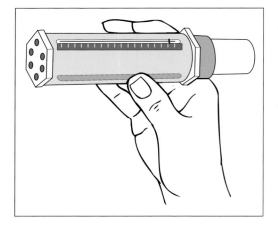

Figure 3.3 Measurement of PEF. The subject takes a *full inspiration*, applies their lips to the mouthpiece and makes a sudden maximal expiratory blast. A piston is pushed down the inside of the cylinder, progressively exposing a slot in the top, until a position of rest is reached. The position of the piston is indicated by a marker and PEF is read from a scale. It is customary to take the best of three properly performed attempts as the PEF.

in this context (Fig 3.5), the abnormality is not so striking as when observed in the flow/volume loop (Fig 3.6 d,e). Without the flow/volume loop, large airway obstruction may be overlooked. By comparing the relative effects on the expiratory and inspiratory limbs, it is also possible to determine whether the large airway obstruction is inside (e.g. tracheal stricture) or outside (e.g. compression by a goitre in the neck) the thorax (Fig. 3.7).

Total lung capacity

The measurement of TLC is not considered in detail here; the interested reader is referred to the reading list at the end of the chapter.

Whereas VC and its subdivisions can be measured directly by spirometry, measurement of residual volume and TLC requires the use of **helium dilution** or **plethysmography** methods. In the dilution technique, a gas of known helium concentration is breathed through a closed circuit and the volume of gas in the lungs is calculated from a measure of the dilution of the helium, which, being an inert gas, is neither absorbed nor metabolised. This dilution method measures only gas in communication with the airways and tends to underestimate TLC in patients with severe airway obstruction, because of the presence of poorly ventilating bullae.

The body plethysmograph is a large airtight box that allows pressure–volume relationships in the thorax to be determined. When the plethysmograph is sealed, changes in lung volume are reflected by a change in pressure within the box. Plethysmography tends to overestimate TLC, because it measures all intrathoracic gas, including that in the bullae, cysts, stomach and oesophagus. **Chest X-ray** can be used to give a rough estimate of TLC. In airway disease, TLC is increased as a manifestation of hyperinflation and as a result of increased lung compliance in emphysema (see Chapter 1). TLC is reduced in restrictive lung disease.

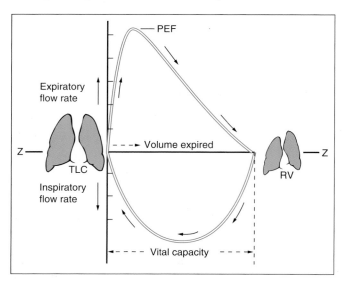

Figure 3.4 Flow/volume loop. Airflow is represented on the vertical axis and lung volume on the horizontal axis. The line Z–Z represents zero flow. Expiratory flow appears above the line; inspiratory flow, below. PEF, peak expiratory flow; RV, residual volume; TLC, total lung capacity.

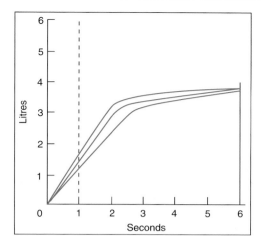

Figure 3.5 Large (central) airway obstruction. Typical tracing obtained with a spirometer. The subject has made three maximal forced expirations. Each shows a striking straight section, which then changes relatively abruptly, at about the same volume, to follow the expected curve of the forced expiratory spirogram. The straight section is not as reproducible as a normal spirogram. A 'family' of similar tracings is thus obtained, each with straight and curved sections. Explanation: over the straight section, flow is limited by the fixed intrathoracic localised obstruction. This is little influenced by lung recoil, so the critical flow is similar during expiration and the spirogram appears straight. A lung volume is eventually reached at which maximum flow is even lower than that permitted by the central obstruction. The ordinary forced expiratory spirogram is described after this point. In the example shown, there must be an element of diffuse airway obstruction, as forced expiratory time is somewhat prolonged (see Fig. 3.2c).

Respiratory muscle function tests

Weakness of the respiratory muscles causes a **restrictive ventilatory defect**, with reduced TLC and VC. Comparison of VC in the erect and supine positions is useful, because the pressure of the abdominal contents on a weak diaphragm typically causes a fall of around 30% in **supine VC**. Chest X-ray often shows small lung volumes with basal atelectasis and high hemi-diaphragms. **Ultrasound screening** may show paradoxical upward movement of a paralysed diaphragm during inspiration. Global respiratory muscle function may be assessed by measuring **mouth pressures**. Maximum inspiratory mouth pressure, P_I **max**, is measured during maximum inspiratory effort from residual volume against an obstructed airway using a mouthpiece and transducer

device, and maximum expiratory mouth pressure, P_E **max**, is measured during a maximal expiratory effort from TLC. When there is severe respiratory muscle weakness, ventilatory failure develops with **hypercapnia**.

Transfer factor for carbon monoxide

At one time, the rate at which gases diffused across the alveolar–capillary membrane was thought to be the principal factor limiting gas exchange. The term **diffusing capacity** was thus coined, defined as 'The quantity of gas transported across in each minute for every unit of pressure gradient'. Although the measurement proved to be very useful clinically, it was later realised that it was affected by many other factors in addition to diffusion, particularly V/Q matching. It was therefore renamed **transfer factor**.

Clearly, it is the transfer of oxygen that is of most interest to clinicians. This is very difficult to measure in practice, however, as transfer of oxygen into the blood quickly becomes limited by the saturation of haemoglobin. Carbon monoxide is thus used as a surrogate for oxygen in this measurement. Very low concentrations are used so that haemoglobin remains avid for the gas as it passes through the alveolar capillary.

The term 'diffusion capacity' ($D_L$co) can still be found in some texts; this is synonymous with 'transfer factor' ($T_L$co).

To measure $T_L$co, we need to know:

1 the amount of CO transferred per minute; and
2 the pressure gradient across the alveolar membrane (in effect, the alveolar partial pressure, as the partial pressure in blood is zero).

Single-breath method

The single-breath method is shown in Fig. 3.8. The patient inspires a gas mixture of helium and carbon monoxide, holds their breath for 10 seconds and then breathes out. An initial volume equivalent to the dead space (the part of the respiratory tract not involved in gas exchange) is discarded and a sample of the expired gas is collected and analysed for alveolar concentrations of helium and carbon monoxide. The change in concentration of helium (which, being an inert gas, is neither absorbed nor metabolised) between the inspired and alveolar samples is the result of gas dilution and gives a measurement of the

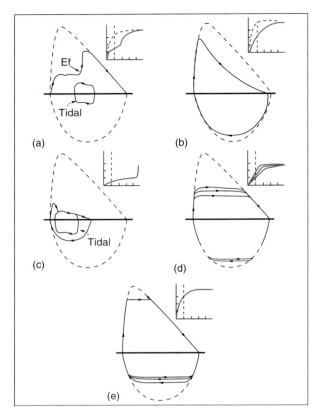

Figure 3.6 Further flow/volume loops. The dotted outline represents a typical normal loop. The small graphs show the appearances of a forced expiration on a spirometer (as in Fig. 3.2). (a) Demonstration of maximum flow. A normal individual makes an unhurried expiration from full inspiration and then, about halfway through the VC, makes a maximal expiratory effort (Ef). The flow/volume tracing rejoins the maximum flow/volume curve, which describes the maximum flow that can be achieved at that lung volume. Also shown in is the flow/volume loop of typical tidal breathing. At the resting lung volume, an abundant reserve of both inspiratory and expiratory flow is available. (b) Moderate airway obstruction (asthma or COPD). Maximum expiratory flow is reduced. The declining portion of the expiratory limb has a characteristic curvilinearity. Inspiration is less severely affected. (c) Very severe airway obstruction. Maximum expiratory flow is very severely reduced. There is a brief peak, followed by an abrupt fall in flow rate (probably caused by some airway closure), after which flow falls very slowly. Also shown in is a loop representing quiet tidal breathing. It is clear that every expiration is limited by maximum flow. Expiratory wheezing or pursed-lip breathing would be expected. The tidal loop has been obliged to move to the left, as the patient is ventilating at a higher lung volume. This has obviated, to some degree, the airway narrowing, but adds to the work of breathing and contributes to the sensation of breathlessness (see Chapter 1). (d) Intrathoracic large airway obstruction. Here the peak inspiratory and expiratory flows have been truncated in a characteristic pattern. Intrathoracic lesions (e.g. tracheal compression by a mediastinal tumour) have a more pronounced effect on the expiratory limb than the inspiratory limb. (e) Extrathoracic obstruction (e.g. tracheal compression by a goitre in the neck). This results in inspiratory collapse of the airway below the obstruction (but still outside the thorax), attenuating maximum inspiratory flow rate to a greater degree than maximum expiratory flow rate.

1. Intrathoracic large airway obstruction

(a)

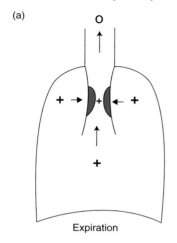

(b)

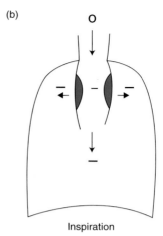

2. Extrathoracic large airway obstruction

(c)

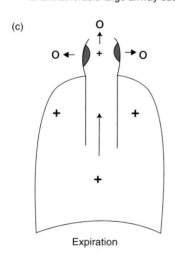

(d)

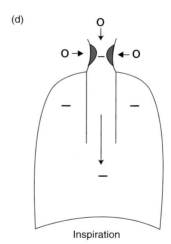

Figure 3.7 Relative effects on expiratory and inspiratory flow of intra- and extrathoracic large airway obstruction. Top: Large airway obstruction within the thorax. (a) Positive intrathoracic (alveolar) pressure generated during expiration acts to compress the airway and further narrow the point of obstruction. (b) Negative intrathoracic pressure during inspiration acts to reduce narrowing at the point of obstruction. Therefore, in large airway obstruction within the thorax, expiratory flow is diminished to a greater degree than inspiratory flow (see Fig. 3.6d). Bottom: Large airway obstruction outside the thorax. (c) Positive pressure within the airway during expiration in relation to atmospheric ('zero') pressure outside acts to reduce narrowing at the point of obstruction. (d) Negative pressure within the airway during inspiration acts to compress the airway and further narrow the point of obstruction. Therefore, in large airway obstruction outside the thorax, inspiratory flow is diminished to a greater degree than expiratory flow (see Fig. 3.6e).

alveolar gas volume (V_A). The expired concentration of carbon monoxide is also lower than the inspired level, but the fall is proportionately greater than in the case of helium because some of the carbon monoxide is absorbed into the bloodstream. The rate of uptake of carbon monoxide can then be calculated as the uptake per minute per unit of partial pressure of carbon monoxide (mmol/min/kPa).

Many factors influence $T_L$co, including:

- V/Q imbalance (disturbed in many diseases, affecting lung parenchyma or vasculature);
- the area of the membrane (reduced in emphysema);
- the thickness of the alveolar capillary membrane (increased in fibrotic lung disease);
- the pulmonary capillary blood volume (increased in high cardiac output states); and
- the haemoglobin concentration.

Free blood in the lungs from pulmonary haemorrhage will also avidly absorb carbon monoxide and lead to an elevated $T_L$co.

Transfer co-efficient

Clearly, $T_L$co can be reduced by a number of disease processes within the lung. It is also reduced if there is simply 'less lung' (a reduced lung volume) participating in gas transfer (e.g. respiratory muscle weakness causing restriction or after pneumonectomy). It would be useful to be able to distinguish between these two very different mechanisms.

Transfer co-efficinet (Kco) is the transfer factor divided by V_A. This tells us the transfer factor 'per unit lung volume'. Like $T_L$co, Kco is reduced when there is intrinsic lung disease, but unlike $T_L$co, Kco is not diminished when a healthy lung is reduced in volume by some external factor.

Interpretation

In the presence of normal spirometry, a reduced Kco is a strong indicator of intrinsic lung disease (affecting the pulmonary vasculature or alveoli; consider pulmonary hypertension or a combination of emphysema and fibrosis).

In restrictive conditions, a reduced Kco suggests an intrapulmonary cause (e.g. fibrosis). In extrapulmonary causes (e.g. chest wall deformity, respiratory muscle weakness, obesity), the Kco tends to be elevated. This is because the Kco is effectively telling us about the transfer of CO only in the alveoli that are ventilated. The non-ventilated alveoli are discounted because they don't contribute to V_A. As the V/Q

matching system will divert blood away from the non-ventilated alveoli, the ventilated alveoli will have more than their normal share of blood. The greater blood volume increases CO absorption and thus gas transfer.

In obstructive conditions, a reduced Kco suggests COPD (emphysema). In asthma, the Kco may be elevated. Asthma does not affect every airway to an identical degree; there is therefore an exaggerated heterogeneity of ventilation. As discussed already, Kco is more heavily influenced by the well-ventilated areas, which, because of V/Q matching, have more than their fair share of perfusion.

Arterial blood gases

Normal values are listed in Table 3.1.

A **sample of arterial blood** may be obtained from any artery, but the **radial artery** at the wrist and the **brachial artery** in the antecubital fossa are the sites most commonly used. The blood enters the heparinised needle and syringe under its own pressure with a pulsatile action. The syringe containing the arterial blood is capped, placed in **ice** and analysed in the laboratory within 30 minutes of sampling.

Review of acid/base balance

CO_2 dissolves in H_2O and forms carbonic acid (H_2CO_3), which dissociates into H^+ and HCO_3^- in a constant relationship:

$$K = \frac{[H^+][HCO_3^-]}{[H_2CO_3]}$$

Thus:

$$[H^+]\alpha \frac{[H_2CO_3]}{[HCO_3^-]}$$

As $[H_2CO_3]$ directly relates to the partial pressure of CO_2:

$$[H^+]\alpha \frac{Pco_2}{[HCO_3^-]}$$

In other words, for a given concentration of bicarbonate, Pco_2 has a direct linear relationship with $[H^+]$ (and thus an inverse relationship with pH, which is the negative logarithm of $[H^+]$).

Similarly, for a given Pco_2, there is a direct relationship between $[HCO_3^-]$ and pH.

These relationships can be represented graphically (Fig. 3.9).

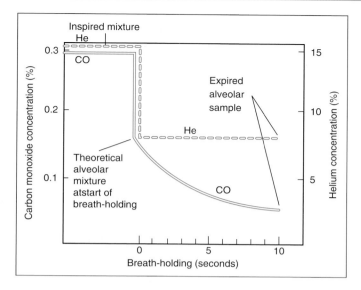

Figure 3.8 Measurement of transfer factor by the single-breath method. Schematic representation of the helium and carbon monoxide concentrations in the inspired mixture and in alveolar air during breath holding.

Bicarbonate concentration

Most blood gas analysers provide two different measurements of bicarbonate – 'actual bicarbonate' and 'standard bicarbonate' – in addition to another value, 'base excess'. This can cause confusion, although it needn't. The analyser measures the bicarbonate level in the blood sample. This actual measurement is (conveniently) known as the **actual bicarbonate**

($aHCO_3^-$). As can be seen in Fig. 3.9, the actual level is directly dependant on the P_{CO_2} (for a given pH: the higher the P_{CO_2}, the higher the $aHCO_3^-$; the lower the P_{CO_2} the lower the $aHCO_3^-$). If pH and P_{CO_2} are known, the bicarbonate level can be calculated. For a given pH, the level of bicarbonate can be calculated for a 'standard' P_{CO_2} (5.3 kPa). This calculated value is (conveniently) known as the **standard bicarbonate** ($sHCO_3^-$). There is little to choose between these

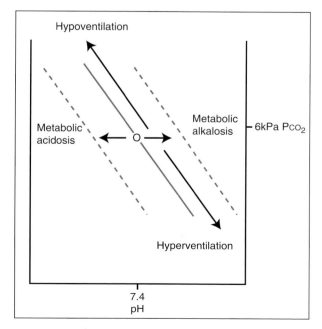

Figure 3.9 Bicarbonate isopleths (diagonal lines; the bicarbonate level is constant along the lines). It can be seen that, if the bicarbonate level and P_{CO_2} are known, the pH can be calculated. Indeed, if any two of the three values of bicarbonate, pH and P_{CO_2} are known then the other value can be calculated. These values are yoked together. A change in ventilation will move the arterial point up or down an isopleth as shown, changing pH (bicarbonate level does not change). A pure metabolic disturbance (before any respiratory response) changes the bicarbonate level, moving from one bicarbonate isopleth to another and changing pH.

Table 3.1 Normal values for arterial blood gases whilst breathing normal room air at sea level

pH	7.35–7.45
Pco$_2$	4.5–6.0 kPa, 34–45 mmHg
Po$_2$	11–14 kPa, 83–105 mmHg
Actual bicarbonate (aHCO$_3^-$)	22–26 mmol/l
Standard bicarbonate (sHCO$_3^-$)	22–26 mmol/l
Base excess	–2 to +2 mmol/l
Oxygen saturation	96–98%

two indices, but the sHCO$_3^-$ takes out the immediate effect of CO$_2$ on the bicarbonate level and can loosely be regarded as giving a more direct indication of the metabolic activity influencing acid/base balance. The **base excess** takes into account the fact that there are other buffers apart from bicarbonate in the blood. It tells a similar story to the bicarbonate level in terms of acid/base disturbance. Its principal advantage is the ease with which its normal range can be remembered. As one might anticipate from the name, the 'excess' should be zero (normal range is 0 ± 2 mmol/l). There aren't many numbers easier to remember than zero.

Acid/base disturbances

The three variables pH, Pco$_2$ and bicarbonate are yoked together as just described. Analysis of their values provides information on the acid/base balance of the body and the broad nature of its cause. It may also provide information about the chronicity of an abnormality.

Changes in the acid/base status caused by changes in Pco$_2$ (hyper- or hypoventilation) are termed **respiratory**. Changes in acid/base status caused by changes in bicarbonate are termed **metabolic.** A disturbance in one system tends to prompt a compensatory response in the other. When needed, the respiratory system responds promptly, and changes are evident within seconds to minutes. The metabolic system, largely regulated via renal excretion, is much slower, taking between hours and days to equilibrate. In respiratory disturbances, therefore, the degree of correction achieved by the metabolic

system can tell us something about the duration of the abnormality.

As a general principal, **physiological compensatory mechanisms don't overcompensate**; in fact, they often stop just short of total correction. This is a useful fact to remember when trying to interpret a blood gas result that displays both respiratory and metabolic changes. If the pH is in the normal range, it may be difficult to determine which is the primary abnormality and which the compensatory response. Look again at the pH. If the pH is towards the higher end of the normal range, the primary abnormality is probably an alkalosis; if at the lower end then the primary disturbance is an acidosis.

In reading the following examples of acid/base disturbance, refer to the diagrams in Figs 3.9 and 3.10.

Respiratory acidosis (acute): pH reduced, Pco$_2$ raised, bicarbonate normal

A reduction in alveolar ventilation causes an increase in arterial Pco$_2$. The pH falls. In the short term, there is insufficient time for metabolic (renal) correction, so the bicarbonate concentration remains almost unchanged. This pattern is seen where there is a sudden reduction in ventilation, such as obstruction of the airway, overdose of sedative drugs or acute neurological damage.

Respiratory acidosis (chronic): pH normal (lower half of normal range), Pco$_2$ raised, bicarbonate high

If underventilation, from whatever cause, is sustained beyond a few days, renal tubular reabsorption of bicarbonate will achieve a significant elevation in plasma bicarbonate level, which will correct the acidosis caused by the underventilation. This can be caused by any process that results in sustained hypoventilation (commonly seen in COPD).

Respiratory alkalosis (cases are usually acute, as the causes are rarely sustained): pH raised, Pco$_2$ reduced, bicarbonate normal

Alveolar hyperventilation causes a fall in Pco$_2$ and a corresponding rise in pH. Bicarbonate concentration is virtually unchanged. This pattern is seen in any form of acute hyperventilation, including pulmonary embolism, acute severe asthma, anxiety-related hyperventilation and salicylate poisoning.

Metabolic acidosis: pH reduced, Pco$_2$ reduced, bicarbonate reduced

The primary disturbance is generally an increase in acid. This has an effect on the equilibrium $H^+ + HCO_3^- \rightleftharpoons H_2O + CO_2$, pushing it to the right. The CO_2 produced is removed by increased ventilation and the net result is a lowering of plasma bicarbonate. In practice, the fall in pH causes further respiratory stimulation, so that CO_2 is promptly blown off, and the pH changes are therefore much less dramatic than they would have been. The arterial point moves in the direction indicated in Fig. 3.10. This respiratory compensation is an inevitable accompaniment of metabolic acidosis – acute and chronic – unless there is some other factor limiting ventilatory function or responsiveness.

This pattern is seen in diabetic ketoacidosis, renal tubular acidosis, acute circulatory failure, sepsis and other forms of lactic acidosis.

Metabolic alkalosis: pH raised, Pco$_2$ high normal or slightly raised, bicarbonate raised

An increase in bicarbonate concentration causes a rise in pH. To compensate, ventilation is reduced in order to accumulate CO_2. This occurs despite the inevitable fall in Po$_2$. For this reason, however, scope for correction is limited; the compensatory fall in alveolar ventilation is modest and correction in pH may not be complete.

This pattern is seen where there has been administration of excessive alkali, loss of acid through vomiting or reabsorption of bicarbonate (e.g. in hypokalaemia).

Mixed disturbances

Mixed respiratory and metabolic disturbances are common. There are usually a number of possible explanations, so it is essential to consider all the clinical details before interpreting the acid/base data. Fig. 3.10 shows the situations that may arise in complex acid/base disturbances. For example:

- Fig. 3.10a (low pH, normal Pco$_2$, low bicarbonate) indicates a mixed metabolic and respiratory acidosis. The metabolic disturbance is perhaps obvious and the respiratory component can be deduced, as the Pco$_2$ is higher than might have been suspected had this been a pure metabolic problem. This pattern could arise in a number of different clinical scenarios, such as a patient with acute severe pulmonary oedema with low cardiac output and ventilatory compromise or a patient in renal failure given a narcotic sedative suppressing ventilatory response to acidosis. Blood gas results should be interpreted in light of clinical data.

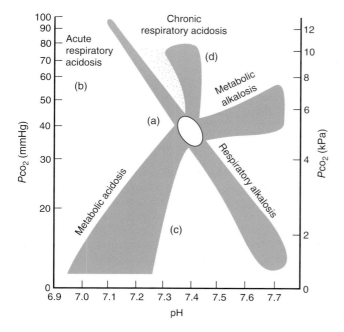

Figure 3.10 Acid/base disturbances. The oval indicates the normal position, the shaded areas indicate the directions of observed 'pure' or uncomplicated disturbances of acid/base balance. Bicarbonate levels are omitted for clarity. Letters (a)–(d) are referred to in the section on mixed disturbances.

- Fig. 3.10b could represent the situation soon after a cardiac arrest, where severe lactic acidosis exists and ventilation has been insufficient.
- Fig. 3.10c could represent the situation in severe aspirin poisoning, where aspirin-induced hyperventilation has been complicated by aspirin-induced metabolic acidosis.
- Fig. 3.10d could represent the situation in an individual with chronic ventilatory failure as a result of COPD who is stimulated to increase ventilation by a pulmonary embolism.

Arterial oxygenation

In addition to the acid/base balance, arterial blood gas analysis provides valuable information on arterial oxygen tension (P_aO_2).

Respiratory failure

'Respiratory failure' is a clinical term used to describe a failure to maintain oxygenation (usually taken as an arbitrary cut-off point of Po_2 8.0 kPa (60 mmHg)).

- Type I respiratory failure is hypoxaemia in the absence of hypercapnia. Overall alveolar ventilation is therefore normal. This pattern of abnormality usually indicates a disturbance of the V/Q matching system within the lung. Such a disturbance can be caused by any intrinsic lung disease affecting the airways, parenchyma or vasculature (e.g. acute asthma, lung fibrosis or pulmonary embolism).
- Type II respiratory failure is hypoxaemia with hypercapnia and indicates alveolar hypoventilation. Note this is *not* merely a severe form of type I respiratory failure; it is brought about by an entirely different mechanism. This may occur from reduced ventilatory drive (e.g. sedative overdose), reduced neuromuscular power (e.g. myopathy) or resetting of the chemoreceptors that drive ventilation in chronic lung disease (e.g. COPD).

Of course, type I and type II respiratory failure can coexist (and commonly do). These matters are dealt with in more detail in Chapter 1.

Oxygen saturation can be measured noninvasively and continuously using a **pulse oximeter**. Oxygenated blood appears red, whereas reduced blood appears blue (clinical sign of cyanosis). An oximeter measures the ratio of oxygenated to total haemoglobin in arterial blood using a probe placed on a finger or earlobe, which comprises two light-emitting diodes – one red and one infrared – and a detector. The light absorbed varies with each pulse, and measurement of light absorption at two points on the pulse wave allows the oxygen saturation of arterial blood to be determined. The accuracy of measurement is reduced if there is reduced arterial pulsation (e.g. low-output cardiac states) or increased venous pulsation (e.g. tricuspid regurgitation, venous congestion). Skin pigmentation or the use of nail varnish may interfere with light transmission. Oximetry is also inaccurate in the presence of carboxyhaemoglobin (e.g. in carbon monoxide poisoning), which the oximeter detects as oxyhaemoglobin. The relationship of Po_2 to oxygen saturation is described by the **oxyhaemoglobin dissociation curve** (see Fig. 1.9). This curve is sigma-shaped, so that oxygen saturation is closely related to Po_2 only over a short range of about 3–7 kPa. Above this level, the dissociation curve begins to plateau and there is only a small increase in oxygen saturation as the Po_2 rises. Oximetry can reduce the need for arterial puncture, but arterial blood gas analysis is necessary to determine accurately the Po_2 on the plateau part of the oxyhaemoglobin dissociation curve, to measure CO_2 level and to assess acid/base status.

A simple algorithm for reviewing blood gas results

Most blood results in medicine are relative easy to make sense of: there's one value, and it's either high or low. When faced with the results of an arterial blood gas measurement, the clinician has to handle six different values, which must be drawn together and interpreted as one. The inexperienced often find their attention skipping from one number to the next, declaring each as either high or low, before becoming utterly confused and giving up. A simple stepwise system for interpreting blood results would help. The following algorithm is easy to follow and will make sense of most of the results you'll come across in clinical practice:

1 **Look at the pH.** Decide whether this is an acidosis or alkalosis. Once that fact is determined, don't be diverted from it after reviewing the other values. It won't change. If the pH is in the normal range, note whether it is erring towards one end of the range or the other. If there is a compensated abnormality, the position of the pH within the range may indicate the nature of the primary disturbance. Remember that physiological compensatory mechanisms don't over compensate.

2 **Look at the Pco2.** Ask whehter the Pco_2 is contributing to or attempting to compensate for the abnormality identified in the pH. That will allow you to know whether the primary disturbance is

respiratory (contributing) or metabolic (attempting to compensate).

3 **Look at the bicarbonate.** I would suggest either the $sHCO_3^-$ or base excess. In the case of a primary metabolic problem, the bicarbonate may hold no surprises. In a metabolic acidosis, it will be low; in a metabolic alkalosis, high. In the case of a primary respiratory problem, the bicarbonate may be: normal (suggesting the problem is acute, having not had time to change), attempting to correct the respiratory effect on the pH (suggesting the problem is chronic) or compounding the problem (suggesting a mixed disturbance).

4 **Look at the Po_2.** Knowing the inspired partial pressure of oxygen, ask whether the Po_2 is what you'd expect given the level of ventilation (i.e. given the Pco_2) or lower than expected. This may be difficult to gauge, in which case the alveolar gas equation should be applied (see Chapter 1). You can then determine whether type I respiratory failure, type II respiratory failure or both are present.

 KEY POINTS

- A reduced FEV_1/VC ratio indicates airways obstruction (e.g. asthma, COPD).
- A reduced Kco indicates disease of the lung parenchyma or its blood supply (e.g. emphysema, lung fibrosis, pulmonary embolism).
- Type I respiratory failure is hypoxia without hypercapnia and may occur in any disease intrinsic to the lung (e.g. asthma, pulmonary oedema, pulmonary embolism, lung fibrosis).
- Type II respiratory failure is hypoxia with hypercapnia and indicates hypoventilation (e.g. sedative overdose, neuromuscular disease or moderate to severe COPD where it occurs in conjunction with a type I respiratory failure).
- An elevated alveolar–arterial gradient implies a problem intrinsic to the lung.

FURTHER READING

Cotes JE. *Lung Function: Assessment and Application in Medicine*. Oxford: Blackwell Scientific Publications, 1993.

Flenley DC. Interpretation of blood-gas and acid–base data. *Br J Hosp Med* 1978; **20**: 384–94.

Gibson GJ. *Clinical Tests of Respiratory Function*. Oxford: Oxford University Press: 2009.

Gibson GJ. Measurement of respiratory muscle strength. *Respir Med* 1995; **89**: 529–35.

Hanning CD, Alexander-Williams JM. Pulse oximetry: a practical review. *BMJ* 1995; **311**: 367–70.

Multiple choice questions

3.1 The volume of gas in the lungs after a normal tidal inspiration is:

A residual volume

B total lung capacity minus residual volume

C functional residual capacity

D tidal volume plus functional residual capacity

E vital capacity minus residual volume

3.2 Lung function test results of FEV_1 reduced, FEV_1/VC normal, T_Lco normal, Kco increased would be most in keeping with:

A kyphoscoliosis

B idiopathic pulmonary fibrosis

C pulmonary hypertension

D asthma

E COPD

3.3 Arterial blood gases of pH 7.33, Pco_2 8.4 kPa, Po_2 12.6 kPa, $sHCO_3$ 28 mmol/L, O_2 saturation 97% are most in keeping with:

A a chronic metabolic acidosis

B an acute on chronic metabolic acidosis

C an overcompensated metabolic alkalosis

D an acute on chronic respiratory acidosis

E a chronic respiratory acidosis

3.4 Given arterial blood gases of pH 7.33, Pco_2 8.4 kPa, Po_2 12.6 kPa, $sHCO_3$ 28 mmol/L, O_2 saturation 97%, one could confidently conclude that:

A the patient is breathing supplemental oxygen

B the patient has COPD

C the patient needs to be transferred to ITU

D the condition is chronic and stable

E the lungs are normal

3.5 A 24-year-old woman presents to hospital as an emergency with breathlessness. Her arterial blood gases while breathing room air are pH 7.49, Pco_2 3.3 kPa, Po_2 11.9 kPa, $sHCO_3$ 24 mmol/L, O_2 saturation 97%. This presentation is most in keeping with:

A pulmonary embolism

B anxiety

C opiate overdose

D excess vomiting

E pneumonia

3.6 A 46-year-old man has an FEV1 that is only 80% of the predicted value:

A his exercise capacity will be approximately 80% of age/height-matched peers

B he will be 20% more breathless than age/height-matched peers

C he has airway obstruction

D this is consistent with the absence of any lung disease at all

E it is likely that he smoked

3.7 A reduced forced vital capacity (FVC):

A implies a restrictive defect

B is expected in airway obstruction

C cannot be present if slow (relaxed) vital capacity is normal

D suggests lung fibrosis

E is a bad prognostic marker

3.8 In diseases causing weakness of the respiratory muscles, the pattern of lung function disturbance expected would be:

A reduced FEV1, relatively normal FVC

B normal FEV1/FVC ratio, reduced kCO

C reduced FEV1 and FVC, increased kCO

D normal lung function

E increased FEV1/FVC ratio

3.9 Transfer coefficient (Kco) would be reduced in the following conditions:

A pneumonia

B COPD

C pulmonary haemorrhage

D asthma

E pulmonary fibrosis

3.10 In kyphoscoliosis, the following physiological findings would be expected:

A reduced FEV1

B reduced FVC

C reduced TLco

D reduced Kco

E reduced TLC

Multiple choice answers

3.1 D

See Figure 3.1.

3.2 A

The normal FEV/VC and reduced FEV_1 implies restriction. The elevated Kco suggests the cause is extra-pulmonary.

3.3 D

The pH is low, so this is an acidosis. The Pco_2 is high, so this is a respiratory acidosis. The bicarbonate is high, suggesting there has been time to attempt to compensate (chronic). However, the pH would be in the normal range had this been a chronic stable state, so there must be an acute component. Remember, too, that physiological compensatory mechanisms don't overcompensate.

3.4 A

If you assume the patient is breathing room air ($P_Io_2 = 21$ kPa), then the alveolar–arterial gradient will be negative, suggesting the patient is a net contributor of oxygen to the environment. This seems unlikely. The inspired Po_2 therefore must be greater than 21 kPa.

The condition is clearly not stable; the pH is outside the normal range. As we aren't given the P_Io_2, we can't conclude the lungs are normal. The A–a gradient may be very high.

3.5 A

This is a primary respiratory alkalosis, so the answer must be either anxiety-driven hyperventilation or pulmonary embolism. The alveolar arterial gradient is increased, implying a problem within the lungs (affecting V/Q matching), which anxiety cannot explain.

3.6 D

At 80% of the predicted value, the result is still well within the normal range and therefore can be found within the normal population (of course, this doesn't mean you can conclude that there is no disease present).

3.7 B

In airway obstruction, although there is a greater proportionate reduction in FEV1 than FVC, because closure of the terminal airways occurs a little earlier (preventing the expulsion of any more air), FVC is also reduced.

3.8 C

Muscle weakness is an example of an extra-pulmonary restrictive defect. Therefore, FEV1 and FVC will be reduced (approximately in proportion) and the gas transfer per unit lung volume (kCO) will be elevated (see text).

3.9 A,B,E

In pulmonary haemorrhage and asthma, Kco is typically elevated.

3.10 A,B,C,E

Kco is increased in restrictive defects caused by extra-pulmonary factors.

4

Radiology of the chest

Chest X-ray

The chest X-ray plays a key role in the investigation of respiratory disease. It is routinely performed on every patient with any symptom even vaguely related to the chest (and many who don't). Yet, for such a ubiquitous investigation, it remains strangely alien and enigmatic to most medical students (and many doctors). It is often intimidating to see an experienced radiologist make immediate sense of the nebulous shadows that have left you perplexed and floundering for so long. Don't be fooled. There is no mysterious perception that only you lack. Start with the premise that X-ray interpretation is difficult (at least to begin with). Don't expect 'the answer' to be obvious. Work through the X-ray in a systematic way. You will at least be able to say something sensible in your report and you may be left with a number of possible explanations for the appearances you observe. There are many occasions on which even an experienced radiologist can do no more than that.

The standard view of a chest X-ray is the erect, **postero-anterior (PA) chest X-ray** taken at full inspiration, with the X-ray beam passing from back to front. A **lateral X-ray** gives a better view of lesions lying behind the heart or diaphragm, which may not be visible on a PA X-ray, and allows abnormalities to be viewed in a further dimension. Supine and **antero-posterior (AP) views** are usually taken at the bedside using mobile equipment in patients who are too ill to be brought to the X-ray department. AP films are less satisfactory in defining many abnormalities, producing magnification of the cardiac outline, for example.

The main landmarks of the normal chest X-ray are shown in Figs 4.1 and 4.2.

X-rays should be examined both close up and from a short distance in an area with reduced background lighting. It is important to confirm the name and date on the X-ray and to check the technical quality of the film. Symmetry between the medial ends of both clavicles and the thoracic spinous processes confirms that the film has been taken without any rotation artefact. If the film has been taken in full inspiration, the right hemidiaphragm is normally intersected by the anterior part of the sixth rib. The vertebral bodies are usually visible through the cardiac shadow if the X-ray exposure is satisfactory. It is helpful to examine the film systematically in order to avoid missing useful information. The shape and bony structures of the chest wall should be surveyed and the positions of the hemidiaphragms and trachea noted. The shape and size of the heart and the appearances of the mediastinum and hilar shadows should be examined. The size, shape and disposition of the vascular shadows should be noted and the patterns of the lung markings in different zones should be compared. Remember, as in clinical examination, to make full use of the fact that we have two lungs. Determining whether an isolated appearance is abnormal may be difficult; spotting, for example, that one lung apex looks different to the other, is easy. Compare the equivalent areas on each side systematically. It is advisable to focus attention on areas of the chest X-ray where lesions are commonly missed, such as the hila, the area behind the heart and the lung apices. Any abnormality detected should be analysed in detail and interpreted in the context of all clinical information. It is often helpful to obtain previous X-rays or to monitor the evolution of abnormalities over time on follow-up X-rays. Some of the radiological features of the major lung diseases are shown in individual chapters. In some circumstances, chest X-ray abnormalities follow a specific pattern that allows a differential diagnosis to be outlined.

Respiratory Medicine Lecture Notes, Ninth Edition. Stephen J. Bourke and Graham P. Burns.
© 2015 John Wiley & Sons, Ltd. Published 2015 by John Wiley & Sons, Ltd.
Companion Website: www.lecturenoteseries.com/Respiratory

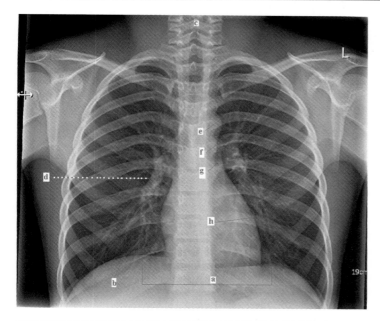

Figure 4.1 Diagram of chest X-ray (PA view). The right hemidiaphragm is 1–3 cm higher than the left (a) and on full inspiration is intersected by the shadow of the anterior part of the sixth rib (b). The trachea (c) is vertical and central. The horizontal fissure (d) is found in the position shown and should be truly horizontal. It is a very valuable marker of a change in volume of any part of the right lung but is not always visible. The left border of the cardiac shadow comprises: (e) aorta, (f) pulmonary artery, (g) concavity overlying the left atrial appendage and (h) left ventricle. The right border of the cardiac shadow normally overlies the right atrium (i) and sits above that of the superior vena cava.

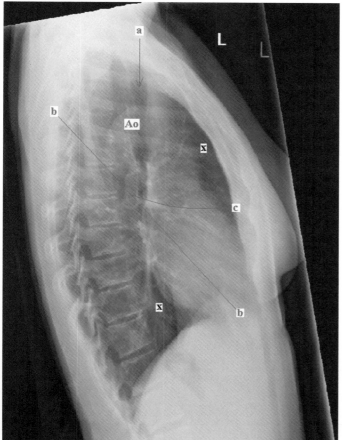

Figure 4.2 Diagram of chest X-ray (lateral view). (a) Trachea. (b) Oblique fissure. (c) Horizontal fissure. It is useful to note that in a normal lateral view, the radiodensity of the lung field above and in front of the cardiac shadow is about the same as that below and behind (x). Ao, aorta.

Abnormal features

Collapse

Obstruction of a bronchus by a carcinoma, foreign body (e.g. inhaled peanut) or mucus plug causes loss of aeration with **'loss of volume'** and collapse of the lung distal to the obstruction. Collapse of each individual lobe of the lung produces its own particular appearance on chest X-ray (Figs 4.3 and 4.4), with **shift of landmarks** such as the mediastinum resulting from loss of volume. Obstruction of a main bronchus usually causes obvious asymmetry (Fig. 4.5). **Compensatory expansion** of other lobes may result in increased transradiency of adjacent areas of the lung. In right middle lobe collapse, there may be little to see on a PA X-ray apart from a lack of definition of the right heart border. This is a useful sign that helps to distinguish it from lower lobe collapse, where the right border of the heart remains clearly defined. Left lower lobe collapse manifests as a triangular area of increased density behind the heart shadow, often with a shift of the heart shadow to the left and increased transradiency of the left hemithorax due to compensatory expansion of the left upper lobe (Fig. 4.4). Collapse is a sinister sign, often indicating an obstructing carcinoma, which may be confirmed by bronchoscopy.

Consolidation

Air in the lungs appears black on X-ray. Consolidation appears as **areas of opacification**, sometimes conforming to the outline of a lobe or a segment of lung in which the air has been replaced by an inflammatory exudate (e.g. pneumonia), fluid (e.g. pulmonary oedema), blood (e.g. pulmonary haemorrhage) or tumour (e.g. adenocarcinoma with lepidic growth). Bronchi containing air passing through the consolidated lung are sometimes clearly visible as black tubes of air against the white background of the consolidated lung (**air bronchograms**; see Fig. 17.2). Structures such as the heart, mediastinum and

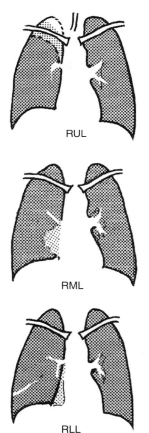

RUL

RML

RLL

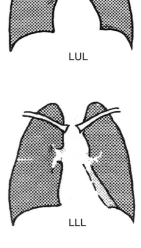

LUL

LLL

Figure 4.3 Radiographic patterns of lobar collapse. Collapsed lobes occupy a surprisingly small volume and are commonly overlooked on the chest X-ray. Helpful information may be provided by the position of the trachea, the hilar vascular shadows and the horizontal fissure. LLL, left lower lobe; LUL, left upper lobe; RLL, right lower lobe; RML, right middle lobe; RUL, right upper lobe.

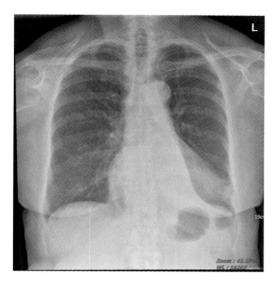

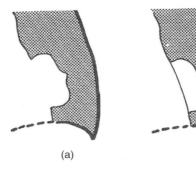

(a)   (b)

Figure 4.6 The silhouette sign, showing abnormal lung shadowing in the left lower zone. Where the sharp outline of mediastinal structures or diaphragm is lost because of normal lung opacification, it can be concluded that the shadow is immediately adjacent to the structure (and vice versa). In example (a), the shadow must be anterior and next to the heart as the sharp outline of the heart is lost. In (b), it must be posterior, as the heart outline is preserved.

Figure 4.4 The left lower lobe has collapsed medially and posteriorly and appears as a dense white triangular area behind the heart, close to the mediastinum. The remainder of the left lung appears hyperlucent because of compensatory expansion. Bronchoscopy showed an adenocarcinoma occluding the left lower lobe bronchus.

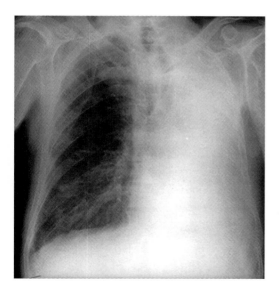

Figure 4.5 Left lung collapse. There is complete opacification of the left hemithorax, with a shift of the mediastinum to the left. Bronchoscopy showed a small-cell carcinoma occluding the left main bronchus.

diaphragm are usually clearly outlined as a silhouette on an X-ray because of the contrast between the blackness of aerated lung and the whiteness of these structures. When there is abnormal shadowing in the lung adjacent to these structures, there is loss of the sharp outline; this is often referred to as the **silhouette sign** (Figure 4.6).

Pulmonary masses

Various descriptive terms, such as 'rounded opacity', 'nodule' and 'coin lesion' are used to refer to pulmonary masses. Carcinoma of the lung is the most important cause of a mass on chest X-ray, but several other diseases may cause a similar appearance (Table 4.1, Fig. 4.7). Features such as **cavitation, calcification, rate of growth**, the presence of **associated abnormalities** (e.g. lymph node enlargement) and whether the lesion is **solitary** or **multiple** lesions are present may provide clues to diagnosis. However, these features are often not reliable indicators of aetiology, and the X-ray appearance must be interpreted in the context of all of the clinical information. Further investigations, such as computed tomography (CT) and biopsy (bronchoscopic, percutaneous, surgical), are often necessary.

Cavitation

Cavitation is the presence of an area of radiolucency within a mass lesion. It is a feature of **bronchial**

Table 4.1 Causes of pulmonary masses

	Typical appearance (not always consistent)
Neoplastic	
• Primary bronchial carcinoma	Spiculated or lobulated
• Metastatic carcinoma	Smooth outline, single or multiple, variable size
• Benign tumours (hamartoma)	Usually solitary, smooth outline, may contain calcium
Non-neoplastic	
• Tuberculoma	Rounded, well-defined, often densely calcified
• Lung abscess	Thick-walled cavity
• Hydatid cyst	Rounded, cystic, variably filled, may be very large
• Pulmonary infarct	'Wedge'-shaped, pleural-based
• Arteriovenous malformation	Homogeneous, well-defined, non-calcified nodule with draining vessels
• Encysted interlobar effusion ('pseudotumour')	Smooth, round or elliptical, in fissures
• Rheumatoid nodule	Rounded, subpleural, multiple, cavitating

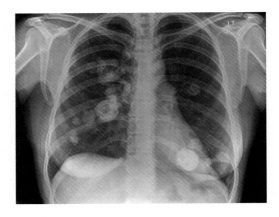

Figure 4.7 Chest X-ray showing multiple partially calcified rounded masses in both lungs, caused by benign chondromas.

carcinoma (particularly squamous carcinoma) (Fig. 4.8), **tuberculosis**, **lung abscess**, **pulmonary infarcts**, **granulomatosis with polyangiitis** (GPA) (formally known as Wegener's granulomatosis) and some **pneumonias** (e.g. *Staphylococcus aureus*, *Klebsiella pneumoniae*).

Fibrosis

Localised fibrosis produces **streaky shadows** with evidence of **traction** upon neighbouring structures. Upper lobe fibrosis causes traction upon the trachea and elevation of the hilar vascular shadows. Generalised interstitial fibrosis produces a hazy shadowing with a **fine reticular (netlike)** or **nodular pattern** (see Chapter 13). Advanced interstitial fibrosis results in a honeycomb pattern with diffuse opacification containing multiple circular translucencies a few millimetres in diameter, best seen on CT scan.

Mediastinal masses

Metastatic tumour and lymphomatous involvement of the mediastinal lymph nodes are the most common causes of mediastinal masses, but there are a number of other diseases that may produce them (Fig. 4.9). Thymic tumours, thyroid masses and dermoid cysts are most commonly situated in the anterior mediastinum, whereas neural lesions (e.g. neurofibroma) and oesophageal cysts are often situated posteriorly. Aneurysmal enlargement of the aorta or ventricle may produce masses in the middle compartment of the mediastinum. CT scans are helpful in delineating the anatomy of mediastinal lesions. Thoracotomy with surgical excision is often necessary.

Ultrasonography

Normal air-filled lung does not transmit high-frequency sound waves, so ultrasonography is not useful in assessing disease of lung parenchyma. It is helpful in assessing lesions of the pleura and is particularly useful for localising loculated pleural effusions and guiding chest tube insertion (see Chapter 16).

Computed tomography

CT scanning uses multiple projection to reconstruct an image from X-ray detectors, so that structures can be displayed in cross-section. A number of different techniques can be used, depending on the area of

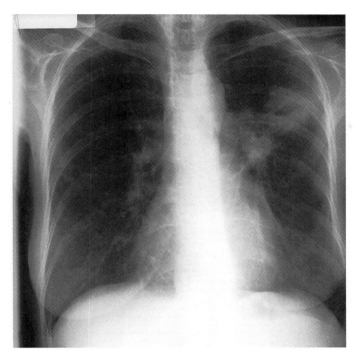

Figure 4.8 A cavitating lesion in the left upper lobe. A cavity appears as an area of radiolucency (black) within an opacity (white). Sputum cytology showed cells from a squamous carcinoma. CT showed left hilar and subcarinal lymphadenopathy.

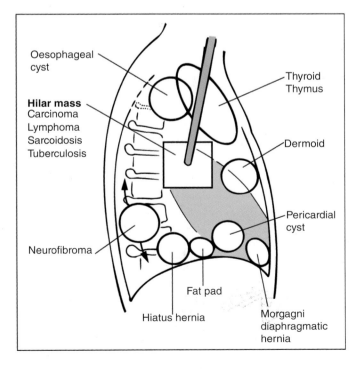

Figure 4.9 Mediastinal masses. Diagram of lateral view of the chest, indicating the sites favoured by some of the more common mediastinal masses.

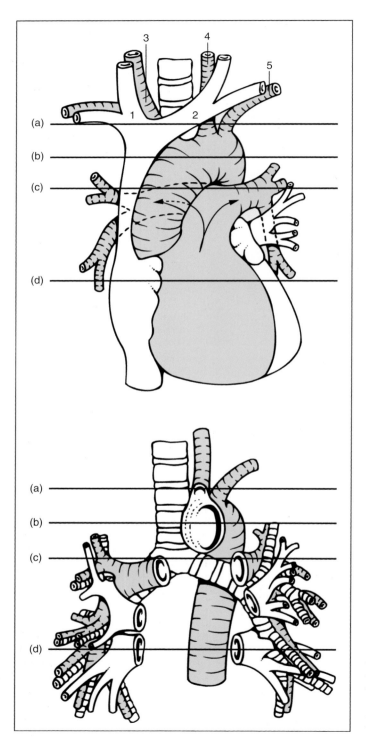

Figure 4.10 Mediastinal structures; principal blood vessels and airways. Top: heart and major blood vessels, showing the aorta curling over the bifurcation of the pulmonary trunk into left and right pulmonary arteries (arrows). The horizontal lines (a)–(d) indicate the levels of the CT sections illustrated in Fig. 4.11. 1, right brachiocephalic vein; 2, left brachiocephalic vein; 3, innominate or brachiocephalic artery; 4, left common carotid artery; 5, left subclavian artery. Bottom: structures with the heart removed. The aorta curls over the left main bronchus, which lies behind the left pulmonary artery. Pulmonary arteries are shown shaded, pulmonary veins are shown unshaded and bronchi are shown striped. In general, the arteries loop downwards, like a handlebar moustache. Veins radiate towards a lower common destination: the left atrium. The veins are applied to the fronts of the arteries and bronchi and take a slightly different path to the respective lung segments. On the right, the order of structures from front to back is vein–artery–bronchus; on the left, the pulmonary artery loops over the left upper lobe bronchus and descends behind, so that the order is vein–bronchus–artery.

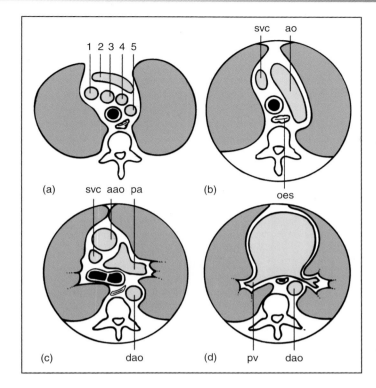

Figure 4.11 Principal mediastinal structures on CT. Sections (a)–(d) are at levels (a)–(d) in Fig. 4.10. The sections should be regarded as being viewed from below **(i.e. the left of the thorax is on the right of the figure)**. (a) *Section above the aortic arch*. Many large vessels and an anterior sausage shape are seen; the trachea has not bifurcated (black circle). Numerals refer to Fig. 4.10 and its legend. (b) *Section at the level of the aortic arch*. A large oblique sausage shape representing the aortic arch is seen (ao). oes, oesophagus (visible in all of the sections); svc, superior vena cava. (c) *Section below the aortic arch*. Both ascending (aao) and descending (dao) aortas are visible. The trachea is bifurcating and the pulmonary arteries are seen. pa, left pulmonary artery. (d) *Section at the level of pulmonary veins (pv)*. Lower lobe intrapulmonary arteries and bronchi are not shown in the diagram.

interest. CT scanning is particularly useful in providing a detailed cross-sectional image of mediastinal disease, which is often difficult to assess on plain chest X-ray. Figure 4.10 shows the principal mediastinal structures, with horizontal lines indicating the levels of the CT sections illustrated diagrammatically in Fig. 4.11. CT scanning is a key investigation in the staging of lung cancer (see Chapter 12) and in detecting and determining the extent of bronchiectasis (see Chapter 8). High-resolution CT scans are much more sensitive than plain X-ray in assessing the lung parenchyma and can provide a detailed image of emphysema (see Chapter 11) and interstitial lung disease. A 'ground glass' appearance on a high-resolution CT scan of a patient with interstitial lung disease may correspond to alveolar inflammation, although it is nonspecific in indicating changes beyond the resolution of the technique. A 'reticular honeycomb pattern' indicates advanced fibrosis with less active inflammation, which is less likely to respond to steroids (see Chapter 13). A **CT pulmonary angiogram** combines a rapid CT sequence with injection of radio-contrast material into a peripheral vein and can be used to identify emboli in central pulmonary arteries in thromboembolic disease (see Chapter 15).

Positron emission tomography

Positron emission tomography (PET) scanning is used in the diagnosis and staging of lung cancer. It is based on the concept that neoplastic cells have greater metabolic activity and a higher uptake of glucose than normal cells. ^{18}F-fluoro-2-deoxy-glucose (FDG) is a glucose analogue that is preferentially taken up by neoplastic cells after intravenous injection and then emits positrons. PET scanning is particularly helpful in the **staging of lung cancer**, where it is used to detect metastases and determine the involvement of lymph nodes in patients being considered for radical treatment such as surgical resection or high-dose radiotherapy (see Chapter 12). It is also particularly useful in the differential diagnosis of an indeterminate **solitary pulmonary nodule**. Often, such a nodule is small and not amenable to biopsy. Calcification or lack of growth of the lesion over time suggests that the nodule is benign (e.g. hamartoma, healed tuberculous granuloma). If the patient is a smoker at high risk of cancer but otherwise fit, it may be advisable to proceed directly to surgical resection of such a lesion, without preoperative histological confirmation. Active accumulation of FDG in the lesion on PET scanning suggests malignancy. False-negative findings can occur in tumours <1 cm and false-positive uptake can occur in inflammatory conditions such as tuberculosis, sarcoidosis, histoplasmosis and coccidioidomycosis.

 KEY POINTS

- The chest X-ray has a key role in the investigation of lung disease. It should be studied in a systematic way and interpreted in the context of all clinical information.
- Ultrasonography is useful in assessing pleural effusions and is used to guide placement of a chest tube when draining a pleural effusion.
- CT is more sensitive than the chest X-ray and is crucial in the staging of lung cancer, assessing interstitial lung disease and diagnosing pulmonary emboli.
- PET is helpful in diagnosing and staging lung cancer.

 FURTHER READING

Hansell DM. Thoracic imaging. In: Gibson GJ, Geddes DM, Costabel U, et al. eds, *Respiratory Medicine*. London: WB Saunders Co, 2003: 316–51.

Lynch DA, Godwin JD, Safrin S, et al. High-resolution computed tomography in idiopathic pulmonary fibrosis. *Am J Respir Crit Care Med* 2005; **172**: 488–93.

MacMahon H, Austin JHM, Gamsu G, et al. Guidelines for the management of small pulmonary nodules on CT scans: a statement from the Fleischner Society. *Radiology* 2005; **237**: 395–400.

Remy-Jardin M, Ghaye B, Remy J. Spiral computed tomography angiography of pulmonary embolism. *Eur Respir Monograph* 2004; **27**: 124–43.

Vansteenkiste JF. Imaging in lung cancer: position emission tomography scan. *Eur Respir J* 2002; **19** (Suppl. 35): 49–60.

Verschakelen JA, DeWever W, Bogaert J, Stroobants S. Imaging: staging of lung cancer. *Eur Respir Monograph* 2004; **30**: 214–44.

Multiple choice questions

4.1 Cavitation is a characteristic feature of:

A a hamartoma

B fibrotic lung disease

C *Haemophilus influenzae* pneumonia

D dermoid cysts

E squamous carcinoma

4.2 An air bronchogram in an area of consolidation suggests:

A bronchial obstruction due to carcinoma

B infarction secondary to a pulmonary embolism

C an arteriovenous malformation

D pneumonia

E sarcoidosis

4.3 A 1 cm peripheral lung nodule with avid uptake of ^{18}F-fluoro-2-deoxy-glucose on PET-CT scan is most likely to be a:

A tuberculous granuloma

B hamartoma

C carcinoma

D neurofibroma

E rheumatoid nodule

4.4 A 65-year-old smoker presents with cough, purulent sputum and left chest pain. Chest X-ray shows features of left lower lobe collapse. The most likely diagnosis is:

A pneumonia

B pneumonia with a parapneumonic effusion

C mucus plugging of the left lower lobe bronchus

D bronchial carcinoma

E an inhaled foreign body in the left lower lobe bronchus

4.5 A 60-year-old woman is found to have an anterior mediastinal mass on chest X-ray and CT. The most likely cause is a:

A hiatus hernia

B thymoma

C oesophageal cyst

D pericardial cyst

E neurofibroma

4.6 On a a chest X-ray there is an indistinct border to the lower right side of the medistinum. The X-ray is otherwise unremarkable. The most likely explanation is a:

A collapse of the right lower lobe

B variation of normal, which can be disregarded

C consolidation in the right middle lobe

D pericardial effusion

E mediastinal shift to the left

4.7 A chest X-ray reveals a total 'white out' of the left hemithorax, with a normally aerated lung on the right. Possible explanations include:

A congenital absence of the left lung

B complete consolidation of the left lung

C a left-sided pleural effusion

D complete collapse of the left lung

E massive pulmonary embolism

4.8 In the X-ray descibed in 4.7, the most useful feature in distinguishing between the the two MOST likely explantions for the 'white out' would be:

A visibility of the left hemidiaphragm

B presence of the silohette sign on the left mediastinum

C position of the trachea

D height of the right hemidiaphragm

E presence of vascular markings on the right

4.9 On a plain chest X-ray, the appearance of a dense white triangluar opacity 'behind' the left heart border suggests:

A pnemothorax

B pleural effusion

C pericardial effuciaon

D collapse of the left lower lobe

E collapse of the left middle lobe

4.10 The following can be identified on an X-ray be a convexity (bulge) on the left heart border:

A aorta

B left pulmonary aretery

C left arial appendage

D left ventricle

E right atrium

Multiple choice answers

4.1 E

Cavitation is the presence of an area of radiolucency within a mass lesion. It is a feature of bronchial carcinoma (particularly squamous carcinoma), tuberculosis, lung abscess, pulmonary infarcts, Granulomatosis with polyangiitis (formerly known as Wegener's granulomatosis) and some pneumonias (e.g. *Staphylococcus aureus, Klebsiella pneumoniae*).

4.2 D

An air bronchogram is visible as a black tube of air against the white background of consolidated lung. It indicates that the bronchus is patent and not occluded. It is a feature of pneumonic consolidation.

4.3 C

Avid uptake of FDG on PET scanning is a feature of bronchial carcinoma, but can also occur in inflammatory conditions such as tuberculosis, sarcoidosis, histoplasmosis and coccidioidomycosis.

4.4 D

Collapse of a lobe is a sinister feature suggesting occlusion of the bronchus by a mass lesion such as a carcinoma.

4.5 B

Thymic tumours, thyroid masses and dermoid cysts are most commonly situated in the anterior mediastinum, whereas neurofibromas and oesophageal cysts are often situated posteriorly.

4.6 C

Absence of the normal 'silhouette' between the right heart border and the adjacent lung (middle lobe) implies there is consolidation in the lung.

4.7 C and D are possible and need to be considered

Congenital problems leading to poor development of the lung tend to leave a radiolucent X-ray on that side. Pulmonary embolism may leave no sign or a subtle diminution of vascular markings. 'Complete' consolidation of an entire lung – with no involvement of the other lung – is an extremely unlikely finding.

4.8 C

In a large effusion, the trachea (and mediastinum) will be pushed 'away' to the other side. In collapse, the tracheal (and mediastinum) will be pulled to that side.

4.9 D

There is no middle lobe on the left.

4.10 A,B,D

The position of the left atrial appendage is indicated by a concavity just below the pulmonary artery.

Part 3

Respiratory diseases

5

Upper respiratory tract infections and influenza

Introduction

Acute upper respiratory tract infections (URTIs) are a very common cause of morbidity, visits to doctors and absence from school or work. They are the most common respiratory complaint, accounting for about **9% of all consultations in general practice**. A child suffers about eight, and an adult about four respiratory infections each year. Although unpleasant, most URTIs are mild and self-limiting, but a small number give rise to serious problems, most notably acute epiglottitis in children and influenza A in elderly patients debilitated by chronic underlying disease. Difficulties arise in distinguishing URTIs from more serious lower respiratory tract infections, such as pneumonia (Fig. 5.1), and alertness combined with careful assessment and clinical judgement is required. Most URTIs are of viral origin, but a variety of viruses and bacteria may produce the same clinical pattern of illness (e.g. pharyngitis, sinusitis).

Common cold

The common cold (coryza) is an acute illness characterised by rhinorrhoea, sneezing, nasal obstruction and sore throat (pharyngitis), with minimal fever or systemic symptoms. It may be caused by about 200 different strains of viruses, including **rhinoviruses**, **coronaviruses**, **respiratory syncytial**, **parainfluenza** and **influenza viruses**. Infection is transmitted by droplet spread, and attack rates are highest in young children attending school, who then transmit infection to their parents and siblings at home. The multiplicity of viral strains prevents the development of immunity. The bacterial flora of the nasopharynx remains unchanged for the first few days of the illness but may then show an increase in the number of *Haemophilus influenzae* and *Streptococcus pneumoniae* organisms, and there is the potential for secondary bacterial infection to occur, with extension of infection beyond the nasopharynx, giving rise to sinusitis, otitis media, bronchitis or pneumonia. Most people with the common cold do not need to see their general practitioner and can be encouraged to manage the condition themselves or to seek advice from a pharmacist. No specific treatment is possible for the common cold, but symptoms are often alleviated by use of paracetamol or aspirin.

Pharyngitis

Pharyngitis may occur as part of the common cold or as a separate illness. Most cases are caused by **viruses** (Table 5.1), but pharyngitis may also be caused by group A **β-haemolytic streptococci**, *Mycoplasma pneumoniae* or *Chlamydophila pneumoniae*, for example. The patient complains of a sore throat and there is erythema of the pharynx, often with enlargement of the tonsils. **Infectious mononucleosis** (glandular fever) often involves pharyngitis but is also associated with lymphadenopathy and splenomegaly, and is caused by the Epstein–Barr (EB) virus. A blood film may show atypical mononuclear cells and the Monospot or heterophile antibody test is positive. Characteristically, patients with infectious mononucleosis develop a rash if given amoxicillin as treatment for pharyngitis. It is not possible to

Respiratory Medicine Lecture Notes, Ninth Edition. Stephen J. Bourke and Graham P. Burns.
© 2015 John Wiley & Sons, Ltd. Published 2015 by John Wiley & Sons, Ltd.
Companion Website: www.lecturenoteseries.com/Respiratory

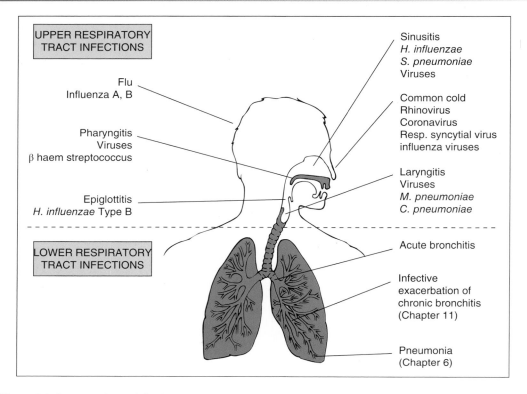

UPPER RESPIRATORY
TRACT INFECTIONS

Flu
Influenza A, B

Pharyngitis
Viruses
β haem streptococcus

Epiglottitis
H. influenzae Type B

LOWER RESPIRATORY
TRACT INFECTIONS

Sinusitis
H. influenzae
S. pneumoniae
Viruses

Common cold
Rhinovirus
Coronavirus
Resp. syncytial virus
influenza viruses

Laryngitis
Viruses
M. pneumoniae
C. pneumoniae

Acute bronchitis

Infective
exacerbation of
chronic bronchitis
(Chapter 11)

Pneumonia
(Chapter 6)

Figure 5.1 Acute respiratory infections.

distinguish between viral and bacterial pharyngitis on clinical grounds. β-haemolytic streptococci may be found on microbiology of a throat swab, but this does not differentiate between active infection and a carriage state. Even when pharyngitis is caused by bacterial infection, antibiotics are not usually necessary, as the illness tends to be self-limiting. Local extension of infection may result in otitis media, tonsillitis or quinsy (peritonsillar abscess). Streptococcal infection may be complicated by glomerulonephritis or rheumatic fever, but these are rare nowadays. Antibiotic treatment of pharyngitis is usually only given to severe or complicated cases. Streptococci are sensitive to phenoxymethylpenicillin or amoxicillin. *Mycoplasma pneumoniae* or *Chlamydophila pneumoniae* requires a tetracycline or macrolide antibiotic (e.g. clarithromycin).

by fever and malaise. A variety of organisms may cause sinusitis, including respiratory **viruses**, **_Haemophilus influenzae_**, **_Streptococcus pneumoniae_**, **_Staphylococcus aureus_** and **anaerobic bacteria**. In chronic sinusitis, X-rays may show mucosal thickening, opacification or the presence of a fluid level in the sinus. Recurrent sinusitis may be accompanied by more widespread respiratory tract infection in patients with bronchiectasis caused by cystic fibrosis, hypogammaglobulinaemia or ciliary dyskinesia. Post-nasal drip from sinusitis is irritating to the larynx and may cause a persistent cough. Sinusitis is usually treated with antibiotics (e.g. amoxicillin, trimethoprim), nasal decongestants (e.g. ephedrine) and analgesia (e.g. paracetamol). Surgical drainage may be necessary for relief of chronic sinusitis.

Sinusitis

Infection of the maxillary sinuses causes facial pain, nasal obstruction and discharge, often accompanied

Acute laryngitis

The term 'acute laryngitis' is used when temporary hoarseness or loss of voice occurs with pharyngitis

Table 5.1 **Principal respiratory viruses**

Virus	Disease	Notes
Rhinovirus	Common cold, pharyngitis, chronic bronchitic exacerbations	More than 100 serotypes; identification and study difficult
Coronavirus	Common cold	Numerous serotypes; identification difficult
Severe acute respiratory syndrome (SARS)	SARS coronavirus (see Chapter 6)	
Adenovirus	Pharyngitis, conjunctivitis, severe bronchitis in childhood, rarely severe pneumonia	About 30 serotypes
Respiratory syncytial virus	Bronchiolitis in infants, common cold in adults	One serotype, winter epidemics
Influenza A	Influenza – may be severe	Epidemics, continuous antigenic variation
Influenza B	Influenza	Milder illness, minor epidemics
Parainfluenza	Croup, other URTIs, some bronchiolitis	Serotypes 1–4, A and B
Measles	Measles, severe illness with pneumonia in immunocompromised	Vaccination effective
Cytomegalovirus	Silent infection or minor respiratory illness, pneumonia in immunosuppressed	One serotype
Herpes simplex	Stomatitis, rarely pharyngitis, pneumonia in immunosuppressed	One serotype, severe infection treatable with aciclovir or vidarabine
Herpes zoster	Pneumonia in adult infection	Severe infection treatable with aciclovir, leaves scattered calcific lesions
Coxsackie, enteroviruses and enteric cytopathic human organ (ECHO) viruses	Minor part in respiratory infection; Coxsackie A may cause herpangina; B causes 'pleurodynia' and pericarditis/myocarditis	Local epidemics
EB virus	Pharyngitis, lymphadenitis, infectious mononucleosis	Heterophile antibody test, typical blood picture

or the common cold, and is caused by oedema of the vocal cords. No treatment is necessary.

Croup

Croup (acute laryngotracheobronchitis) is usually caused by **viruses** such as parainfluenza virus, respiratory syncytial virus, influenza A and B, rhinoviruses, adenovirus and measles. Characteristically, a child develops a harsh barking cough with an upper respiratory infection, which may progress to stridor. Often, no treatment is required, but some children develop more severe lower respiratory infections and progressive respiratory distress, requiring intubation and ventilation. Oral prednisolone is sometimes beneficial in severe croup and nebulised high-dose budesonide may be associated with more rapid recovery in less severely affected patients.

Pertussis

Pertussis (whooping cough) is an infectious disease of the respiratory tract caused by *Bordetella pertussis*. In the initial phase of the illness, there is nasal discharge, pharyngitis and conjunctivitis. This is followed by a severe cough, with spasms of coughing that typically end with a deep inspiration (whoop). The bacteria is difficult to culture but can be grown from nasopharyngeal secretions and an antibody response can be detected on serology. It is treated by macrolide antibiotics (e.g. clarithromycin, erythromycin). In the past, it typically occurred in young children and had a significant mortality rate, due to secondary bacterial pneumonia, and long-term sequelae in the form of bronchiectasis. The incidence was greatly reduced by a successful vaccination programme for infants. Vaccine-induced immunity wanes after about 5–10 years and pertussis can be a cause of a troublesome cough in adults.

Acute epiglottitis

Epiglottitis is a very serious disease that is usually caused by virulent strains of *Haemophilus influenzae* **type B**, and there is often an accompanying septicaemia. Death may result from occlusion of the airway by the inflamed oedematous epiglottis. It is most common in children of about 2–3 years of age, but cases have also occurred in adults. The patient is ill with pyrexia, sore throat, laryngitis and painful dysphagia. Symptoms of upper airway obstruction may develop rapidly, with stridor and respiratory distress. A lateral neck X-ray may show epiglottic swelling. Blood cultures often isolate *Haemophilus influenzae* type B. Patients with suspected epiglottitis should be admitted to hospital and attempts at examining the upper airway should only be made when facilities are available for tracheal intubation and ventilation. Because of possible amoxicillin resistance, chloramphenicol or cefuroxime is an appropriate antibiotic. The widespread use of vaccination against *Haemophilus influenzae* in childhood is making epiglottitis increasingly rare.

Influenza

Seasonal influenza

Influenza is an acute illness characterised by pyrexia, malaise, myalgia, headache and prostration, as well as upper respiratory symptoms. Lethargy and depression may persist for several days afterwards. Although the term 'flu' is used very loosely by the public, it is the systemic features that characterise true infection with the influenza viruses. Influenza virus type A undergoes frequent spontaneous changes in its haemagglutinin and neuraminidase surface antigens. Minor changes, referred to as '**antigenic drift**', result in outbreaks of seasonal influenza in the winter months each year. Major changes, referred to as '**antigenic shift**', result in epidemics and **pandemics** of infection, reflecting the lack of immunity in the population to the new strain. Type B is more antigenically stable and produces less severe disease. Type C causes only mild sporadic cases of upper respiratory infection.

Influenza is highly infectious, so that all members of a household often become ill together. Outbreaks of influenza cause considerable morbidity even in healthy adults. It is usually a self-limiting illness, but it can be complicated by bronchitis, otitis media and secondary bacterial pneumonia (e.g. *Staphylococcus aureus*, *Streptococcus pneumoniae* or *Haemophilus influenzae*). The greatest morbidity and mortality occur in patients who are elderly or who have underlying cardiac or respiratory disease, and seasonal influenza outbreaks cause an average annual excess mortality of about 12 000 deaths in the UK.

The diagnosis of influenza can be confirmed by immunofluorescent microscopy of nasal secretions or by serology. **Oseltamivir** and **zanamivir** are drugs that reduce the replication of influenza viruses by inhibiting viral neuraminidase. Oseltamivir is given orally, whereas zanamivir is only available by inhalation. These drugs have to be given within 48 hours of the onset of symptoms to be effective. They reduce the duration of illness by about 1 day and they may reduce complications in at-risk patients with severe influenza. They can also be given for post-exposure prophylaxis in at-risk adults not protected by vaccination. Vaccination remains the most effective way of preventing illness from seasonal influenza. However, if new pandemic strains of influenza emerge, it will take time to develop vaccines. **Amantadine** is an older antiviral agent that blocks the ion-channel function of a protein in the influenza virus, but some strains are resistant to this drug and it is not currently recommended for the treatment of influenza in the UK. Use of aspirin or paracetamol relieves symptoms. Antibiotics are used when there are features of secondary bacterial infection (e.g. otitis media, sinusitis). Pneumonia associated with influenza may be severe and requires treatment with broad-spectrum antibiotics, including antibiotics against *Staphylococcus aureus* (e.g. co-amoxiclav, cefuroxime, flucloxacillin).

Influenza vaccination

The influenza vaccine is prepared annually using the virus strains most likely to be prevalent that year. The vaccine contains inactivated virus and is about 70–80% effective in protecting against infection. Where infection occurs despite vaccination, it is usually less severe and associated with less morbidity and mortality than the disease seen in unvaccinated patients. Selective immunisation is recommended to protect those most at risk of serious illness or death from influenza. Annual vaccination is recommended for those over the age of 65 years, those with chronic respiratory disease (e.g. chronic obstructive pulmonary disease, asthma, bronchiectasis etc.), chronic heart disease, renal failure, diabetes mellitus or immunosuppression and those living in care homes. Vaccination is recommended for pregnant women, as they are at increased risk from complications of flu, and flu during pregnancy is associated with premature births and reduced birth size and weight. Vaccination during pregnancy also provides passive immunity to infants in the first few months of life. Vaccination is also recommended for healthcare workers, to reduce the risk of their contracting influenza and spreading the infection to their patients, colleagues and family members.

Adverse reactions to influenza vaccine are usually mild, consisting of fever and malaise in some patients and local reactions at the site of injection. The vaccine is contraindicated in patients with egg allergy. Patients should be advised that the vaccine will not protect them from all respiratory viruses.

Pandemic influenza

Influenza pandemics have occurred sporadically and unpredictably over the last century. They arise when there are major changes in the haemagglutinin (H) and neuraminidase (N) surface antigens of the influenza A virus. In 1918, a pandemic of influenza caused by the H1N1 strain (Spanish flu) killed about 30 million people worldwide. In this pandemic, the mortality was particularly high in those aged 20–40 years. There were further pandemics in 1957, caused by the H2N2 strain (Asian flu), and in 1968, caused by the H3N2 strain (Hong Kong flu), each killing about 1 million people worldwide. In recent years, there has been concern about the transmission of an avian strain of influenza (H5N1) from birds such as ducks and poultry to humans. This has occurred mainly in South East Asia and has produced severe influenza pneumonia in humans, with a high death rate. Spread of infection was contained by slaughtering large numbers of birds in affected areas. In 2009/10, a further pandemic occurred, caused by H1N1 ('swine flu'). It first appeared in Mexico but then spread globally. This virus was not particularly pathogenic and therefore the number of deaths was relatively low. In 2013, there was an outbreak of influenza in China caused by a new strain of avian influenza (H7N9). There is potential for influenza viral strains to undergo mutations that might increase their virulence and capacity for transmission from human to human. During pandemics, the number of patients with influenza can overwhelm the normal healthcare systems. Contingency plans have been developed for such circumstances.

 KEY POINTS

- Most upper respiratory infections are self-limiting and caused by viruses; antibiotics are not usually indicated.
- Seasonal influenza A causes an acute systemic illness with substantial morbidity and mortality, particularly in elderly at-risk patients.
- Influenza A vaccine is prepared every year for the prevalent strains and gives effective protection against seasonal influenza.
- Pandemic influenza occurs when there are major mutations in the virus that result in increased virulence and a lack of immunity in the population.

 FURTHER READING

British Infection Society, British Thoracic Society, Health Protection Agency in collaboration with the Department of Health. Pandemic flu: clinical management of patients with an influenza-like illness during an influenza pandemic. *Thorax* 2007; **62** (Suppl. 1): 1–46.

Gueris D, Strebel PM, Bardenheir B, et al. Changing epidemiology of pertussis in the United States: increasing reported incidence among adolescents and adults. *Clin Infect Dis* 1999; **28**: 1230–7.

Husby S, Agertoft L, Mortensen S, Pedersen S. Treatment of croup with nebulised steroid (budesonide): a double-blind placebo controlled study. *Arch Dis Child* 1993; **68**: 352–6.

Lagace-Wiens PR, Rubinstein E, Gurnel A. Influenza epidemiology – past, present and future. *Crit Care Med* 2010; **38** (Suppl.): e1–9.

Little PS, Williamson I, Shvartzman P. Are antibiotics appropriate for sore throats? *BMJ* 1994; **309**: 1010–12.

Nguyen-Van-Tam JS, Openshaw PJ, Hashim A, et al. Risk factors for hospitalization and poor outcome with pandemic A/H1N1 influenza. *Thorax* 2010; **65**: 645–51.

Vernon DD, Sarnaik AP. Acute epiglottitis in children: a conservative approach to diagnosis and management. *Crit Care Med* 1986; **14**: 23–5.

Watts G. Pandemic flu: A/H1N1 infleunza virus, the basics. *BMJ* 2009; **339**: 368–9.

Wilson R. Influenza vaccination. *Thorax* 1994; **49**: 1079–80.

Wong SSY, Yuen KY. Avian influenza virus infections in humans. *Chest* 2006; **129**: 156–68.

Multiple choice questions

5.1 Acute epiglottitis is usually caused by:
A *Streptococcus pneumoniae*
B *Mycoplasma pneumoniae*
C infectious mononucleosis
D *Haemophilus influenzae* type B
E *Staphylococcus aureus*

5.2 Contact with birds is a risk factor for infection with:
A *Chlamydophila pneumoniae*
B *Mycoplasma pneumoniae*
C *Coxiella burnetti*
D *Legionella pneumophila*
E *Chlamydophila psittaci*

5.3 Severe seasonal influenza is usually caused by:
A influenza virus type A
B *Haemophilus influenzae*
C influenza virus type B
D influenza virus type C
E *Staphylococcus aureus*

5.4 Recurrent sinusitis is a characteristic feature of:
A cystic fibrosis
B chronic obstructive pulmonary disease
C atopic asthma
D chronic bronchitis
E obstructive sleep apnoea syndrome

5.5 Influenza pandemics occur because of:
A emergence of new coronaviruses
B antigenic shift in influenza viral antigens
C overuse of antibiotics
D lack of uptake of influenza vaccination
E antigenic drift in influenza viral antigens

5.6 Influenza vaccination is contraindicated in patients with:
A egg allergy
B atopic asthma
C HIV infection
D diabetes
E pregnancy

5.7 Whooping cough is caused by:
A respiratory syncytial virus
B influenza B
C rhinovirus
D *Bordatella pertussis*
E Epstein–Barr virus

5.8 It is estimated that influenza causes an average annual excess number of deaths in the UK of:
A 2000
B 6000
C 12 000
D 20 000
E 50 000

5.9 It is estimated that the number of deaths caused by the pandemic of H1N1 influenza (Spanish flu) in 1918 was:
A 1 million
B 5 million
C 10 million
D 20 million
E 30 million

5.10 Outbreaks of avian flu (H5N1) were controlled by:
A vaccination programmes
B Oseltamivir
C Zanamivir
D Amantadine
E slaughter of birds

Multiple choice answers

5.1 D

Acute epiglottitis is a serious illness that is usually caused by virulent strains of *H. influenzae* type B. It typically affects young children, may cause occlusion of the airway and is often accompanied by septicaemia.

5.2 E

Chlamydophila psittaci is primarily a disease of birds that is transmitted to humans as a zoonosis. *Chlamydophila pneumoniae* typically causes mild upper respiratory tract infections and is spread from person to person.

5.3 A

Influenza A is the main cause of seasonal influenza, which is characterised by systemic symptoms of headache, malaise, myalgia and prostration, in addition to upper respiratory tract symptoms.

5.4 A

Recurrent sinusitis is a feature of cystic fibrosis, hypogammaglobulinaemia and ciliary dyskinesia, all of which also cause bronchiectasis.

5.5 B

Influenza A undergoes frequent changes in its surface antigens. Minor changes, referred to as 'antigenic drift', result in outbreaks of seasonal influenza, but major changes, referred to as 'antigenic shift', result in epidemics and pandemics.

5.6 A

Many flu vaccines are prepared in hens' eggs and may contain ovalbumin (egg). The latest guidance and the product characteristics should be consulted when the vaccines for each season are released.

5.7 D

Whooping cough is caused by *Bordatella pertussis*. Vaccination programmes for infants have greatly reduced the incidence of infection.

5.8 C

Seasonal outbreaks of influenza cause an average excess mortality of about 12 000 deaths each year, particularly in the elderly and those with chronic diseases. Vaccination programmes are therefore targeted at those over the age of 65 years, those with chronic lung disease (e.g. COPD, asthma, bronchiectasis) and those with other chronic diseases (e.g. heart disease, diabetes, patients who are immunosuppressed, renal failure).

5.9 E

The 1918 pandemic of influenza caused by the H1N1 strain (Spanish flu) killed about 30 million people worldwide. In that pandemic, the mortality was particularly high in those aged 20–40 years.

5.10 E

The H5N1 strain of influenza was transmitted from birds such as ducks and poultry to humans. This occurred mainly in South East Asia, where people lived in close proximity to poultry. Spread of infection was contained by slaughtering large numbers of birds in affected areas.

6

Pneumonia

Lower respiratory tract infections

The lower respiratory tract, below the larynx, is normally sterile. Infections can reach the lungs by a number of routes: **inhalation**, **aspiration**, **direct inoculation** (e.g. stab wound to chest) and **blood-borne** (e.g. from intravenous drug misuse). In some situations, lower respiratory tract infection may be regarded as a **primary exogenous event**, in which inhalation of a large dose of a virulent pathogen produces a severe infection in a previously healthy person. Thus, *Legionella pneumophila* may be inhaled from a contaminated water system, or *Chlamydophila psittaci* from an infected bird, resulting in a severe pneumonia. In other circumstances, infection is a **secondary endogenous event**. Thus, a patient who is debilitated by major trauma and requires endotracheal ventilation in an intensive therapy unit (ITU) may develop pneumonia. Typically, in these circumstances, the patient's oropharynx becomes colonised by Gram-negative enteric bacteria, which are usually acquired from endogenous sources within the patient, such as the upper gastrointestinal tract, subgingival dental plaque or periodontal crevices. These bacteria may then reach the lower airway by microaspiration.

Pneumonia

'Pneumonia' is a general term denoting inflammation of the gas-exchange region of the lung. Usually, it implies **parenchymal lung inflammation caused by infection**, and the term 'pneumonitis' is sometimes used to denote inflammation caused by physical, chemical or allergic processes. Pneumonia is an important cause of morbidity and mortality in all age groups. Globally, it is estimated that 5 million children under the age of 5 years die from pneumonia each year (95% in developing countries). In the UK, about 1 in 1000 of the population is admitted to hospital with pneumonia each year, and the mortality in these patients is about 18%. There are about 3000 deaths from pneumonia each year in the age group 15–55 years. About 25% of all deaths in elderly people are related to pneumonia, although this is often the terminal illness in a patient with serious concomitant disease.

Classification in relation to clinical context

A microbiological approach to pneumonia focuses primarily on identification of the pathogen and its susceptibility to antibiotics. However, many of the major respiratory pathogens may be present in the oropharynx in a normal person, so that identification of an organism in respiratory tract secretions may not be sufficient to implicate it as the cause of the illness. Conversely, the same pathogen can cause various illnesses at different levels in the respiratory tract, such as sinusitis, bronchitis or pneumonia, and different bacteria may cause an identical clinical syndrome, such as pneumonia. A clinical approach to pneumonia focuses on the clinical context of the illness, the patient's previous health status and the circumstances of the illness (Fig. 6.1). Pneumonia is the result of a complex interaction between the **patient**, the **environment** and the **infecting organism**, and the pattern of the disease depends on the **virulence** of the pathogen and the **vulnerability** of the patient. The circumstances of the illness include the following:

- site of infection;
- age of the patient;

Respiratory Medicine Lecture Notes, Ninth Edition. Stephen J. Bourke and Graham P. Burns.
© 2015 John Wiley & Sons, Ltd. Published 2015 by John Wiley & Sons, Ltd.
Companion Website: www.lecturenoteseries.com/Respiratory

- community- or hospital-acquired infection;
- concurrent disease;
- environmental and geographical factors; and
- severity of the illness.

Site of infection

The term 'chest infection' is an imprecise term, often used by lay people to refer to nonspecific respiratory symptoms. In assessing and treating respiratory tract infections, it is important to define the site of infection as clearly as possible. **Upper respiratory tract infections** (UTRIs; above the larynx) are often viral in origin and self-limiting, not requiring treatment (see Chapter 5). **Lower respiratory tract infections** may affect the bronchial tree, such as **bronchitis**, or the lung parenchyma, such as **pneumonia**. Infective exacerbations of chronic bronchitis (see

Previously well infant
1 RSV
2 Adenovirus and other viruses
3 Bacterial

Previously ill infant
1 Staphylococcus
2 *E. coli* and Gram-negative bacteria
3 Viruses and opportunistic organisms

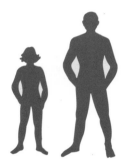

Children
1 Viruses
2 Pneumococcus
3 Mycoplasma
4 Others

Previously fit adults
1 Pneumococcus
2 Mycoplasma
3 *H. influenzae*
4 Viruses
5 Staphylococcus
6 *Legionella*
7 Others

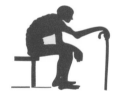

Previous respiratory illness;
elderly and debilitated
1 Pneumococcus
2 *H. influenzae*
3 Staphylococcus
4 *Klebsiella* and
   Gram-negative organisms

If no response think of:
TB, *Mycoplasma, Legionella,*
carcinoma

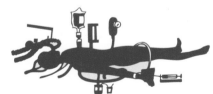

Severely immunocompromised
and AIDS
1 Pneumocystis pneumonia
2 Cytomegalovirus
3 Adenovirus
4 Herpes simplex
5 Bacteria (*Legionella,*
   Staphylococcus, Pneumococcus)
6 Opportunistic mycobacteria;
   tuberculosis

Hospital-acquired pneumonia
1 Gram-negative bacteria
   (*Pseudomonas, Klebsiella,*
   Proteus)
2 Staphylococcus
3 Pneumococcus
4 Anaerobic bacteria, fungi
5 NB aspiration pneumonia
6 Others

Figure 6.1 Likely causes of pneumonia in different clinical circumstances. Age and previous health are important factors.

Chapter 11) are often caused by organisms of low virulence (e.g. non-typeable *Haemophilus influenzae*) when the patient's defences against infection are compromised by smoking-induced damage to the bronchial mucosa. Penetration of antibiotics into the scarred mucosa and viscid secretions may be difficult. Extension of bronchial infection into the surrounding lung parenchyma is often referred to as **bronchopneumonia**. Infection of the lung parenchyma with extensive consolidation of a lobe of a lung – **lobar pneumonia** – is usually caused by organisms of greater virulence (e.g. *Streptococcus pneumoniae*). Infection may spread to the pleura, resulting in **empyema**, or to the bloodstream, causing **septicaemia**.

Age of the patient

In **children** under the age of 2 years, pneumonia is commonly caused by viruses such as respiratory syncytial virus (RSV), adenovirus, influenza and parainfluenza viruses. *Chlamydia trachomatis* infection may be transmitted to an infant from the mother's genital tract during birth, resulting in pneumonia. In older children and **adults** of all ages, *Streptococcus pneumoniae* is the most common cause of primary pneumonia. *Mycoplasma pneumoniae* infection is rare in elderly people and particularly affects young adults. The incidence of pneumonia increases greatly in **elderly people** and the high frequency of underlying chronic diseases (e.g. chronic obstructive pulmonary disease (COPD), heart failure) in this group is associated with a high mortality.

Community- or hospital-acquired infection

The characteristics of the patient and the spectrum of pathogens differ greatly depending on whether pneumonia is contracted in the community or in hospital. When pneumonia is acquired in the community, it may be a primary infection in a previously healthy individual or it may occur in association with concomitant disease (e.g. COPD), but a few pathogens (notably *Streptococcus pneumoniae*) account for the majority of cases and Gram-negative organisms are rare. Most patients are treated at home, with only about 25% needing hospital admission. The most important organisms identified as causing **community-acquired pneumonia** are as follows:

- *Streptococcus pneumonia*: 50–60%
- *Mycoplasma pneumoniae*: 10%
- *Chlamydophila pneumonia*: 10%
- Viruses (e.g. influenza): 10%
- *Haemophilus influenzae*: 5%

- *Staphylococcus aureus*: 3%
- *Legionella pneumophila*: 2%
- Other: 2%

Hospital-acquired (nosocomial) pneumonia is defined as pneumonia developing 2 or more days after admission to hospital for some other reason. It is therefore a secondary infection in patients with other illnesses. In those with milder pneumonia on general wards, the causative organisms may be similar to those found in the community. However, pneumonia in the context of endotracheal ventilation on ITU or in those who have already received antibiotics is different. In these circumstances, Gram-negative organisms (e.g. *Pseudomonas aeruginosa*, *Escherichia coli*) are the most important pathogens, and meticillin-resistant *Staphylococcus aureus* (MRSA) is an increasing problem. A variety of factors, including the use of broad-spectrum antibiotics and impaired host defences, promote the colonisation of the nasopharynx of hospitalised patients with Gram-negative organisms. Aspiration of infected nasopharyngeal secretions into the lower respiratory tract is facilitated by factors that compromise the defence mechanisms of the lung (e.g. endotracheal intubation in ITU), impaired cough associated with anaesthesia, surgery and cerebrovascular disease. The spectrum of causative organisms varies depending on the exact circumstances, but the most common pathogens in hospital-acquired pneumonia are as follows:

- Gram-negative bacteria: 50%
- *Staphylococcus aureus*: 20%
- *Streptococcus pneumonia*: 15%
- Anaerobes and fungi: 10%
- Other (e.g. *Legionella pneumophila*): 5%

Concurrent disease

Alcohol misuse, **smoking**, **malnutrition**, **diabetes** and underlying **cardiorespiratory disease** predispose to pneumonia and are associated with a greatly increased mortality. Patients with **COPD** have impaired mucociliary clearance, and organisms of quite low virulence (e.g. *Haemophilus influenzae*) may spread from the bronchi into the peribronchial lung parenchyma, causing bronchopneumonia. Mortality from **influenza infection**, either as a cause of primary pneumonia or associated with secondary bacterial pneumonia, is highest in **elderly** people. **Aspiration pneumonia** is likely to occur in patients with impaired swallowing, as a result of oesophageal or neuromuscular disease, or in patients with impaired consciousness (e.g. epileptic fits, anaesthesia). Patients who have undergone

splenectomy are particularly vulnerable to pneumococcal pneumonia and septicaemia and are usually given pneumococcal vaccination and maintained on lifelong penicillin prophylaxis.

Environmental and geographical factors

Although in some cases pneumonia arises by aspiration of endogenous infective organisms from the oropharynx, in others the patient's environment is the source of infection, following the inhalation of infected droplets from **other patients** (e.g. influenza, tuberculosis), an **animal source** (e.g. *Chlamydophila psittaci* from birds, *Coxiella burnetti* from farm animals) or other **environmental sources** (e.g. *Legionella pneumophila* from contaminated water systems).

Some infections have a particular **geographical distribution** (e.g. histoplasmosis in North America, *Burkholderia pseudomallei* in East Asia, typhoid in tropical countries) and need to be considered in patients who live in, or have recently visited, these areas. Knowledge of the **local pattern of prevalent infections** and **antibiotic resistance** in a community is important. For example, *Mycoplasma pneumoniae* infection particularly occurs in outbreaks about every 4 years and requires treatment with tetracycline or a macrolide (e.g. clarithromycin) antibiotic. Although *Streptococcus pneumoniae* in the UK is usually sensitive to penicillin, about 30% of strains isolated in Spain are resistant, and this should be borne in mind when choosing initial antibiotic therapy.

Severity of the illness

Community-acquired pneumonia has a wide spectrum of severity, from a mild self-limiting illness to a fatal disease. It is therefore vital to assess accurately the severity of the pneumonia, as this is an important factor in determining the choice of antibiotics, the extent of investigations and whether a patient should be treated **in hospital** rather than **at home** or in an **ITU** rather than on a general ward. Severe pneumonia can rapidly develop into multiorgan failure with respiratory, circulatory and renal failure. Patients who have certain core adverse prognostic features have a greatly increased risk of death: acute **confusion**, elevated **urea** (>7 mmol/l), increased **respiratory rate** (≥30/min), low **blood pressure** (systolic < 90 mmHg, diastolic < 60 mmHg) and age over 65 years. A **CURB-65 score** (confusion, elevated urea, respiratory rate, blood pressure, age > 65 years) is useful in assessing the severity of pneumonia

(Fig. 6.2). Patients with severe pneumonia are likely to benefit from more intensive monitoring (arterial catheter, central venous catheter, urinary catheter) and treatment (rapid correction of hypovolaemia, inotropic support, ventilatory support) in an ITU.

Clinical features

Patients with pneumonia typically present with **cough**, **purulent sputum** and **fever**, often accompanied by **pleuritic pain** and **breathlessness**. There may be a history of a recent URTI. Diagnosing the site and severity of respiratory tract infection is notoriously difficult, and careful assessment combined with good clinical judgement is important. Early review of the situation is crucial in the event of deterioration, because the severity of the illness is often underestimated by the patient and doctor alike. **Localised chest signs**, such as crackles, dullness or bronchial breathing, indicate pneumonia rather than bronchitis, for example, but may not always be present. Cyanosis and tachypnoea are features of respiratory failure. Rigors, high fever or prostration suggests septicaemia. Elderly patients, in particular, may present with nonrespiratory symptoms, such as confusion.

The initial clinical approach focuses on an **assessment of the circumstances and severity** of the illness, because these guide decisions as to how and where the patient should be treated. Rather than diagnosing a patient as having a 'chest infection', an effort should be made to use an appropriate descriptive phrase, such as 'a previously fit adult with severe community-acquired pneumonia and suspected septicaemia (rigors, prostration)' or 'probable bronchopneumonia (crackles) and respiratory failure (cyanosis) in a patient with COPD'.

Investigation

Patients with mild pneumonia that responds rapidly to antibiotics are usually treated at home, in which situation investigations do not usually influence management or outcome. Nonetheless, microbiology laboratories will often request that general practitioners send sputum and serology samples from some patients treated in the community so as to be able to alert clinicians to outbreaks of influenza or *Mycoplasma pneumoniae*, for example, and to provide information on local patterns of bacterial resistance to antibiotics. More extensive investigations are indicated for patients requiring admission to hospital.

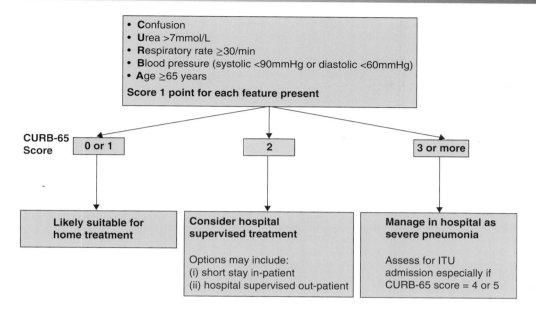

- **C**onfusion
- **U**rea >7mmol/L
- **R**espiratory rate ≥30/min
- **B**lood pressure (systolic <90mmHg or diastolic <60mmHg)
- **A**ge ≥65 years

Score 1 point for each feature present

CURB-65 Score

| 0 or 1 | 2 | 3 or more |

| **Likely suitable for home treatment** | **Consider hospital supervised treatment**

Options may include:
(i) short stay in-patient
(ii) hospital supervised out-patient | **Manage in hospital as severe pneumonia**

Assess for ITU admission especially if CURB-65 score = 4 or 5 |

Figure 6.2 CURB-65 severity score. The severity of pneumonia can be assessed using a scoring system based on the key parameters of new-onset confusion, an elevated urea, respiratory rate, blood pressure and age >65 years, giving a CURB-65 score. Patients with a score of >3 are at high risk of death and may need to be treated in an ITU. Patients with a score <1 may be suitable for treatment at home. Clinical judgement, social circumstances and the stability of comorbid illness are also important in assessing disease severity.

General investigations

- **Chest X-ray** (Fig. 6.3) confirms the diagnosis of pneumonia by demonstrating consolidation, detects complications such as lung abscess or empyema and helps to exclude any underlying disease (e.g. bronchial carcinoma).
- **Haematology and biochemistry tests** are useful in assessing the severity of disease.
- **Oxygenation** is assessed by pulse **oximetry**; those with O_2sat <94% should have **arterial blood gas** measurements.

Further investigations may be indicated if alternative diagnoses are being considered (e.g. computed tomographic angiography for pulmonary embolism). Where there is a suspicion of aspiration pneumonia, a radiocontrast oesophagogram (e.g. 'gastrografin swallow') is useful in assessing swallowing problems. Recurrent pneumonia may be an indication of an immunodeficiency state, and tests for immunoglobulin levels or human immunodeficiency virus (HIV) should be performed as appropriate. Measurement of C-reactive protein may help in differentiating pneumonia from noninfective diseases and in monitoring response to treatment.

Specific investigations

Specific investigations are aimed at detecting the pathogen causing the pneumonia:

- **Sputum Gram stain** may give a valuable and rapid clue to the responsible organism in an ill patient.
- **Sputum culture** is the main test used to detect bacterial causes of pneumonia, but contamination of the sample by oropharyngeal organisms, prior use of antibiotics and inability to produce sputum limit its sensitivity and specificity.
- **Blood cultures** should be performed on all patients admitted to hospital with moderate or severe pneumonia but are positive in only about 15% of cases.
- **Pleural fluid** should be aspirated in all patients with pleural effusions and may yield a causative organism or reveal empyema (see Chapter 16).
- **Antigen-detection tests** are available for some pathogens. Pneumococcal antigen may be identified in sputum, urine, pleural fluid or blood and may be positive in cases where prior antibiotics limit the sensitivity of cultures. Direct fluorescent antibody staining may detect *Legionella pneumophila* in bronchoalveolar lavage fluid, and tests for *Legionella* antigen in urine are available.

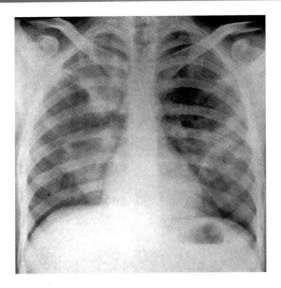

Figure 6.3 This 60-year-old man was admitted to hospital with a 2-week history of myalgia, headache, dyspnoea and cough without sputum. He was severely ill, cyanosed and confused, with a fever of 39°C, tachycardia 110/min, respiratory rate 40/min and blood pressure 110/60 mmHg. Po_2 was 5.7 kPa (43 mmHg), Pco_2 4.9 kPa (37 mmHg), white cell count 4.6×10^9/l and urea 31 mmol/l. He had received amoxicillin for 6 days before admission, without improvement. The chest X-ray shows extensive bilateral multilobar consolidation. He kept birds as a hobby and one of his budgerigars had died recently. The clinical diagnosis of psittacosis was subsequently confirmed by serology tests. He was treated with intravenous fluids, oxygen and tetracycline, and recovered fully.

Pneumococcal and Legionella urine antigen tests should be performed in those with severe pneumonia.

- **Serological tests** allow a retrospective diagnosis of the infecting organism if a rising titre is found between acute and convalescent samples. This is most useful for some viruses and for pneumonia caused by atypical organisms, such as *Mycoplasma pneumoniae* and *Chlamydophila pneumoniae*.

Invasive investigations, such as bronchoscopy with bronchoalveolar lavage, may be indicated in severe pneumonia and in immunocompromised patients.

Treatment

General

Mild pneumonia in a fit patient can be treated **at home**. Admission to **hospital** is necessary for patients who demonstrate features of severe pneumonia, who have concomitant disease or who do not have adequate family help at home. The severity of the pneumonia should be formally assessed at the time of admission to hospital and elective transfer to an **ITU** should be considered for patients with severe disease.

Sufficient **oxygen** should be given to maintain arterial $Po_2 > 8$ kPa (60 mmHg) and an oxygen saturation of 94–98%. Adequate nonsedative **analgesia** (e.g. paracetamol or nonsteroidal anti-inflammatory drugs) should be given to control pleuritic pain. **Fluid balance** should be optimised, using intravenous rehydration as required for dehydrated patients. Chest physiotherapy may be beneficial to patients with COPD and copious secretions but is not helpful in patients without underlying lung disease. Nutritional support (e.g. oral dietary supplements, nasogastric feeding) should be given in prolonged illnesses. The patient's general condition, pulse, blood pressure, temperature, respiratory rate and oxygen saturation should be monitored frequently and any deterioration should prompt reassessment of the need for transfer to ITU. Prophylaxis of venous thromboembolism with low-molecular-weight heparin should be given to patients who are not fully mobile.

Antibiotics

The initial choice of antibiotics is based upon an assessment of the circumstances and severity of the pneumonia. Treatment is then adjusted in accordance with the patient's response and the results of microbiology investigations. Careful patient selection for treatment and appropriate antibiotic choice are important in reducing the risks of antibiotic resistance, MRSA and *Clostridium difficile* infection. Hospitals often have their own antibiotic policies, based on their particular circumstances, and specialist advice should be sought for complex problems. For **community-acquired pneumonia**, *Streptococcus pneumoniae* is the most likely pathogen and **amoxicillin** 500 mg t.d.s. orally is an appropriate antibiotic. **Doxycycline** and clarithromycin are alternatives for those allergic to penicillins. Where there is a suspicion of an 'atypical pathogen' (e.g. *Mycoplasma pneumoniae*, *Chlamydophila psittaci*), addition of a macrolide antibiotic, such as **clarithromycin** 500 mg b.d., is required. In **severe pneumonia**, the initial antibiotic regimen must cover all likely pathogens and allow for potential antibiotic resistance, and intravenous **co-amoxiclav** 1.2 g t.d.s. and **clarithromycin** 500 mg b.d. are appropriate.

Cefuroxime is an alternative for those with allergy to penicillin. In severe **hospital-acquired pneumonia**, Gram-negative bacteria are common pathogens, and a combination of an **aminoglycoside** (e.g. tobramycin) and a **third-generation cephalosporin** (e.g. ceftazidime) or an **antipseudomonal penicillin** (e.g. piperacillin with tazobactam) is commonly used.

Patients should be reviewed frequently and switched from intravenous to oral antibiotics when improving. Failure to respond or failure of the C-reactive protein level to fall by 50% within 4 days suggests the occurrence of a complication (e.g. empyema), infection with an unusual pathogen (e.g. *Legionella pneumophila*), the presence of antibiotic resistance or incorrect diagnosis (e.g. pulmonary embolism).

Specific pathogens

Pneumococcal pneumonia

Streptococcus pneumoniae is the causative organism in about **60% of community-acquired pneumonias** and in about 15% of hospital-acquired pneumonias (Fig. 6.4). Research studies using tests for pneumococcal antigen suggest that it may account for many cases in which no organism is identified. It is a Gram-positive coccus and can cause infections at all levels in the respiratory tract, including sinusitis, otitis media, bronchitis and pneumonia. Up to 60% of people carry *Streptococcus pneumoniae* as a **commensal in the nasopharynx** and infection is transmitted in airborne droplets. Nasopharyngeal carriage may progress to infection where there is a breach in the respiratory tract defences, and smoking and viral infections are important factors disrupting surface defence mechanisms. There are many **different serotypes, which vary in their virulence**, but virulent strains can render a previously fit and healthy person critically ill within a few hours.

Pneumococcal infection in asplenic patients (e.g. post-splenectomy) is severe, with a high mortality, such that these patients are usually given pneumococcal vaccination and long-term prophylactic phenoxymethylpenicillin 500 mg b.d. *Streptococcus pneumoniae* is usually **sensitive to penicillin antibiotics** (e.g. amoxicillin or benzylpenicillin) but **antibiotic resistance is an emerging problem**, particularly in certain countries (such as Spain, where about 30% of isolates are resistant). It is necessary to give broad antibiotic cover to a patient who has acquired pneumonia in a country with a high

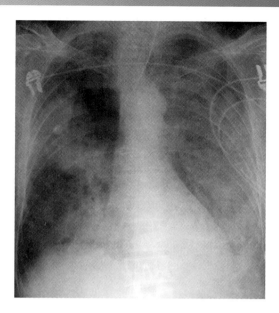

Figure 6.4 Pneumococcal pneumonia. This 70-year-old man was admitted to hospital with severe community-acquired pneumonia. He was confused, with a fever of 39 °C, respiratory rate 32/min, blood pressure 90/50 mmHg and urea 22 mmol/l. His CURB-65 score was 5, indicating severe pneumonia. He was admitted to the ITU but died despite treatment with antibiotics, mechanical ventilation and full supportive care. Blood cultures isolated *Streptococcus pneumoniae*. In the UK, about 1 in 1000 of the population is admitted to hospital each year with community-acquired pneumonia and about 18% of these patients die.

prevalence of antibiotic-resistant pneumococcus. **Pneumococcal vaccine** is recommended for those above 65 years of age and for patients with chronic lung disease, diabetes, renal and cardiac disease and those who are asplenic or immunodeficient (e.g. hypogammaglobulinaemia, HIV).

Haemophilus influenzae pneumonia

Haemophilus influenzae is a **Gram-negative bacillus**. Virulent strains are encapsulated and divided into six serological types. *Haemophilus influenzae* **type B (Hib)** is a virulent encapsulated form that causes **epiglottitis, bacteraemia, meningitis** and **pneumonia**. Hib vaccine is given to children to reduce the risk of meningitis and also provides protection against epiglottitis. However, it is the less virulent form of the organism – **non-typeable** unencapsulated *Haemophilus influenzae* – that is a common cause of respiratory tract infection, predominantly where there has been damage to the bronchial mucosa by smoking or viral infection. *Haemophilus influenzae* often forms part of the normal pharyngeal flora. Deficient mucociliary clearance in patients with smoking-induced chronic bronchitis facilitates spread of the organism to the lower respiratory tract, where it gives rise to **exacerbations of COPD**. Spread of infection into the lung parenchyma causes **bronchopneumonia**. It is usually treated with **amoxicillin**, but about 10% of strains are resistant; alternative antibiotics include co-amoxiclav (amoxicillin with clavulanic acid), doxycycline, trimethoprim and moxifloxacin.

Staphylococcal pneumonia

Staphylococcus aureus is a **Gram-positive coccus** that forms clusters resembling bunches of grapes. Although it is a relatively uncommon cause of either community- or hospital-acquired pneumonia, it may produce a very **severe illness with a high mortality**. It particularly occurs as a **sequel to influenza**, so that antistaphylococcal antibiotics should be given to patients who develop pneumonia following influenza. Infection may also reach the lungs via the bloodstream when staphylococcal bacteraemia arises from intravenous cannulae in hospitalised patients or from intravenous drug misuse. The production of toxins (e.g. Panton–Valentine leukocidin) may cause tissue necrosis with cavitation, pneumatocele formation and pneumothoraces. It is usually sensitive to flucloxacillin, co-amoxiclav or cefuroxime. MRSA is an increasing problem. Most isolates are susceptible to vancomycin and linezolid.

Klebsiella pneumonia

Klebsiella pneumoniae is a **Gram-negative organism** that generally causes pneumonia only in **patients who have impaired resistance** to infection (e.g. **alcohol misuse, malnutrition, diabetes**) or **underlying lung disease** (e.g. bronchiectasis). It often produces severe infection with destruction of lung tissue, **cavitation** and **abscess formation**. Treatment requires examination of the underlying disease state and prolonged antibiotic therapy, guided by the results of microbiology culture and sensitivity. Often, a **third-generation cephalosporin** (e.g. ceftazidime) or piperacillin with tazobactam is appropriate.

Pseudomonas aeruginosa pneumonia

Pseudomonas aeruginosa is a **Gram-negative bacillus** that is a common cause of **pneumonia in hospitalised patients**, particularly those with neutropenia and those receiving endotracheal ventilation in ITU. It is usually treated with a combination of an aminoglycoside (e.g. gentamicin, tobramycin) and a third-generation cephalosporin (e.g. ceftazidime) or **antipseudomonal penicillin** (e.g. meropenem or piperacillin with tazobactam).

Pneumonia caused by 'atypical pathogens'

'Atypical pathogens' is an imprecise term that is sometimes used in clinical practice to refer to certain pathogens that cause pneumonia, such as *Mycoplasma pneumoniae*, chlamydial organisms and *Legionella pneumophila*. Characteristically, these organisms are **not sensitive to penicillins** and require treatment with **tetracycline or macrolide (e.g. clarithromycin)** antibiotics. These organisms are **difficult to culture** in the laboratory and the diagnosis is often made retrospectively by demonstrating a rising antibody titre on serological tests.

Mycoplasma pneumonia

Mycoplasma pneumoniae is a small, free-living organism that does not have a rigid cell wall and is therefore not susceptible to antibiotics that act on bacterial cell walls, such as penicillin. Infection is transmitted from person to person by infected respiratory droplets. It **particularly affects children and young adults**, although any age group may contract it. Infection typically occurs in **outbreaks every 4 years** and spreads throughout families, schools and colleges. *Mycoplasma pneumoniae* typically causes an initial URTI with pharyngitis, sinusitis and otitis, followed by pneumonia in about 30% of cases. A variety of **extrapulmonary syndromes** can occur, which may be related to immune responses to infection. These include lymphocytic meningoencephalitis, cerebellar ataxia, peripheral neuropathy, rashes, arthralgia, splenomegaly and hepatitis. **Cold agglutinins** to type O red cells are often present and haemolytic anaemia may occur. *Mycoplasma pneumoniae* causes significant protracted morbidity but is rarely life-threatening.

Chlamydial respiratory infections

There are three chlamydial species that cause respiratory disease:

1 *Chlamydophila psittaci* is primarily an infection of **birds** that is transmitted to humans as a **zoonosis** (a disease contracted from animals) by inhalation of contaminated droplets. 'Psittacosis' or 'ornithosis' is the name given to the resultant illness, which is often severe and is characterised by high fever, headache, delirium, a macular rash and severe pneumonia.
2 *Chlamydophila pneumoniae* was identified as a respiratory pathogen in 1986. Infection is confined to **humans** and there is no avian or animal reservoir. It is extremely common in all age groups and spreads directly from **person to person**, with **outbreaks occurring in families, schools and colleges**. It typically produces upper respiratory disease, including pharyngitis, otitis and sinusitis, but it may also cause pneumonia, which is usually mild. Other bacterial pathogens (e.g. *Staphylococcus pneumoniae*) are often identified at the same time, so that the direct pathogenic role of *Chlamydophila pneumoniae* is uncertain.
3 *Chlamydia trachomatis* is a common cause of sexually transmitted genital tract infection and **infants** may acquire respiratory tract infection with this organism from their mother's genital tract during birth.

Legionella pneumonia

Legionella pneumophila is a **Gram-negative bacillus** that is widely distributed in nature in **water**. The organism was first identified in 1976, when an outbreak of severe pneumonia affected delegates at a convention of the American Legion, who contracted infection from a contaminated humidifier system (**Legionnaires' disease**). In sporadic cases, there is often no apparent source for the infection. Sometimes infection can be traced back to a **contaminated water system**, such as a shower in a hotel room, and epidemics may occur from a common source, such as a contaminated humidification plant, water storage tanks or heating circuits. Infection does not spread from patient to patient. *Legionella pneumophila* typically causes a **severe pneumonia** with prostration, confusion, diarrhoea, abdominal pain and respiratory failure, with an associated high mortality. Direct fluorescent antibody staining may detect the organism in bronchoalveolar lavage fluid, and tests to detect *Legionella* antigen in urine are available, allowing rapid diagnosis. A combination of clarithromycin or a fluoroquinolone (e.g. levofloxacin, moxifloxacin, ciprofloxacin) and rifampicin is often used to treat severe *Legionella* pneumonia.

Severe acute respiratory syndrome

In 2003, there was a global epidemic of a severe acute respiratory syndrome (SARS), characterised by a severe pneumonia with a high mortality. The causative organism was identified as a new coronavirus that was named **SARS coronavirus**, which is likely to have evolved from coronaviruses that infect bats. The epidemic seems to have emerged from the Guandong province of China and then spread explosively, with outbreaks in Hong Kong, Beijing, Taiwan, Singapore, Hanoi and Toronto. A particular feature of the epidemic was the very rapid global spread of infection by **aeroplane travel**. For example, an infected person travelled by plane from Hong Kong to Toronto, resulting in spread of infection to a new continent. Passengers on the plane and taxi drivers in contact with the index case developed infection. The SARS coronavirus is very virulent and highly infectious, spreading from person to person by direct aerosol transmission or by indirect aerosolisation from contaminated surfaces. Secondary spread of infection from patients to **healthcare workers** and medical students was a major feature of the epidemic. Tertiary cases then occurred in the families of healthcare workers. Aerosolising procedures (e.g. nebulisation, suctioning of secretions, tracheal intubation) are particularly hazardous for transmission of infection from patients to healthcare workers. Many of the patients also had diarrhoea, and in some outbreaks transmission may also have occurred by aerosolisation from sewage drainage systems. In total, during 2003, approximately 8500 cases of SARS occurred in 29 countries, with 916 deaths, giving a global case fatality of 11%. Patients presented with fevers, rigors, myalgia, cough, vomiting and diarrhoea and typically had peripheral consolidation on chest X-ray. Treatment mainly consisted of supportive care, and 20% of patients required care on an ITU. Broad-spectrum antibiotics were given for potential secondary bacterial infections and some patients seemed to benefit from corticosteroids. Currently available antiviral drugs do not seem to be effective against the SARS coronavirus. The global epidemic was brought to an end by late 2003 using **public health measures** including rapid case detection, case isolation, contact tracing and strict **infection control procedures**, such as isolation of patients in negative-pressure cubicles and use of respiratory protective masks, gowns, goggles and gloves. In 2012, there was an outbreak of severe pneumonia in patients from Saudi Arabia, Jordan and Qatar, termed 'Middle East respiratory syndrome' (MERS). A further novel coronavirus, the **MERS coronavirus**, was identified, which is suspected to have originated in camels.

Immunocompromised patients

An increasing number of patients are severely immunocompromised by a variety of diseases and by use of immunosuppressive drugs. Patients with neutropenia are particularly vulnerable to **bacterial infections** (e.g. *Streptococcus pneumoniae*, Gram-negative bacteria) and invasive **fungal infections** (e.g. *Aspergillus fumigatus*, *Candida albicans*), and patients with depressed T-lymphocyte function are vulnerable to **pneumocystis pneumonia (PCP), tuberculosis and cytomegalovirus (CMV) infection**, for example.

There are three particular situations in which profound immunosuppression commonly arises:

1 Patients with cancer receiving **antineoplastic chemotherapy**.
2 Patients with inflammatory diseases (e.g. rheumatoid disease, connective tissue diseases, inflammatory bowel disease) receiving **immunosuppressive drugs** (e.g. corticosteroids, cyclophosphamide, methotrexate, infliximab).
3 Patients **post-organ transplantation** (bone marrow, renal, lung, etc.) receiving immunosuppressive drugs (e.g. ciclosporin, azathioprine).

The problem is often that of a patient with one of these conditions presenting with pulmonary infiltrates on chest X-ray accompanied by breathlessness, and sometimes fever. The infiltrates in these circumstances may be caused by pulmonary involvement by the underlying disease process, a reaction to drug treatment, infection resulting from immunosuppression or other coincidental disease processes. Treatment is crucially dependent upon accurate diagnosis.

Assessment involves a careful clinical history and examination, focusing on the clinical context and clues to aetiology (Table 6.1). Microbiology of sputum, urine and blood may identify specific pathogens. Induced sputum is particularly useful in diagnosing PCP. If these initial tests are not diagnostic, it is often advisable to proceed directly to bronchoscopy with bronchoalveolar lavage for detailed microbiology. Transbronchial lung biopsy is useful in obtaining tissue for histological diagnosis but carries the risk of pneumothorax or haemorrhage. Occasionally, surgical lung biopsy is warranted.

Pulmonary complications of HIV infection

HIV is a retrovirus that binds to the CD4 molecule of T-lymphocytes, resulting in a progressive fall in the number and function of CD4 lymphocytes. The occurrence of various infections reflects the CD4 T-lymphocyte count and depends on the patient's previous and current exposure to pathogens (e.g. reactivation of previous tuberculosis or reinfection with tuberculosis in areas with a high prevalence, such as Africa) (Table 6.2). As the CD4 T-lymphocyte count falls, there is first an increase in the frequency of infection with common **standard pathogens** (e.g. *Streptococcus pneumoniae*, *Mycobacterium tuberculosis*), followed by infection with **opportunistic pathogens** (e.g. *Pneumocystis jirovecii*) as the CD4 count drops below about 200/mm^3. These are infections that do not usually cause disease in immunocompetent people. In the later stages of acquired immune deficiency syndrome (AIDS), **neoplastic diseases** (e.g. Kaposi's sarcoma, B-cell lymphomas) occur. There is an increased incidence of **airway** disease and **emphysema** in HIV patients, due to pathogenic synergy between HIV and smoking. These patients also have an increased risk of lung cancer, often occurring at a young age.

Bacterial respiratory infections

Patients with HIV have an increased incidence of respiratory tract infections, with **sinusitis, bronchitis, bronchiectasis** and **pneumonia** occurring as a result of standard bacterial pathogens. Infection with *Streptococcus pneumoniae*, *Haemophilus influenzae* or *Staphylococcus aureus* is common, and may precede

Table 6.1 Differential diagnosis of pulmonary infiltrates in immunocompromised patients

Chest X-ray infiltrates

- Is it the underlying disease?
- Is it a reaction to drugs?
- Is it infection?
- Is it some other disease process?

Disease	*Cancer*	*Inflammatory disease*	*Organ transplant*
	(e.g. lymphoma, carcinoma)	(e.g. rheumatoid disease)	(e.g. bone marrow, renal)
	Lymphangitis	Interstitial lung disease	Graft-versus-host disease
	Lung metastases		
Drugs	Lung fibrosis or pneumonitis (e.g. bleomycin, busulfan, cyclophosphamide, methotrexate, gold, penicillamine)		
Infection	Bacterial or opportunistic infections (PCP, CMV)		
Other process	Pulmonary oedema, haemorrhage, embolism etc.		

Pulmonary infiltrates

Clinical assessment

Microbiology of sputum, urine, blood (e.g. TB, bacteria)

Induced sputum (e.g. PCP)

Bronchoscopy and bronchoalveolar lavage (CMV, PCP, TB)

Transbronchial lung biopsy

Surgical lung biopsy (histology)

Diagnosis ⟶ **Specific treatments**

PCP, pneumocystis pneumonia; CMV, cytomegalovirus; TB, tuberculosis.

the diagnosis of HIV infection or the onset of opportunistic infections. Infection with Gram-negative organisms (e.g. *Pseudomonas aeruginosa*) occurs in more advanced disease. The clinical features may be unusual, with a higher frequency of complications such as bacteraemia, abscess formation, cavitation and empyema. Pneumococcal and influenza vaccination may be helpful and sometimes long-term prophylactic antibiotics are used. With the advent of highly active antiretroviral treatment (HAART), HIV is now a treatable condition with a good prognosis, but it is estimated that in the UK one-third of people do not know that they are infected and so do not get the benefits of HAART. Late diagnosis is a major factor in HIV-related morbidity and mortality. Patients with a wide range of conditions (e.g. pneumonia, bronchiectasis, tuberculosis) should now be offered HIV testing.

Pneumocystis pneumonia

Pneumocystis jirovecii (formerly known as *carinii*) is a fungus that only causes disease in immunocompromised individuals, and in HIV infection it typically occurs at the stage at which the CD4 T-lymphocyte count has fallen to below 200/mm^3. PCP typically presents as a subacute illness over a few weeks, with cough, dyspnoea, fever, hypoxaemia, reduced transfer factor for carbon monoxide and bilateral perihilar interstitial infiltrates on chest X-ray (Fig. 6.5). These clinical features are not specific to PCP and can be caused by a variety of other infections, and more than one pathogen may be present. The chest X-ray may be normal in early PCP, and high-resolution computed tomography (CT) is more sensitive. Sometimes, the radiological features are unusual, showing unilateral consolidation, nodules or upper lobe consolidation,

Table 6.2 Pulmonary complications of HIV infection

Infectious diseases

- Bacterial infections
  - *Streptococcus pneumoniae*
  - Haemophilus influenzae
  - *Pseudomonas aeruginosa*
  - Tuberculosis
- Opportunistic infections
  - Fungal
    - *Pneumocystis jirovecii*
    - Aspergillus fumigatus
    - *Candida albicans*
  - Viral
    - Cytomegalovirus
    - Herpes simplex
  - Mycobacterial
    - *Mycobacterium avium* complex

Immune reconstitution syndromes

- Sarcoid-like syndrome
- Paradoxical deterioration of pneumonia

Noninfectious diseases

- Neoplastic
  - Kaposi's sarcoma
  - B-cell lymphoma
  - Primary effusion cell lymphoma
- Inflammatory
  - Lymphocytic alveolitis ($\downarrow T_L$co)
  - Nonspecific interstitial pneumonitis
  - Lymphocytic interstitial pneumonitis
  - Airway disease and emphysema
  - Primary pulmonary hypertension

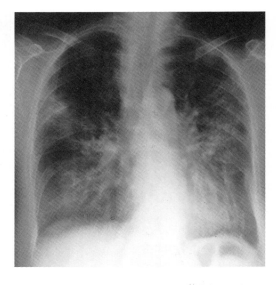

Figure 6.5 Pneumocystis pneumonia (PCP). This 28-year-old woman, who was an intravenous drug misuser, presented with fever, dyspnoea and hypoxaemia (Po$_2$ 8.2 kPa (62 mmHg)). The chest X-ray shows diffuse bilateral perihilar and lower zone shadowing. HIV antibody test was positive and CD4 T-lymphocyte count was 100/mm^3 (normal 600–1600/mm^3). Induced sputum was positive for *Pneumocystis jirovecii* on immunofluorescent monoclonal antibody testing. The patient responded fully to high-dose intravenous co-trimoxazole, prednisolone and oxygen, and she was then commenced on long-term secondary prophylaxis with oral co-trimoxazole 3 days/week. When her PCP had been fully treated, highly active antiretroviral therapy (HAART) was started.

for example. Cavitating lesions may occur and pneumothorax is a recognised complication.

The **diagnosis** is usually confirmed by detecting *Pneumocystis jirovecii* using a monoclonal antibody immunofluorescent technique on specimens obtained by **sputum induction** or by bronchoscopy and **bronchoalveolar lavage**. To induce sputum, the patient is given 3–7% hypertonic saline by nebulisation followed by chest physiotherapy. If this test is negative, it is usual to proceed to bronchoalveolar lavage, whereby a bronchoscope is advanced into a subsegmental bronchus and 60 ml aliquots of warmed sterile saline are instilled and aspirated. More invasive procedures, such as **transbronchial** or **surgical lung biopsy**, are usually only performed in complex cases where the aetiology of lung infiltrates cannot be determined by other tests and where a histological diagnosis is considered essential for guiding treatment decisions.

Treatment of PCP consists of high-dose intravenous **co-trimoxazole** (trimethoprim 15 mg/kg/day and sulfamethoxazole 75 mg/kg/day in four divided doses), subsequently converted to oral therapy, usually continued for 3 weeks. Side effects (e.g. allergic rashes, nausea, marrow suppression) are common and intravenous **pentamidine** or **clindamycin with primaquine** are alternatives. Patients with moderate or severe PCP (e.g. Po$_2$ < 9.5 kPa (70 mmHg)) benefit from the addition of **corticosteroids** (e.g. prednisolone 40 mg/day) to reduce the pulmonary inflammatory response. High-flow **oxygen** is often required, and use of **continuous positive airway pressure (CPAP)** may reduce the need for **ventilation** in severe cases.

Primary prophylaxis is given to HIV-infected patients whose CD4 T-cell count is <200/mm³, in order to prevent first infection. **Secondary prophylaxis** is given to prevent recurrence in patients who have already suffered an episode of PCP. Co-trimoxazole (trimethoprim and sulfamethoxazole) 960 mg given on 3 days/week is the regimen of choice. Nebulised pentamidine given once monthly, atovaquone and a combination of oral pyrimethamine and dapsone are alternatives for patients who cannot tolerate co-trimoxazole. PCP prophylaxis may be stopped in patients who have responded well to HAART, with control of viral replication and recovery of CD4 cell counts.

Mycobacterial infection

Mycobacterium tuberculosis

Patients with HIV infection and impaired CD4 lymphocyte function are highly susceptible to developing **reactivation** of previously acquired latent tuberculosis and to **contracting the disease from an exogenous source**, with rapid **progression to active disease**. Early in HIV disease, tuberculosis resembles the typical disease seen in non-HIV patients, with upper lobe consolidation and cavitation. In severely immunocompromised patients, the clinical features may be very nonspecific, with fever, weight loss, malaise, diffuse shadowing on chest X-ray and a high incidence of extrapulmonary disseminated disease. Standard antituberculosis treatment is given using isoniazid, rifampicin, pyrazinamide and ethambutol (see Chapter 7). Bacillus Calmette–Guérin (BCG) vaccination is contraindicated in HIV infection because of the risk of active infection developing with the live attenuated vaccine bacillus in severely immunocompromised patients. Because of their impaired cellular immunity, patients with HIV are very susceptible to contracting and transmitting tuberculosis, so that strict isolation precautions are warranted, particularly for patients with multidrug-resistant tuberculosis.

Mycobacterium avium complex

This is an opportunistic mycobacterium that does not usually cause disease in normal subjects but commonly infects patients with advanced AIDS, particularly when their CD4 count is <100/mm³. Extrapulmonary disease is more common than pulmonary disease and the diagnosis of disseminated *Mycobacterium avium* complex (MAC) is usually made when the organism is cultured from blood, bone marrow, lymph node or liver biopsy.

The organism is not usually responsive to standard antituberculosis drugs and is treated with a combination of rifabutin, ethambutol, ciprofloxacin and clarithromycin or azithromycin.

Viral infections

Cytomegalovirus (CMV) infection is common in AIDS, usually causing systemic infection with hepatitis, retinitis, encephalitis and colitis, rather than overt pulmonary infection. CMV is often isolated from the lungs of AIDS patients but it is not always pathogenic, sometimes being present as a commensal. It is treated with ganciclovir. **Epstein–Barr (EB) virus**, **adenovirus**, **influenza** and **herpes simplex virus** may cause pneumonia in AIDS patients. Herpes simplex virus is frequently present in the mouth of HIV-infected patients, so that its isolation from the respiratory tract often indicates colonisation rather than infection.

Fungal pulmonary infections

Invasive pulmonary infections with *Aspergillus fumigatus* or *Candida albicans* are unusual but may occur late in the course of AIDS. **Cryptococcal** pneumonia may occur as part of a disseminated infection, but usually meningoencephalitis dominates the clinical picture. Treatment is with fluconazole, flucytosine and amphotericin. Pulmonary **histoplasmosis** and **coccidioidomycosis** may occur in areas where these fungi are endemic (e.g. the United States).

HIV-related neoplasms

Kaposi's sarcoma

This is the most common malignancy in HIV-infected patients. Characteristically, it occurs in HIV-infected homosexual men and it is thought that it may relate to **co-infection with human herpes virus 8**. Pulmonary Kaposi's sarcoma is nearly always accompanied by lesions in the skin or buccal mucosa. Chest X-ray appearances are variable, as the tumour may affect the bronchi, lung parenchyma, pleura or mediastinal lymph nodes. At bronchoscopy, Kaposi's sarcoma appears as red or purple lesions. The diagnosis is usually made on the basis of the visual appearances in the context of mucocutaneous Kaposi's sarcoma, as biopsy of the bronchial lesions is often nondiagnostic and may cause haemorrhage. Antiretroviral therapy (HAART) may lead to regression of Kaposi's sarcoma, but antineoplastic chemotherapy (e.g. doxorubicin, paclitaxel) is often needed.

Lymphoma

Late in the course of AIDS, high-grade **B-cell lymphomas** arise. The lungs are often involved as part of multiorgan involvement. **Primary effusion lymphoma** can occur and may present with pleural, pericardial or peritoneal effusions. The response to chemotherapy is often poor.

Interstitial pneumonitis

Patients with HIV infection may develop **nonspecific interstitial pneumonitis (NSIP)**. This presents as episodes of dyspnoea with pulmonary infiltrates, reduced gas diffusion and hypoxaemia. Bronchoalveolar lavage is negative for infection and lung biopsy shows evidence of lymphocytic inflammation. NSIP may be a manifestation of direct HIV infection of the lung. It is often self-limiting, but prednisolone may be beneficial.

Lymphoid interstitial pneumonitis is usually seen only in children with HIV infection, and the pneumonitis may be part of a more widespread lymphocytic infiltration of liver, bone marrow and parotid glands with hypergammaglobulinaemia. Its aetiology is uncertain but it may be related to EB virus co-infection.

Primary pulmonary hypertension

Primary pulmonary hypertension is a rare complication of HIV infection and may result from the effect of inflammatory mediators and cytokines – produced by infection of the lung with the HIV virus – on the pulmonary circulation (see Chapter 15).

Immune reconstitution syndromes

When antiretroviral therapy (HAART) inhibits viral replication, there is a corresponding increase in the population of T-cells, enhancement of lymphoproliferative responses and increase in IL-2 receptor expression. These proinflammatory effects may give rise to certain syndromes associated with immune reconstitution. Some patients develop a **sarcoid-like granulomatous disorder**, with diffuse opacities on chest X-ray, lymphadenopathy, salivary gland enlargement and elevated serum angiotensin-converting enzyme (ACE) levels. **Pulmonary hypersensitivity** reactions to antiretroviral drugs have also been described. **Paradoxical deterioration** of opportunistic pneumonia (e.g. PCP, tuberculosis), despite antibiotic therapy, may occur as the patient mounts an inflammatory response. This may be severe enough to cause acute respiratory failure and require corticosteroid therapy. In patients presenting with HIV infection and low CD4 counts, opportunistic infections should be sought and treated before starting HAART.

Respiratory emergencies Pneumonia

- Urgent chest X-ray is key in confirming the diagnosis.
- Enquire about travel, recent influenza, contact with animals, allergy to antibiotics.
- Full blood count, urea/electrolytes, C-reactive protein.
- Assess severity: CURB-65 score (confusion, elevated urea, respiratory rate, blood pressure, age > 65 years).
- Assess oxygenation (O_2sat/blood gases), social circumstances, comorbid illness.
- In severe pneumonia, send blood and sputum for microbiology cultures and urine for pneumococcal and legionella antigen.
- Give antibiotics urgently: mild = amoxicillin 500 mg t.d.s. orally; moderate/severe = IV co-amoxiclav 1.2 g t.d.s. + clarithromycin 500 mg b.d.
- Consider prophylaxis for venous thrombosis, e.g. tinzaparin 3500 units subcutaneously daily.
- Monitor respiratory rate, O_2sat, pulse, blood pressure, temperature.
- Review frequently. Switch from intravenous to oral antibiotics when improving. If not improving, consider other diagnoses (e.g. pulmonary embolism) or complications (e.g. empyema).
- Arrange clinical review and chest X-ray 6 weeks after discharge from hospital.

 KEY POINTS

- Pneumonia is an important cause of morbidity and mortality in all age groups.
- About 1 in 1000 of the UK population is admitted to hospital each year with pneumonia and the mortality is 18%.
- *Streptococcus pneumoniae* is the most common cause of community-acquired pneumonia, but atypical pathogens (e.g. *Mycoplasma pneumoniae*) are also important, such that treatment is often with a combination of amoxicillin and a macrolide antibiotic (e.g. clarithromycin).

- Gram-negative organisms (e.g. *Pseudomonas aeruginosa*) are the main cause of hospital-acquired pneumonia, such that treatment is often with antibiotics such as ceftazidime, meropenem or piperacillin with tazobactam.
- The severity of community-acquired pneumonia should be assessed using the CURB-65 score (confusion, elevated urea, respiratory rate, blood pressure, age > 65 years).
- Patients with HIV are initially vulnerable to lung infections with bacteria (e.g. *Streptococcus pneumoniae*, *Mycobacterium tuberculosis*). When the CD4 count falls below 200/mm^3, opportunistic infections (e.g. PCP) develop.

 ## FURTHER READING

American Thoracic Society. Guidelines for the management of adults with hospital-acquired, ventilation-associated and healthcare-associated pneumonia. *Am J Respir Crit Care Med* 2005; **171**: 388–416.

Assiri A, McGeer A, Perl TM, et al. Hospital outbreak of Middle East respiratory syndrome coronavirus. *N Engl J Med* 2013; **369**: 407–16.

Barlow G, Nathwani D, Davey P. The CURB65 pneumonia severity score outperforms generic sepsis and early warning scores in predicting mortality in community- acquired pneumonia. *Thorax* 2007; **62**: 253–9.

Benito N, Moreno A, Miro JM, Torres A. Pulmonary infections in HIV-infected patients: an update in the 21st century. *Eur Respir J* 2012; **39**: 730–45.

British Society for Antimicrobial Chemotherapy. Report of the working party on hospital-acquired pneumonia of the British Society for Antimicrobial Chemotherapy. *JAC* 2008; **62**: 5–34.

British Thoracic Society Community Acquired Pneumonia in Adults Guideline Group. Guidelines for the management of community acquired pneumonia in adults: update 2009. *Thorax* 2009; **64**(Suppl. III): 1–61.

Brown JS. Community-acquired pneumonia. *Clin Med* 2012; **12**: 538–43.

Winstone TA, Man SFP, Hull M, et al. Epidemic of lung cancer in patients with HIV infection. *Chest* 2013; **143**: 305–14.

Woodhead M, Blasi F, Ewig S, et al. European Society Task Force. Guidelines for the management of adult lower respiratory tract infections. *Eur Respir J* 2005; **26**: 1138–80.

World Health Organization. Consensus document on the epidemiology of severe acute respiratory syndrome (SARS). WHO, 2003 (http://www.who.int/csr/sars/en/WHOconsensus.pdf, last accessed 29 December 2014).

Multiple choice questions

6.1 The most common cause of community-acquired pneumonia is:

A *Mycoplasma pneumoniae*
B *Haemophilus influenzae*
C *Pseudomonas aeruginosa*
D *Streptococcus pneumoniae*
E *Staphylococcus aureus*

6.2 *Chlamydophila psittaci*:

A is associated with contaminated water
B is associated with foreign travel
C is a zoonosis
D is associated with recent influenza infection
E is a common cause of hospital-acquired pneumonia

6.3 A 40-year-old man presents with cough, fever and purulent sputum. Chest X-ray shows consolidation in the right lower lobe. He is alert, with respiratory rate of 22/min, blood pressure of 122/78 mmHg, urea of 5.6 mmol/l, white cell count $18.4 \times 10^9/l$. His CURB-65 score is:

A 0
B 1
C 2
D 4
E 5

6.4 Severe acute respiratory syndrome (SARS) is caused by:

A *Legionella pneumophila*
B a coronavirus
C meticillin-resistant *staphylococcus aureus* (MRSA)
D a retrovirus
E *Chlamydophila pneumoniae*

6.5 A 28-year-old man is admitted to hospital with severe respiratory failure (Po$_2$ 7.5 kPa) and diffuse bilateral consolidation in the perihilar areas on chest X-ray. His HIV test is positive and his CD4 count is 100/mm^3. The most likely cause of his lung consolidation is:

A pneumocystis pneumonia
B Kaposi's sarcoma
C *Mycobacterium avium* complex infection
D HIV pneumonitis
E *Streptococcus pneumoniae*

6.6 A suitable choice of antibiotics for a patient admitted to hospital with community-acquired pneumonia with a CURB score of 2 is:

A co-amoxiclav (amoxicillin and clavulanic acid)
B amoxicillin and clarithromycin
C metronidazole
D ceftazidime
E co-trimoxazole

6.7 A 40-year-old man with left lower lobe pneumonia and a pleural effusion continues to be febrile and has a white cell count of $17 \times 10^9/l$ (normal 4–11) and a C-reactive protein of 322 mg/l (normal 0–5) despite 5 days of antibiotics. The most likely diagnosis is:

A parapneumonic effusion
B pulmonary embolism
C HIV infection
D empyema
E tuberculosis

6.8 The mortality for patients admitted to hospital with community-acquired pneumonia is about:

A 1%
B 5%
C 12%
D 18%
E 25%

6.9 Middle East respiratory syndrome (MERS) is caused by:

A histoplasmosis
B H2N1 influenza A
C *Burkhoderia pseudomallei*
D *Coxiella burnetti*
E a coronavirus

6.10 The most common cause of hospital-acquired pneumonia is:

A Gram-negative bacteria
B *Clostridum difficile*
C Legionella pneumonia
D *Haemophilus influenzae*
E *Moraxella catarrhalis*

Multiple choice answers

6.1 D

Streptococcus pneumoniae is the most common cause of community-acquired pneumonia.

6.2 C

Chlamydophila psittaci is primarily an infection of birds but can be transmitted to humans as a zoonosis.

6.3 A

This patient's CURB-65 score is zero. He is not **C**onfused, his **U**rea is normal at 5.6 mmol/l, his **R**espiratory rate is not elevated above 30/minute, his **B**lood pressure is normal and he is not over **65** years of age. This indicates a low risk for developing complications and he is likely to be suitable for treatment at home, rather than in hospital.

6.4 B

SARS is a very severe pneumonic illness caused by a newly identified coronavirus. It caused a global pandemic in 2003, which was brought to an end by public health measures including rapid case detection, case isolation, contact tracing and strict infection-control procedures.

6.5 A

Pneumocystis pneumonia is likely to occur in patients with HIV infection whose CD4 count is <200/mm³. The diagnosis may be confirmed by detecting *Pneumocystis jirovecii* in induced sputum or in bronchoalveolar lavage fluid. The patient requires treatment with high-dose intravenous co-trimoxazole, prednisolone and oxygen.

6.6 B

Community-acquired pneumonia is usually treated by a combination of amoxicillin and clarithromycin.

6.7 D

He continues to have features of sepsis despite antibiotics and is likely to have developed a complication of pneumonia in the form of empyema. Ultrasound-guided pleural aspiration is advisable.

6.8 D

The British Thoracic Society audit of community-acquired pneumonia in 2009/10 showed a high mortality rate, with about 18% of patients dying in hospital within 30 days. Many patients are elderly, with substantial concomitant disease.

6.9 E

In 2012, there was an outbreak of severe pneumonia in patients from Saudi Arabia, Jordan and Qatar. A novel coronavirus (MERS coronavirus) was identified as the cause.

6.10 A

Hospital-acquired pneumonia is defined as pneumonia developing 2 or more days after admission to hospital for some other reason. It is most common in patients in ITU. Gram-negative bacteria (e.g. *Pseudomonas aeruginosa*, *E. coli*) are the most commonly involved organisms.

7

Tuberculosis

Tuberculosis is an infection caused by *Mycobacterium tuberculosis* that may affect any part of the body but most commonly affects the lungs. It is spread by inhalation of the bacterium in droplets coughed or exhaled by someone with infectious tuberculosis.

Epidemiology

Tuberculosis continues to be a major global health problem. The World Health Organization estimates that **2 billion people (one-third of the world's population) have latent infection with *Mycobacterium tuberculosis*, 8.6 million people develop active disease and 1.3 million die each year** from tuberculosis. In the UK in the 19th century, more than 30 000 people died from tuberculosis each year (about the same as for lung cancer at present). Mortality and notification rates declined steadily from 1900 onwards due to improvements in nutritional and social factors, with a sharper decline occurring from the late 1940s onwards following the introduction of effective treatment. Notification rates in England and Wales reached a low point of about 5000 a year in 1987 but have increased again to about 9000 a year recently, and about 5% of these patients die from the disease. This increased incidence of tuberculosis is mainly seen in those born abroad and in ethnic minority groups. The notification rates for tuberculosis are highest in the Indian (155 per 100 000 population), Pakistani (132 per 100 000) and black African (97 per 100 000) ethnic groups and lowest in those born in the UK (4 per 100 000). The recent increase in notification rates is partly the result of patterns of immigration and increasing international travel. Other groups of people with a high incidence of tuberculosis are the homeless, those misusing drugs and alcohol and those co-infected with human immunodeficiency virus (HIV). In younger age groups, tuberculosis is often a newly acquired infection, whereas in the older age groups it is often a reactivation of latent infection acquired many years previously. Factors that reduce resistance and precipitate reactivation include ageing, alcohol misuse, poor nutrition, debility from other diseases, use of immunosuppressive drug therapy and co-infection with HIV. In the UK, overlap between the population with HIV infection (mainly young white men) and the population with tuberculosis (mainly older white people and younger immigrants from the Indian subcontinent) is limited, so that only 5% of patients with acquired immune deficiency syndrome (AIDS) have tuberculosis and about 6% of patients with tuberculosis are identified as having HIV infection. However, **15 million people worldwide are estimated to be co-infected with HIV and tuberculosis**.

Clinical course

The clinical course of tuberculosis (Fig. 7.1) often evolves over many years and represents a complex interaction between the infecting organism (*Mycobacterium tuberculosis*) and the patient's specific immune response and nonspecific resistance to infection. Traditional descriptions of tuberculosis divide the disease into two main patterns, **primary** and **post-primary** tuberculosis, although these are mainly based upon the characteristic evolution of the disease in the days before effective chemotherapy.

Primary tuberculosis

Primary tuberculosis is the pattern of disease seen with **first infection** in a patient (often a child) **without specific immunity** to tuberculosis. Infection is acquired by inhalation of organisms from an infected individual, and the initial lesion typically develops in the peripheral subpleural region of the lung, followed

Respiratory Medicine Lecture Notes, Ninth Edition. Stephen J. Bourke and Graham P. Burns.
© 2015 John Wiley & Sons, Ltd. Published 2015 by John Wiley & Sons, Ltd.
Companion Website: www.lecturenoteseries.com/Respiratory

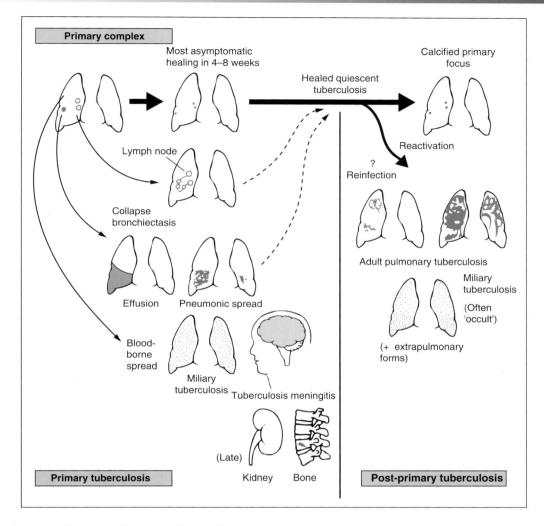

Figure 7.1 Summary of the natural history of tuberculosis.

by a reaction in the hilar lymph nodes. The **primary complex** appears on chest X-ray as a peripheral area of consolidation (Gohn focus) with hilar adenopathy. Occasionally, erythema nodosum develops at this stage. An immune response develops, the tuberculin test becomes positive and **healing** often takes place. This stage of the disease is often asymptomatic but can leave calcified nodules on chest X-rays, representing the healed primary focus. Active **progression** of first infection may occur. Bronchial spread of infection can cause progressive consolidation and cavitation of the lung parenchyma, and pleural effusions may develop. Lymphatic spread of infection may cause progressive lymph node enlargement, which in children may compress bronchi with obstruction,

distal consolidation and the development of collapse and bronchiectasis. Bronchiectasis of the middle lobe is a very typical outcome of hilar node involvement by tuberculosis in childhood. Haematogenous spread of infection results in early generalisation of disease, which may cause miliary tuberculosis and the lethal complication of tuberculous meningitis (particularly in young children). Infection spread during this initial illness may lie **dormant** in any organ of the body (e.g. bone, kidneys), only to **reactivate** many years later.

Post-primary tuberculosis

Post-primary tuberculosis is the **pattern of disease seen after the development of specific immunity**. It may occur following direct progression of the initial infection or result from endogenous **reactivation** of infection or from exogenous **re-infection** (inhalation of *Mycobacterium tuberculosis* from another infected individual) in a patient who has had previous contact with the organism and has developed a degree of specific immunity. Reactivation particularly occurs in old age and in circumstances where immunocompetence is impaired (e.g. illness, alcohol misuse, immuno-suppressive drug treatment). The lungs are the most usual site of post-primary disease and the apices of the lungs are the most common pulmonary site.

Diagnosis

Clinical features

Definitive diagnosis requires identification of *Mycobacterium tuberculosis*, because the clinical features of the disease are nonspecific. The most typical **chest symptoms** are persistent cough, sputum production and haemoptysis. **Systemic symptoms** include fever, night sweats, anorexia and weight loss. A range of **chest X-ray** abnormalities occur (Figs 7.2 and 7.3). Cavitating apical lesions are characteristic of tuberculosis, but such lesions may also be caused by lung cancer. Irregular mottled shadowing (particularly of the lung apices), streaky fibrosis, calcified granuloma, miliary mottling, pleural effusions and hilar gland enlargement may all be features.

Diagnosis depends on the doctor having a high level of awareness of the many presentations of tuberculosis and undertaking appropriate investigations (e.g. sputum **acid- and alcohol-fast bacilli (AAFB) staining** and culture for tuberculosis) in patients with persistent chest symptoms or abnormal X-rays. A high index of suspicion is required in assessing patients who have recently immigrated from a high-prevalence area (e.g. Africa, the Indian subcontinent) and in patients at risk for reactivation of infection because of factors that lower their resistance (age, alcohol misuse, debilitating disease, use of immunosuppressive drugs).

Although tuberculosis most commonly affects the lungs, **any organ in the body may be involved** and the diagnosis needs to be considered in patients with a **pyrexia of unknown origin** and those with a variety of indolent chronic lesions (e.g. in bone, kidney or lymph nodes). The term **miliary tuberculosis** refers to a situation in which there has been widespread haematogenous dissemination of tuberculosis, usually with multiple 'millet seed'-sized nodules

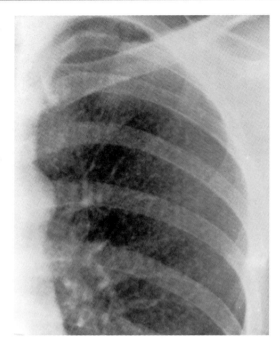

Figure 7.2 This 24-year-old man presented with malaise, fever and weight loss without any respiratory symptoms. He had immigrated to the UK from Pakistan 6 months previously. The X-ray shows multiple 1–2 mm nodules throughout both lungs, characteristic of miliary tuberculosis. Sputum and bronchoalveolar lavage did not show AAFB. Transbronchial biopsies, however, showed caseating granulomas characteristic of tuberculosis. His symptoms resolved and the chest X-ray appearances returned to normal after 6 months of antituberculosis chemotherapy.

evident on chest X-ray. Chest symptoms are often minimal and typically the patient is ill and pyrexial with anaemia and weight loss.

Laboratory diagnosis

Identification of *Mycobacterium tuberculosis* by laboratory tests can take some time and antituberculosis treatment may have to be commenced based on clinical and radiological features while awaiting the results. Once the diagnosis is suspected, repeated **sputum** samples should be examined by the **Ziehl–Neelsen** (ZN) method, looking for AAFBs, which appear as red rods on a blue background. **Sputum cultures** require special media (e.g. Löwenstein–Jensen medium) and the tubercle bacillus grows slowly, taking 4–7 weeks to give a positive culture and a further 3 weeks for in vitro

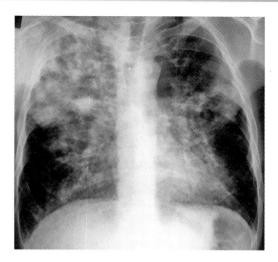

Figure 7.3 This 68-year-old man was persuaded to consult a doctor because of a 6-month history of cough, haemoptysis, night sweats and weight loss. He suffered from alcoholism and lived in a hostel for homeless men. His chest X-ray shows cavitating consolidation throughout the right upper lobe, with further areas of consolidation in the left upper and right lower lobes. Sputum AAFB stains were positive and cultures yielded *Mycobacterium tuberculosis* sensitive to standard drugs. He was treated with directly observed antituberculosis therapy. On contact tracing, 6 of 38 residents of the hostel were found to have active tuberculosis. DNA fingerprinting techniques showed that this cluster of cases was caused by three different strains of *Mycobacterium tuberculosis*, arising as a result of both reactivation of latent tuberculosis in debilitated elderly men and spread of infection within the hostel.

techniques make it possible to distinguish different strains of *Mycobacterium tuberculosis*, which can give useful insights into the likely source and spread of infection and help assess the relative contributions of newly acquired and reactivated infections in different populations.

Treatment

Before effective antibiotics became available in the late 1940s, about 50% of patients with sputum-positive tuberculosis died of the disease. Patients were admitted to sanatoria for bed rest, 'sunshine and fresh air' therapy and nutritional support, in an attempt to enhance their innate resistance to the disease. When large tuberculous cavities developed in the lungs, attempts were made to collapse them by inducing an artificial pneumothorax, crushing the phrenic nerve, putting various materials outside the pleura to compress the lung (plombage) or performing thoracoplasty, whereby the ribs were excised and the lung compressed against the mediastinum (Fig. 7.4). In the

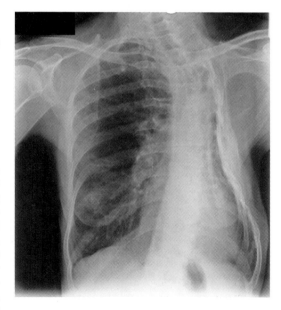

Figure 7.4 Thoracoplasty. Before effective antibiotics became available in the late 1940s, about 50% of patients with sputum-positive tuberculosis died of the disease. At that time, attempts were sometimes made to collapse large tuberculous cavities by performing a thoracoplasty, an operation in which the ribs were resected and the lung was compressed against the mediastinum

testing of antibiotic sensitivity. **Biopsy** of an affected site (e.g. pleura, lymph node, liver, bone marrow) may show the characteristic features of **caseating granulomas** (central cheesy necrosis of a lesion formed by macrophages, lymphocytes and epithelial cells). Biopsy specimens should also be submitted for mycobacterial cultures. Newer techniques are being developed to improve the speed, sensitivity and specificity of the laboratory diagnosis of tuberculosis. The **Bactec radiometric system**, for example, uses a liquid medium containing a radioactively ^{14}C-labelled substance that releases $^{14}CO_2$ when metabolised, detection of which indicates the growth of *Mycobacterium tuberculosis*. DNA techniques using the **polymerase chain reaction** (PCR) are currently being developed, which may prove useful in detecting evidence of infection in cerebrospinal fluid in tuberculous meningitis. **DNA fingerprint**

late 1940s, **streptomycin** and **para-amino salicylic acid** (PAS) were introduced into clinical practice and the outlook for patients with tuberculosis was revolutionised. It soon became apparent that treatment had to be **prolonged** and that **combinations** of antibiotics had to be used, because of the capacity of the tubercle bacillus to lie dormant in lesions for long periods and to develop resistance to antibiotics.

The current standard treatment of tuberculosis consists of **6 months** of **rifampicin** and **isoniazid**, supplemented by **pyrazinamide and ethambutol** for the first 2 months (Table 7.1). All drugs are usually given in a single daily dose. Rifampicin and isoniazid are bactericidal drugs that kill extracellular bacilli that are actively metabolising. Both rifampicin and pyrazinamide are effective against intracellular bacilli within macrophages. Prolonged treatment is needed to eradicate bacilli lying dormant. The use of a combination of drugs also prevents the emergence of resistance from the small number of bacilli that are naturally resistant to any one of the antibiotics. Ethambutol is bacteriostatic and is included in the treatment regimen to prevent the emergence of resistance to other drugs. Meticulous **supervision** of treatment is essential and patients should be seen at least monthly to prescribe medication, check **adherence** to treatment and monitor for side effects (e.g. liver function tests). Errors in the prescription of medication or failure of the patient to comply with treatment may have serious consequences, with the emergence of resistant organisms. **Directly observed therapy** should be instituted for patients who have difficulty adhering to treatment, watching to ensure that they swallow the medication. This can be achieved by giving high doses of the antituberculosis medication three times per week at the hospital or general practice clinic under the supervision of a doctor or nurse. Flexible strategies are required to ensure compliance of patients with social (e.g. homelessness) or psychological (e.g. alcohol misuse, mental illness) problems, and there is an important role for community health workers or trained laypersons in these circumstances.

At present, **drug-resistant tuberculosis** is rare in the initial treatment of patients from the white ethnic group in the UK but is more common in patients who have had previous treatment or who come from Africa or the Indian subcontinent. Overall, about 6.8% of isolates of *Mycobacterium tuberculosis* are resistant to isoniazid, 1.8% are resistant to rifampicin and 1.6% have multiple drug resistance. **Multidrug-resistant tuberculosis** results from inadequate previous treatment. The development of resistant organisms in a patient failing to comply with treatment may make the tuberculosis very difficult to treat, and such a patient poses a risk to public health as they may infect others with drug-resistant tuberculosis. Some outbreaks of multidrug-resistant tuberculosis have occurred in prisons and hospitals, with high mortality rates.

The most dangerous of the **adverse reactions** to antituberculosis treatment is **hepatotoxicity**, and patients should be advised to stop treatment

Table 7.1 Treatment of tuberculosis

Drug	Dose Children	Adult	Duration	Adverse effects
Isoniazid	10 mg/kg	300mg	6 months	Hepatitis, neuropathy
Rifampicin	10 mg/kg	<50 kg 450mg	6 months	Hepatitis, rashes
		>50 kg 600mg		Enzyme induction
Pyrazinamide	35 mg/kg	<50 kg 1.5 g	Initial	Hepatitis, rashes
		>50 kg 2.0 g	2 months	Elevated uric acid
Ethambutol	15 mg/kg	15 mg/kg	2 months	Optic neuritis

- 6 months of rifampicin and isoniazid, with pyrazinamide and ethambutol for first 2 months
- Monitor treatment meticulously (e.g. monthly review)
- Check compliance
- Use directly observed therapy if problems with compliance
- Notify the diagnosis to Public Health Authorities
- Contact tracing of close family contacts.

and report for medical advice if they develop fever, vomiting, malaise or jaundice. Isoniazid, rifampicin and pyrazinamide may all cause hepatitis and allergic reactions, such as **rashes**. Isoniazid may cause a **peripheral neuropathy**, which is preventable by pyridoxine 10 mg/day; this is given routinely to those at risk of neuropathy (e.g. patients with diabetes or alcohol misuse). Intermittent rifampicin may cause 'flu-like' symptoms, and the **induction of microsomal hepatic enzymes** reduces the serum half-life of drugs such as warfarin, steroids, phenytoin and oestrogen contraceptives, so that patients may need an adjustment in dosage of medications and may require alternative contraceptive measures. Rifampicin produces a reddish discoloration of urine (which can be used to monitor compliance) and may cause staining of soft contact lenses. Pyrazinamide sometimes causes initial facial flushing, and may cause an **elevation of uric acid levels** with arthralgia. Ethambutol causes a dose-related **optic neuritis**, which is rare at doses below 15 mg/kg/day. Patients should have their visual acuity checked before starting treatment and should stop treatment if visual symptoms occur, and the drug should be avoided if possible in patients with impaired renal function or pre-existing visual problems.

Latent tuberculosis

The term **latent tuberculosis** refers to the situation in which a patient has been infected with *Mycobacterium tuberculosis* at some time in the past but does not currently have active disease. The immune response has controlled the primary infection but all viable organisms may not have been eliminated. It is estimated that there is a 5–10% risk of a patient with latent tuberculosis developing active disease at some stage over the course of their life. The greatest risk of progression to disease is within 2 years of the initial infection, and this is particularly relevant when undertaking contact tracing of people who may have acquired infection recently from a patient with active tuberculosis. Factors that increase the risk of reactivation of latent infection include ageing, alcohol misuse, poor nutrition, co-infection with HIV and the use of immunosuppressive drugs. Recently, for example, tumour necrosis factor alpha (TNF-α) antagonists have been used in the treatment of Crohn's disease and rheumatoid arthritis. These drugs are associated with a significant risk of reactivation of latent tuberculous infection, however, and so latent infection should be sought for and treated

before starting TNF-α treatment. People with latent tuberculosis are asymptomatic and usually have a normal chest X-ray. Detection of latent infection depends on demonstrating an immune response to *Mycobacterium tuberculosis* using a tuberculin test or an interferon gamma (IFN-γ)-based blood test.

Tuberculin testing

Hypersensitivity to the tubercle bacillus can be detected by the intradermal injection of a purified protein derivative (PPD) of the organism (Fig. 7.5). The response is of the type IV cell-mediated variety and results in a raised area of induration and reddening of the skin. In the **Mantoux test**, 0.1 ml of tuberculin solution is injected intradermally (not subcutaneously). The test is read at 48–72 hours: a positive result is indicated by redness and induration at least 10 mm in diameter. If active tuberculosis is suspected, the lowest dilution may be used initially to prevent a severe reaction, followed by higher concentrations if there is no reaction. The **Heaf test** is performed with a spring-loaded needled 'gun'. A drop of undiluted PPD (100 000 TU/ml) is placed on the volar surface of the forearm and the 'gun' is used to puncture through the PPD solution. The reaction is graded from I to IV according to the formation of papules and the extent of induration. A positive tuberculin test indicates the presence of hypersensitivity to tuberculin resulting from either previous infection with tubercle bacillus or bacillus Calmette–Guérin (BCG) vaccination. A weak reaction may be nonspecific and indicate contact with other nontuberculous environmental mycobacteria. A strongly positive test in a child who has not received BCG vaccination is likely to indicate primary infection. If there is evidence of active disease, full antituberculosis treatment is required; if there is no evidence of active disease, chemoprophylaxis is advisable. A source must be carefully sought amongst adult contacts of the child. A negative tuberculin test makes active tuberculosis unlikely and indicates a lack of immunity, so that BCG vaccination is recommended.

Interferon-gamma release assays

Tuberculin skin tests lack specificity in diagnosing *Mycobacterium tuberculosis* infection, because a positive reaction may be due to either previous BCG vaccination or exposure to nontuberculous mycobacteria. In recent years, laboratory assays

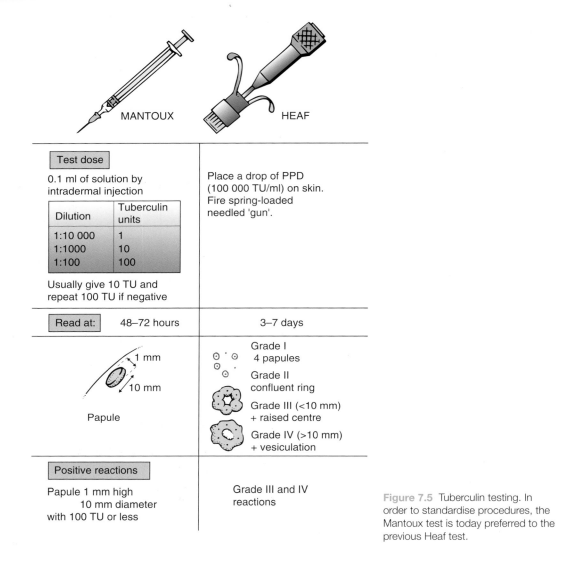

MANTOUX   **HEAF**

Test dose	
0.1 ml of solution by intradermal injection	Place a drop of PPD (100 000 TU/ml) on skin. Fire spring-loaded needled 'gun'.

Dilution	Tuberculin units
1:10 000	1
1:1000	10
1:100	100

Usually give 10 TU and repeat 100 TU if negative

Read at:	48–72 hours	3–7 days

1 mm

10 mm

Papule

Grade I
4 papules

Grade II
confluent ring

Grade III (<10 mm)
+ raised centre

Grade IV (>10 mm)
+ vesiculation

Positive reactions	
Papule 1 mm high 10 mm diameter with 100 TU or less	Grade III and IV reactions

Figure 7.5 Tuberculin testing. In order to standardise procedures, the Mantoux test is today preferred to the previous Heaf test.

have been developed that measure the release of IFN-γ from a patient's T-cells when exposed to specific antigens from *Mycobacterium tuberculosis*. There are currently two such assays available in the UK: the Quantiferon Gold assay (Cellestis Limited, Australia) and the T-spot TB assay (Oxford Immunotec, Oxford, UK). These tests require only a single blood test, but this must be analysed in the laboratory within a few hours. IFN-γ blood tests are most useful in the specific diagnosis of latent *Mycobacterium tuberculosis* infection and should not be used as a routine diagnostic tool for active tuberculosis.

Control

Treating active disease

Prompt **identification** and **treatment** of patients with active tuberculosis limits the spread of infection. Sputum-positive patients (AAFB-positive) should be considered potentially infectious until they have completed 2 weeks of treatment. Their families will already have been exposed to the risk of infection, so segregation of patients from contact with their families at the time of diagnosis is not useful, and most patients can be treated as outpatients. Where patients with suspected or confirmed tuberculosis are admitted to hospital, they should be kept in a single room. Particular care is required if a patient has multidrug-resistant tuberculosis; such patients should be treated in a negative-pressure ventilation room to prevent transmission of infection to other patients or healthcare workers.

Contact tracing

When a diagnosis of tuberculosis is made, there is a statutory requirement in the UK for the doctor to **notify** the patient to the public health authorities, who are then responsible for undertaking **screening of contacts**. The index patient may have acquired infection from, or transmitted infection to, someone in his or her close environment. It is usual to limit contact tracing to household contacts and close friends sharing a similar level of contact with the index patient. If initial investigations reveal a large number of contacts with tuberculosis, consideration should be given to widening the circle of investigation. Typically, about 1–3% of close contacts of smear-positive cases are found to have active disease, and many more have latent infection.

Screening of contacts consists of a combination of checking for symptoms of tuberculosis, **chest X-ray**, **tuberculin testing**, **IFN-γ tests** and assessment of **BCG status**. Most cases of active tuberculosis are found at the first clinic visit in unvaccinated close contacts of smear-positive disease. If a contact has not had **BCG vaccination**, a tuberculin test is performed, and if this is negative, vaccination is recommended. For children, a tuberculin test is the usual initial screening test. Children with a strongly positive tuberculin test should have a chest X-ray. A strongly positive tuberculin test with a normal chest X-ray suggests that the child has been infected with tubercle bacillus and has not developed active disease but remains at risk of doing so in the future. The risk of future activation of such latent infection is reduced by **chemoprophylaxis**, consisting of treatment for 6 months with isoniazid alone or for 3 months with isoniazid and rifampicin. There are many thousands of times fewer bacteria in latent tuberculosis than in active tuberculosis, and treatment with a single drug for 6 months or two drugs for 3 months is sufficient to kill dormant bacteria. Those with a negative tuberculin test should have it repeated 6 weeks later (to ensure they are not in the process of developing immunity to recently acquired infection); if they remain tuberculin-negative then BCG vaccination is advisable.

Screening of immigrants

Immigrants from areas with a high prevalence of tuberculosis (e.g. Africa, the Indian subcontinent) should be screened for tuberculosis on arrival in a country of low prevalence such as the UK. Adults should have a chest X-ray and children should have a tuberculin test. Thereafter, the procedure is the same as for close contacts, with treatment of active disease, chemoprophylaxis of latent infection or BCG vaccination as appropriate.

BCG vaccination

BCG is a live attenuated strain of tuberculosis that **provides about 75% protection against tuberculosis for about 15 years**. It is given by intradermal injection (not subcutaneous injection) and produces a local skin reaction. In the UK, BCG vaccination used to be offered to children at the age of 13 years. In 2005, this policy was changed from routine to **targeted vaccination**, so that BCG vaccination is now offered to infants in communities with a high incidence of tuberculosis (>40 per 100 000) and to unvaccinated individuals who come from, or whose parents come from, countries with a high prevalence of tuberculosis.

Nontuberculous mycobacteria (atypical opportunist mycobacteria)

There are a number of other mycobacteria that can cause pulmonary disease and that do not belong to the *Mycobacterium tuberculosis* complex, which are called 'atypical' or 'opportunist' mycobacteria. The most common are ***Mycobacterium kansasii***, ***Mycobacterium avium*** complex, ***Mycobacterium malmoense***, ***Mycobacterium xenopi***, ***Mycobacterium abscessus*** and ***Mycobacterium chelonae***. They are widespread in nature and can be found in water and soil, so that sometimes contamination of clinical specimens occurs via environmental sources. Atypical mycobacteria act as low-grade pathogens and do not usually pose a risk to normal individuals. Infections occur mainly in patients with impaired immunity (e.g. AIDS; see Chapter 6) or in those with damaged lungs (e.g. advanced emphysema, cystic fibrosis, bronchiectasis). They are often associated with chronic symptoms such as cough, sputum production, haemoptysis and weight loss. Diagnosis is made on the basis of their characteristics on laboratory culture tests. Treatment is often difficult, requiring a prolonged (e.g. 2 years) course of rifampicin and ethambutol, because these organisms often show resistance to some standard antituberculosis antibiotics. Some more recently developed antibiotics (e.g. clarithromycin or ciprofloxacin) may be useful in treatment. These organisms do not pose a threat to contacts of infected patients, so there is usually no need for contact-tracing procedures.

Recently, *Mycobacterium abscessus* infection has been emerging as a common infection in patients with cystic fibrosis, and transmission of infection can occur between these patients.

 KEY POINTS

- Worldwide, 2 billion people have latent infection with *Mycobacterium tuberculosis* and 8.6 million people have active tuberculosis.
- In the UK, the incidence of tuberculosis is highest in the Indian, Pakistani and African ethnic groups, in homeless people and in people with reduced immunity due to ageing, alcohol misuse, poor nutrition, immunosuppressive drug treatment or co-infection with HIV.
- Diagnosis depends on having a high level of awareness of the presentations of tuberculosis and undertaking appropriate investigations (e.g. sputum AAFB staining) to identify *Mycobacterium tuberculosis*.
- Treatment consists of 6 months of rifampicin and isoniazid, with pyrazinamide and ethambutol for the first 2 months.
- Control of tuberculosis involves the detection and meticulous treatment of cases of active tuberculosis, notification of the diagnosis to the public health authorities, contact tracing to detect active or latent infection in contacts of the index case and targeted vaccination of groups with a high incidence of tuberculosis.

 FURTHER READING

Anandaiah A, Dheda K, Keane J, et al. Novel developments in the epidemic of human immunodeficiency virus and tuberculosis coinfection. *Am J Resp Crit Care Med* 2011; **183**: 987–97.

American Thoracic Society/Centers for Disease Control and Prevention/Infectious Diseases Society of America. Controlling tuberculosis in the United States. *Am J Respir Crit Care Med* 2005; **172**: 1169–227.

British Thoracic Society. Recommendations for assessing risk and for managing *Mycobacterium tuberculosis* infection and disease in patients due to start anti-TNF-α treatment. *Thorax* 2005; **60**: 800–5.

British Thoracic Society. Management of opportunist mycobacterial infections: Joint Tuberculosis Committee guidelines. *Thorax* 2000; **55**: 210–18.

British Thoracic Society. Chemotherapy and management of tuberculosis in the United Kingdom. *Thorax* 1998; **53**: 536–48.

National Institute for Health and Care Excellence. *Clinical Guideline 33: Tuberculosis: Clinical Diagnosis and Management of Tuberculosis, and Measures for its Prevention and Control.* London: NICE, 2006 (http://www.nice.org.uk/guidance/CG33, last accessed 29 December 2014).

Panchal RK, Browne I, Monk P, et al. The effectiveness of primary care based risk stratification for targeted latent tuberculosis infection screening in recent immigrants to the UK: a retrospective cohort study. *Thorax* 2014; **69**: 354–62.

Public Health England. Tuberculosis in the UK: 2014 report. London: Public Health England, 2014 (https://www.gov.uk/government/uploads/system/uploads/attachment_data/file/360335/TB_Annual_report__4_0_300914.pdf, last accessed 29 December 2014).

Multiple choice questions

7.1 A 70-year-old man who lives in a hostel for homeless men and has a history of alcohol excess presents with a chronic cough. Chest X-ray shows diffuse consolidation in the left upper lobe, with cavitation. Tuberculosis is suspected but initial sputum AAFB stains are negative. The next definitive investigation to confirm the diagnosis is:
  A interferon gamma release assay
  B Mantoux test
  C Heaf test
  D bronchoscopy and bronchoalveolar lavage
  E gastric washings

7.2 At present, the number of new cases of tuberculosis in England and Wales each year is approximately:
  A 4000
  B 9000
  C 12 000
  D 20 000
  E 30 000

7.3 The main usefulness of interferon gamma release assays for tuberculosis is in:
  A detecting active tuberculosis
  B detecting latent tuberculosis
  C confirming immunity after BCG vaccination
  D detecting non-tuberculosis mycobaterial infection
  E monitoring a response to drug treatment

7.4 The lifetime risk of latent tuberculosis becoming active is approximately:
  A 1%
  B 10%
  C 40%
  D 60%
  E 90%

7.5 The most important adverse effect of ethambutol is:
  A renal toxicity
  B hepatitis
  C rashes
  D peripheral neuropathy
  E optic neuritis

7.6 A 65-year-old woman who has recently arrived in the UK from India presents with cough. Chest X-ray shows bilateral upper zone consolidation. Sputum AAFB stains are positive. Standard treatment consists of:
  A isoniazid, rifampicin, ethambutol and pyrazinamide for 6 months
  B isoniazid for 6 months
  C isoniazid and rifampicin for 3 months
  D isoniazid and rifampicin for 6 months with ethambutol and pyrazinamide for the initial 2 months
  E isoniazid and rifampicin for 9 months with ethambutol and pyrazinamide for the initial 2 months

7.7 The number of close contacts of a patient with smear-positive tuberculosis who have active disease is about:
  A 3%
  B 5%
  C 10%
  D 15%
  E 20%

7.8 At present, the number of isolates of *Mycobacterium tuberculosis* which show multidrug resistance in the UK is about:
  A 1–2%
  B 5%
  C 10%
  D 12%
  E 15%

7.9 The characteristic histopathology feature of tuberculosis on biopsy is:
  A cavitation
  B a Ghon focus
  C caseating granulomas
  D erythema nodosum
  E noncaseating granulomas

7.10 BCG vaccination is:
  A given to HIV infected patients who have a low CD4 lymphocyte count
  B no longer used because of its low efficacy
  C given to all infants at birth in the UK
  D a live attenuated strain of tuberculosis
  E given to patients once a diagnosis of tuberculosis has been established

Multiple choice answers

7.1 D

Obtaining bronchoalveolar lavage fluid will allow rapid diagnosis of active tuberculosis by AAFB staining, and culture will allow tests of sensitivity to drugs.

7.2 B

Notification rates for tuberculosis in England and Wales reached a low point of about 5000 per year in 1987, but then gradually rose and have now stabilised at about 9000 a year.

7.3 B

Interferon gamma release assays are useful in diagnosing latent tuberculosis but are not recommended as a routine test for active tuberculosis.

7.4 B

The term 'latent tuberculosis' refers to the situation where a person has been infected with tuberculosis at some time but does not currently have active disease. There is an approximately 10% risk of the tuberculosis becoming active at some stage. This risk may be reduced by prophy-lactic treatment with isoniazid and rifampicin for 3 months.

7.5 E

Because of the risk of optic neuritis, visual acuity should be tested before starting treatment with ethambutol and patients should be advised to report visual changes. The dose should be reduced in renal impairment (creatinine clearance <30 ml/minute).

7.6 D

Standard treatment consists of isoniazid and rifampicin for 6 months, with ethambutol and pyrazinamide for the initial 2 months.

7.7 A

When a diagnosis of tuberculosis is made, close contacts of the index case are screened. Typically, about 1–3% of close contacts of smear-positive cases are found to have active disease.

7.8 A

At present, in the UK, about 1.8% of isolates of *Mycobacterium tuberculosis* are resistant to both isoniazid and rifampicin, which is defined as multidrug resistance.

7.9 C

Biopsy of an affected site characteristically shows caseating granulomas (central cheesy necrosis of a lesion formed by macrophages, lymphocytes and epithelial cells).

7.10 D

BCG provides about 75% protection for about 15 years. The vaccination programme in the UK is now targeted at infants in communities with a high incidence of tuberculosis. BCG vaccination is contraindicated in HIV infection.

8

Bronchiectasis and lung abscess

Bronchiectasis

Bronchiectasis is a chronic disease characterised by irreversible **dilatation of bronchi** caused by bronchial wall damage resulting from infection and inflammation. These morphological changes are usually accompanied by chronic **suppurative lung disease** with cough productive of purulent sputum. There is now renewed interest in bronchiectasis, with more precise recognition of the disease by high-resolution computed tomography (CT) scanning. The spectrum of causes has changed over the years with the decline in childhood lung infections and tuberculosis, but bronchiectasis is still an important cause of chronic lung disease with significant morbidity and mortality.

Pathogenesis

Bronchiectasis represents a particular type of bronchial injury that may result from a number of different underlying disease processes. Damage to the bronchial wall causes disruption of the mucociliary escalator and allows bacteria to adhere to the respiratory epithelium and colonise the lung. **Adherence of bacteria** to the respiratory epithelium often involves specific interactions between adhesive structures on the bacterial membrane and receptors on the mucosal surface. After injury, the airway epithelium undergoes a process of repair that involves the spreading, migration and proliferation of epithelial cells. During this process, epithelial cells synthesise fibronectin, which is required for cell migration, and integrin, which is important for cell-to-cell adhesion.

These fibronectin and integrin epithelial receptors are used by the outer membrane protein of bacteria such as *Pseudomonas aeruginosa* as sites of bacterial adherence. Thus, key elements in the repair process of epithelium are also major receptors for bacterial adherence. The presence of bacteria at a normally sterile site stimulates an inflammatory response as part of the body's attempt to eradicate infection. However, in bronchiectasis, this inflammatory response is ineffective in eradicating infection and a persistent cycle of chronic infection and inflammation ensues, resulting in further tissue damage.

Bronchiectasis may be confined to one area of the lung if there is a **local** cause (e.g. bronchial obstruction by a foreign body) or may be **diffuse** if there is a generalised cause (e.g. immunoglobulin deficiency). The walls of the bronchi are infiltrated by inflammatory cells and are scarred and dilated with reduced elastin content. The exact mechanisms giving rise to bronchiectasis are not fully understood, but the disease may become self-perpetuating through a vicious circle of steps that can be initiated in a variety of ways (Fig. 8.1):

- **Impaired mucociliary clearance** leads to accumulation of secretions.
- Accumulated secretions predispose to bacterial **infection**.
- Infection provokes an **inflammatory response**, increased mucus production and impaired ciliary function.
- Excessive inflammation causes **tissue damage**.
- Damage to the bronchial wall produces **dilatation of bronchi** and disruption of mucociliary clearance, and the vicious circle of injury progresses.

Respiratory Medicine Lecture Notes, Ninth Edition. Stephen J. Bourke and Graham P. Burns.
© 2015 John Wiley & Sons, Ltd. Published 2015 by John Wiley & Sons, Ltd.
Companion Website: www.lecturenoteseries.com/Respiratory

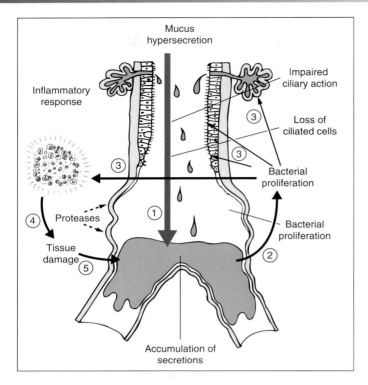

Mucus
hypersecretion

Inflammatory
response

Impaired
ciliary action

③

Loss of
ciliated cells

③

③

Bacterial
proliferation

④ Proteases

①

Bacterial
proliferation

Tissue
damage

②

⑤

Accumulation of
secretions

Figure 8.1 Bronchiectasis is often a progressive disease because bronchial damage results in impaired ciliary function with the accumulation of secretions, secondary bacterial infection, a destructive inflammatory response and further bronchial damage in a vicious self-perpetuating circle.

Aetiology

The aetiology of bronhiectasis is sketched in Table 8.1.

Infections

Severe infections are one of the most common causes of bronchial wall damage and bronchiectasis. In childhood, **pertussis (whooping cough)** and **measles** are important causes, although these are declining in frequency as a result of childhood vaccination programmes. In adults, bronchiectasis may complicate **pneumonia** resulting from virulent organisms such as *Streptococcus pneumoniae*, *Staphylococcus aureus* or *Klebsiella pneumoniae*. Better use of antibiotics has resulted in an overall decline in post-infective bronchiectasis. **Tuberculosis** is still a common cause of bronchiectasis in developing countries. Recurrent aspiration pneumonia may also lead to bronchiectasis. Many adults with **idiopathic** lower lobe bronchiectasis attribute their disease to childhood lung infections.

Bronchial obstruction

Bronchiectasis may develop in an area of lung obstructed by a bronchial **carcinoma**. In children, inhalation of a **foreign body** (e.g. peanut) may give rise to bronchial obstruction and distal bronchiectasis. **Lymph node enlargement** as part of tuberculosis may compress a bronchus and give rise to bronchiectasis. This particularly occurs in the middle lobe.

Immunodeficiency states

Patients with congenital **hypogammaglobulinaemia** or **selective immunoglobulin deficiencies** usually present with recurrent respiratory tract infections in childhood. Sometimes, the diagnosis is not established until adulthood, by when bronchiectasis may have developed. All patients with bronchiectasis should have measurement of immunoglobulins IgG, IgA and IgM with serum electrophoresis. Patients with immunoglobulin deficiencies require specialist immunology assessment with regard to intravenous immunoglobulin replacement therapy. Baseline specific antibody levels to tetanus toxoid and the capsular polysaccharides of *Streptococcus pneumoniae* and *Haemophilus influenzae* type b (Hib) should be measured. If baseline levels are low, the adequacy of the humoral response should be assessed by immunisation with appropriate vaccines and remeasurement of antibody levels after 21 days. Immunoglobulin deficiencies may also arise secondary to malignancies

---

Table 8.1 Aetiology of bronchiectasis

Severe infection

Childhood pertussis
Bacterial pneumonia
Recurrent aspiration pneumonia
Tuberculosis

Bronchial obstruction

Foreign body (e.g. peanut)
Bronchial carcinoma
Lymph node enlargement

Immunodeficient states

Hypogammaglobulinaemia
Immunodeficiency as a result of lymphoma
HIV infection

Allergic bronchopulmonary aspergillosis

Cystic fibrosis (see Chapter 9)

Ciliary dysfunction

Primary ciliary dyskinesia
Kartagener's syndrome

Associated diseases

Ulcerative colitis
Rheumatoid arthritis

Idiopathic bronchiectasis

---

such as **lymphoma** or **myeloma**. Patients with **human immunodeficiency virus (HIV) infection** are also susceptible to recurrent bacterial infections and bronchiectasis, and HIV testing should be offered when appropriate (see Chapter 6).

Allergic bronchopulmonary aspergillosis

Aspergillus fumigatus is a ubiquitous fungus that may **colonise** the respiratory tract as an incidental finding, without giving rise to symptoms (Fig. 8.2). Patients with lung cavities (e.g. post-tuberculosis or sarcoidosis) may develop an **aspergilloma**, which is a ball of fungal hyphae that appears on X-ray as a mass in the centre of a cavity, surrounded by a halo of radiolucency (Fig. 8.3). This is often asymptomatic, but associated inflammation may cause bronchial artery hypertrophy and haemoptysis, requiring surgical resection or therapeutic bronchial

artery embolisation. **Invasive aspergillosis** (e.g. necrotising pneumonia or fungaemia) occurs in immunocompromised patients.

Patients with **asthma** may develop an allergic reaction to *Aspergillus* and demonstrate **precipitating antibodies** to *Aspergillus* in their serum and positive responses to **skin prick tests**. Some of these patients develop **allergic bronchopulmonary aspergillosis**, in which there is intense bronchial inflammation with **eosinophilia** and **high IgE** levels in the blood. Eosinophilic infiltrates in the lung give rise to **fleeting X-ray shadows**. Thick **mucus plugs** cause obstruction of small bronchi and give rise to **bronchiectasis** that is usually proximal in location. All patients with bronchiectasis should have measurement of serum IgE, skin prick testing or specific serum IgE to *Aspergillus fumigatus* and aspergillus precipitins. Treatment requires suppression of the inflammatory immune response by oral prednisolone and high-dose inhaled corticosteroids.

Ciliary dyskinesia

The epithelial cells of the bronchi possess cilia that beat in an organised way so as to move particles in the layer of mucus on their surface upwards and out of the lung. This **mucociliary escalator** is an essential clearance mechanism. Ciliary function is impaired by cigarette smoke and bacterial toxins. Viral infections may cause widespread shedding of ciliated respiratory cells. Bronchial damage of whatever cause often disrupts the mucociliary clearance mechanism, impairing the lung defence mechanisms and perpetuating the vicious circle of bronchiectasis.

Primary ciliary dyskinesia is an autosomal recessive condition in which there is an abnormality of the ultrastructure of cilia throughout the body such that they do not beat in a coordinated fashion. Failure of ciliary function in the respiratory tract gives rise to otitis, sinusitis and bronchiectasis. The tail of sperm is also a ciliary structure and men with primary ciliary dyskinesia are usually infertile or subfertile. Women with impaired ciliary function in the fallopian tubes may have reduced fertility and a higher incidence of ectopic pregnancy, due to delayed transit of the ovum in the fallopian tube. It is thought that cilia are also responsible for the normal rotation of internal structures in embryonic life, so that failure of ciliary function results in random rotation, with about 50% of patients having dextrocardia and situs inversus (e.g. appendix in left iliac fossa). Ciliary dyskinesia with situs inversus is known as **Kartagener's syndrome** (Fig. 8.4).

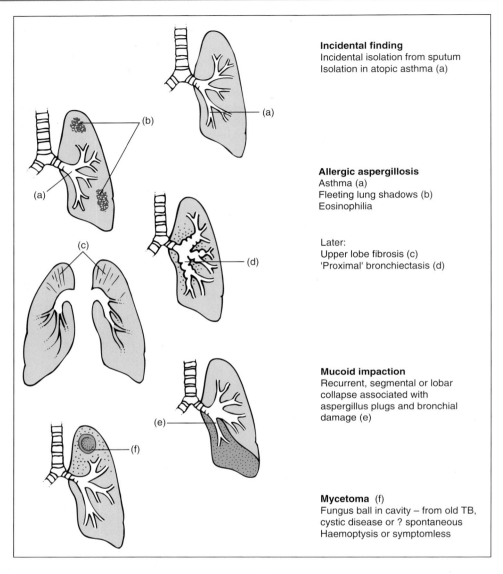

Incidental finding
Incidental isolation from sputum
Isolation in atopic asthma (a)

Allergic aspergillosis
Asthma (a)
Fleeting lung shadows (b)
Eosinophilia

Later:
Upper lobe fibrosis (c)
'Proximal' bronchiectasis (d)

Mucoid impaction
Recurrent, segmental or lobar
collapse associated with
aspergillus plugs and bronchial
damage (e)

Mycetoma (f)
Fungus ball in cavity – from old TB,
cystic disease or ? spontaneous
Haemoptysis or symptomless

Figure 8.2 Summary of the clinical spectrum of *Aspergillus* lung disease. TB, tuberculosis.

An estimate of ciliary function used to be obtained by timing the nasal clearance of saccharin. In this test, a 1 mm cube of saccharin is placed on the inferior turbinate of the nose and the time to the patient tasting the saccharin is recorded, providing a measure of nasal ciliary clearance. In healthy patients, this time is usually less than 30 minutes. However, this test is difficult to perform and a simple cold can disrupt mucociliary clearance for up to 6 weeks. Patients with primary ciliary dyskinesia characteristically have low exhaled nasal nitric oxide levels. In men, sperm motility may be assessed by microscopy of seminal fluid. However, definitive testing for primary ciliary dyskinesia requires referral to a designated specialist centre, where a brush biopsy of nasal mucosa is performed. The ultrastructure of cilia can then be assessed by electron microscopy and ciliary function can be assessed by microscope photometry, which assesses the ciliary beat frequency and pattern.

Cystic fibrosis

Cystic fibrosis usually presents in early childhood with recurrent respiratory infections and failure to

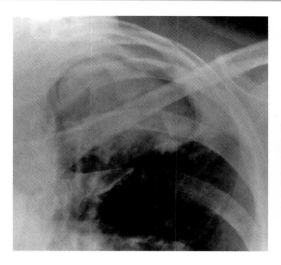

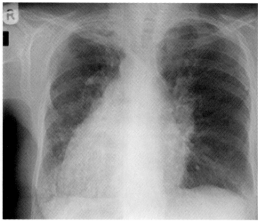

Figure 8.3 This 70-year-old woman had suffered from tuberculosis in the 1950s that had resulted in bilateral apical lung fibrosis and severely impaired lung function (forced expiratory volume in 1 second, 0.5 L; forced vital capacity, 1.1 L). She presented with recurrent major haemoptysis, and chest X-ray showed features characteristic of an aspergilloma with an opacity in the left apex surrounded by a halo of radiolucency. *Aspergillus* hyphae were seen on sputum microscopy and *Aspergillus* precipitins were present in her blood. Tests for carcinoma and tuberculosis were negative. Bronchial arteriography showed marked hypertrophy of the bronchial artery to the left upper lobe and therapeutic embolisation was performed resulting in resolution of the haemoptysis.

Figure 8.4 This 60-year-old woman has primary ciliary dyskinesia, which is an autosomal recessive disorder in which abnormalities of ciliary structure and function give rise to chronic upper and lower respiratory tract infections such as otitis, sinusitis and bronchiectasis. Cilia are also involved in the normal rotation of internal structures in embryonic life and failure of ciliary function results in random rotation such that 50% of these patients have dextrocardia and situs inversus (e.g. heart on the right side and appendix in the left iliac fossa).

thrive due to pancreatic insufficiency (see Chapter 9). It is now usually detected by newborn screening. However, more than 1900 mutations of the cystic fibrosis gene have been described and the clinical spectrum of the disease has been extended to include patients with less severe lung disease and normal pancreatic function. Some of these patients present with bronchiectasis in adulthood. As such, it is recommended that all children and adults up to the age of 40 years should have **sweat tests** and gene analysis for cystic fibrosis. The diagnosis of cystic fibrosis should also be considered in older patients with persistent isolation of *Staphylococcus aureus*, progressive bronchiectasis or associated features such as malabsorption, pancreatitis, nasal polyposis and male infertility.

Associated diseases

Patients with certain diseases, such as rheumatoid arthritis, ulcerative colitis, Crohn's disease and coeliac disease, seem to have an increased incidence of bronchiectasis. The mechanism by which bronchiectasis arises in these diseases is unclear.

Clinical features

The cardinal feature of bronchiectasis is **chronic cough** productive of copious **purulent sputum**. There is considerable variation in the severity of the disease and mild cases are often misdiagnosed as chronic bronchitis. Patients with more severe bronchiectasis are vulnerable to repeated exacerbations characterised by an increase in cough and purulent sputum, sometimes with **fever** and **pleuritic pain**. **Haemoptysis** is common and may occasionally be severe, requiring therapeutic embolisation of hypertrophied bronchial arteries to control the bleeding source. Severe bronchiectasis may cause chronic **malaise**, **fatigue**, **weight loss** and **halitosis** (foul breath). Coarse **crackles** may be audible over affected areas and **clubbing** is sometimes present. Key parameters in assessing the severity of the disease and the effects of treatment include the frequency of exacerbations, hospital admissions, health-related quality of life and mortality. A recent bronchiectasis severity index study showed a 10% mortality rate

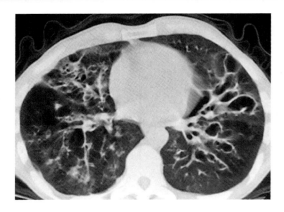

Figure 8.5 This 50-year-old man had suffered pertussis pneumonia at the age of 18 months. He had chronic cough productive of copious purulent sputum isolating *Pseudomonas aeruginosa* on culture. CT showed extensive bilateral bronchiectasis with dilatation of bronchi, cyst formation and patchy peribronchial consolidation. He was treated with postural drainage physiotherapy, salbutamol, long-term nebulised antibiotics (colistin) and intermittent courses of oral ciprofloxacin or intravenous ceftazidime.

over a 4 year period of follow-up. Mortality was significantly related to increasing age, frequent exacerbations, low forced expiratory volume in 1 second (FEV_1) and low body mass index (BMI).

Investigations

A **chest X-ray** may show features of bronchiectasis such as peribronchial thickening, which is evident as parallel tramline shadowing, or cystic dilated bronchi. However, the chest X-ray is often normal in less severe cases and high-resolution **CT** is the key investigation in confirming the diagnosis and in determining the location and extent of the disease (Fig. 8.5). The CT features of bronchiectasis are bronchial dilatation (internal bronchial lumen diameter greater than the accompanying pulmonary artery) and lack of the normal tapering of the bronchi peripherally. Diffuse bronchiectasis is seen in immune deficiency, ciliary dyskinesia and cystic fibrosis. Localised bronchiectasis may follow an episode of pneumonia.

Having confirmed the presence of bronchiectasis, an attempt should be made to diagnose the underlying cause, and further specific tests should be performed as indicated, such as *Aspergillus* **precipitins** and skin-prick tests (allergic bronchopulmonary aspergillosis), **immunoglobulin level** (hypogammaglobulinaemia), **ciliary function tests** (ciliary dyskinesia) and **sweat tests** with genetic

analysis for cystic fibrosis. **Bronchoscopy** is useful in detecting any endobronchial obstruction in cases of localised bronchiectasis. **Sputum microbiology** should be performed to define what infective organisms are present as a guide to antibiotic treatment. Mycobacterial cultures should also be performed, as nontuberculous mycobacteria (e.g. *Mycobacterium avium* complex, MAC) are sometimes associated with bronchiectasis (see Chapter 7). **Lung function tests** define the level of any deficit and help determine whether bronchodilator drugs might be helpful.

Treatment

- **Specific treatment** of the underlying cause is rarely possible, but relief of endobronchial obstruction (e.g. foreign body) is the key treatment for some patients, intravenous immunoglobulin replacement therapy is essential for patients with hypogammaglobulinaemia and suppression of the inflammatory response by oral or inhaled corticosteroids is important in allergic aspergillosis.
- **Chest physiotherapy** is an effective treatment in clearing secretions. Patients should receive instruction from a physiotherapist in airway clearance techniques, such as the active cycle of breathing technique, oscillating positive expiratory pressure devices (e.g. flutter, Acapella devices), autogenic drainage and postural drainage using gravity-assisted positions based on the location of the bronchiectasis on CT scans. Nebulised 7% **hypertonic saline** or **mannitol** as a dry-powder inhaler may be useful in improving sputum clearance. These mucolytic medications sometimes provoke bronchoconstriction, so that pretreatment with a bronchodilator (e.g. salbutamol, terbutaline) is needed. Oral carbocisteine is sometimes used as a **mucolytic agent**, but nebulised DNase, used in cystic fibrosis, is not effective in other forms of bronchiectasis.
- **Antibiotics** are used to suppress chronic infection and to treat exacerbations. High doses are sometimes required to penetrate the scarred bronchial mucosa and purulent secretions, and it is often recommended that treatment should be prolonged for 14 days. The choice of antibiotics is guided by the results of sputum microbiology. *Haemophilus influenzae* and *Streptococcus pneumoniae* are common and are usually sensitive to amoxicillin. Long-term oral antibiotics (e.g. amoxicillin, doxycycline) are sometimes used in severe disease, but there is a risk of promoting antibiotic resistance. *Moraxella catarrhalis* is usually associated with the production of β-lactamase, so that co-amoxiclav or ciprofloxacin may be useful. *Pseudomonas*

aeruginosa is common in severe disease and may be treated by oral ciprofloxacin or intravenous antipseudomonal antibiotics (e.g. meropenem, ceftazidime, tobramycin). Chronic pseudomonas infection is an adverse feature associated with more severe bronchiectasis. When this organism is first identified, an attempt should be made to eradicate it using oral ciprofloxacin 750 mg b.d. for 14 days. If this is not successful, options include a 4-week course of ciprofloxacin with nebulised colistin or a course of intravenous antipseudomonas antibiotics. If pseudomonas is isolated persistently, long-term nebulised antibiotics (e.g. colistin, tobramycin) may be used to suppress the infection and associated inflammation. Long-term treatment with a macrolide antibiotic (e.g. azithromycin) may reduce the frequency of exacerbations of bronchiectasis via an anti-inflammatory rather than an antimicrobial effect. Pneumococcal and influenza vaccinations are recommended for patients with bronchiectasis.

- **Bronchodilator drugs** (e.g. salbutamol, terbutaline) and **inhaled steroids** (e.g. beclometasone, budesonide, fluticasone) are indicated only where there is associated reversible airway obstruction.
- **Surgical excision** is a potential treatment for the few patients who have localised disease and troublesome symptoms. **Lung transplantation** is an option for some patients whose disease has progressed to respiratory failure.

Lung abscess

A lung abscess is a **localised collection of pus within a cavitated necrotic lesion in the lung parenchyma** (Fig. 8.6). The chest X-ray characteristically shows a cavitating lesion containing a fluid level. The patient typically complains of cough with expectoration of large amounts of foul material, often accompanied by haemoptysis, fever, weight loss and malaise. It is important to distinguish between a lung abscess and other causes of cavitating lung lesions, such as a squamous cell carcinoma, and bronchoscopy or percutaneous fine-needle aspiration of the lesion may be required.

The infection giving rise to a lung abscess may arise via a number of routes. Oropharyngeal **aspiration** is the most common cause and occurs in states of unconsciousness (e.g. alcohol excess, epilepsy, anaesthesia) and where there is dysphagia as a result of oesophageal or neuromuscular disease. Infection of the upper airways (e.g. sinusitis, dental abscess) may be an important source of bacteria, and anaerobic organisms (e.g. *Fusobacteria*, *Prevotella*) are common. Infection may arise distal to **bronchial obstruction** caused by a tumour or foreign body (e.g. inhaled peanut). The centre of an area of destructive **pneumonia** may break down to form a lung abscess, particularly when the pneumonia results from *Staphylococcus aureus* or *Klebsiella pneumoniae*. Tuberculosis may present as a lung abscess. **Blood-borne** infection may occur by intravenous injection of infected material by drug addicts. Pulmonary emboli may cause pulmonary infarction, with secondary infection giving rise to an abscess. Penetrating **chest trauma** is an unusual cause of lung abscess. **Trans-diaphragmatic** spread of infection may occur from a subphrenic abscess (e.g. post-cholecystectomy) or a hepatic abscess (e.g. amoebic abscess).

Drainage of pus from the abscess cavity is a key aspect of treatment. This can often be achieved by bronchial drainage using postural drainage physiotherapy. Sometimes, percutaneous drainage is achieved by positioning a catheter drainage tube under radiological guidance. Prolonged **antibiotic** therapy is given in accordance with the likely organism and the results of microbiology tests (e.g. metronidazole for anaerobic infections). **Surgical excision** of the abscess cavity is sometimes required where medical treatment fails.

Necrobacillosis

Necrobacillosis (Lemière's disease) is an unusual cause of lung abscess that is associated with a very characteristic clinical picture first described by Lemière. Typically, a young adult develops a **severe sore throat** with **cervical adenopathy** due to infection with the anaerobe *Fusobacterium necrophorum*. This is associated with a local venulitis, followed by a **septicaemic illness** with haematogenous spread of infection. The lungs are frequently involved, with multiple **abscesses** forming, often with a **pleural empyema** and evidence of infection elsewhere (e.g. **septic arthritis**, **osteomyelitis**). Prolonged anaerobic blood culture is required to identify the organism, which is sensitive to metronidazole.

Bronchopulmonary sequestration

Bronchopulmonary sequestration is a congenital anomaly in which an **area of lung is not connected to the bronchial tree** (i.e. it is 'sequestered') and has

Bronchial obstruction
Foreign body (e.g. peanut)
Tumour

Aspiration
Unconsciousness (e.g. alcohol)
Oropharyngeal sepsis
Oesophageal disease
Neuromuscular disease

Cavitating pneumonia
Staphylococcus aureus
Klebsiella pneumoniae
Streptococcus pneumoniae
Tuberculosis

**Bronchopulmonary
sequestration**

Blood-borne sepsis
IV drug misuse
Infected pulmonary infarct
Necrobacillosis

Transdiaphragmatic
Subphrenic abscess
Hepatic abscess

Trauma
Penetrating chest injury

Figure 8.6 Aetiology of lung abscess.

an **anomalous blood supply**, usually from the aorta. If infection develops in the sequestration, it often progresses to an abscess, because of lack of drainage to the bronchial tree. Surgical resection is required, but preoperative bronchial arteriography is necessary to identify the anomalous blood supply.

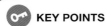

KEY POINTS

- Bronchiectasis is characterised by permanent dilatation of bronchi due to bronchial damage caused by infection and inflammation.
- High-resolution CT is the key investigation in confirming the diagnosis.
- Investigations for specific causes of bronchiectasis include sweat tests (cystic fibrosis), immunoglobulin levels (hypogammaglobulinaemia), *Aspergillus* preciptins (allergic aspergillosis) and ciliary tests (primary ciliary dyskinesia).
- Treatment involves chest physiotherapy, antibiotics, inhaled bronchodilators and specific treatment of any underlying cause.
- A lung abscess is a localised collection of pus within a cavitated necrotic lesion in the lung parenchyma.

FURTHER READING

Chalmers JD, Goeminne P, Aliberti S, et al. The bronchiectasis severity index: an international derivation and validation study. *Am J Respir Crit Care Med* 2014; **189**: 576–85.

DeBoeck K, Wilschanski M, Castellani C, et al. Cystic fibrosis: terminology and diagnostic algorithms. *Thorax* 2006; **61**: 627–35.

Hill AT, Welham S, Reid K, Bucknall CE. British Thoracic Society national bronchiectasis audit. *Thorax* 2012; **67**: 928–30.

Kellett F, Robert NM. Nebulised 7% hypertonic saline improves lung function and quality of life in bronchiectasis. *Respir Med* 2011; **105**: 1831–5.

Knowles MR, Daniels LA, Davis SD, et al. Primary ciliary dyskinesia: recent advances in diagnostics, genetics, and characterization of clinical disease. *Am J Respir Crit Care Med* 2013; **188**: 913–22.

McShane PJ, Naureckas ET, Tino G, Strek ME. Concise clinical review: non-cystic fibrosis bronchiectasis. *Am J Respir Crit Care Med* 2013; **188**: 647–56.

Murray MP, Pentland JL, Hill AT. A randomized crossover trial of chest physiotherapy in non-cystic fibrosis bronchiectasis. *Eur Respir J* 2009; **34**: 1086–92.

Pasteur MC, Bilton D, Hill AT on behalf of the British Thoracic Society Guideline for (non-CF) Bronchiectasis Group. British Thoracic Society guideline for non-CF bronchiectasis. *Thorax* 2010; **65**(Suppl. 1): 1–64.

Primary Ciliary Dyskinesia Family Support Group Web site (www.pcdsupport.org.uk, last accessed 29 December 2014).

Multiple choice questions

8.1 A 32-year-old man has diffuse bronchiectasis, *Pseudomonas aeruginosa* infection, nasal polyps and infertility due to obstructive azoospermia. The main diagnosis to consider is:

A HIV infection

B cystic fibrosis

C allergic bronchopulmonary aspergillosis

D hypogammaglobulinaemia

E primary ciliary dyskinesia

8.2 Allergic bronchopulmonary aspergillosis is characterised by:

A the halo sign on chest X-ray

B low IgG levels

C non-tuberculous mycobaterial infection

D reduced specific antibodies to polysaccahride antigens

E proximal bronchiectasis on CT scans

8.3 Definitive diagnosis of bronchiectasis is made by:

A high-resolution CT scanning

B sputum microbiology

C bronchoscopy

D clinical history

E lung function tests

8.4 In bronchiectasis due to previous pneumonia, sputum clearance is facilitated by:

A nebulised colistin

B oral ciprofloxacin

C nebulised hypertonic saline

D nebulised DNAse

E azithromycin

8.5 A 55-year-old woman has bilateral basal bronchiectasis that is thought to have arisen from childhood pneumonia. She has chronic lung infection with *Pseudomonas aeruginosa*. Her symptoms are troublesome, despite intermittent courses of antibiotics and regular chest clearance physiotherapy. The most appropriate additional treatment to recommend is:

A long-term oral doxycycline

B nebulised colistin or tobramycin

C intravenous immunoglobulin therapy

D long-term prednisolone

E surgery with resection of areas of bronchiectasis

8.6 A characteristic feature of a lung abscess on chest X-ray is:

A anomalous blood supply

B cavitation

C air bronchograms

D halo sign

E pleural effusion

8.7 A low exhaled nasal nitric oxide level is a characteristic feature of:

A allergic aspergillosis

B sinusitis

C primary ciliary dyskinesia

D hypogammaglobulinaemia

E HIV

8.8 A 40-year-old woman with asthma is found to have proximal bronchiectasis on CT scan. She has a high IgE level, eosinophilia and precipitating antibodies to aspergillus. The most likely diagnosis is:

A allergic bronchopulmonary aspergillosis

B ciliary dyskinesia

C mycetoma

D aspergillus colonization

E aspergilloma

8.9 Necrobacillosis is caused by:

A *Aspergillus fumigatus*

B *Mycobacterium tuberculosis*

C *Mycobacterium abscessus*

D *Klebsiella pneumoniae*

E *Fusobacterium necrophorum*

8.10 Dextrocardia is a feature associated with:

A cystic fibrosis

B hypogammaglobulinaemia

C allergic aspergillosis

D Kartagener's syndrome

E Lemiere's disease

Multiple choice answers

8.1 B

Bronchiectasis, pseudomonas infection, nasal polyps and infertility due to obstructive azoospermia (no sperm in ejaculate) are all characteristic features of cystic fibrosis. It is recommended that all children and adults up to the age of 40 years with bronchiectasis should have sweat tests and DNA analysis for cystic fibrosis. About 6–10% of patients with cystic fibrosis are diagnosed in adulthood.

8.2 E

Allergic bronchopulmonary aspergillosis is characterised by severe bronchial inflammation, with mucus plugging and bronchiectasis that is typically proximal in location. The halo sign is a feature of an aspergilloma (a fungal ball within a cavity), rather than allergic bronchopulmonary aspergillosis.

8.3 A

High-resolution CT scanning is the key investigation in diagnosing bronchiectasis. Chest X-ray is not sufficiently sensitive.

8.4 C

Nebulised hypertonic saline improves sputum clearance in patients with bronchiectasis. Nebulised DNase is a treatment for patients with cystic fibrosis but is not effective in other forms of bronchiectasis.

8.5 B

This patient has chronic *Pseudomonas aeruginosa* lung infection and is therefore likely to benefit from nebulised antipseudomonas antibiotics, such as colistin or tobramycin. Doxycycline is not effective against *Pseudomonas aeruginosa*.

8.6 B

A lung abscess is characterised on chest X-ray by a cavitating lesion, which often contains an air fluid level.

8.7 C

Definitive diagnosis of primary ciliary dyskinesia requires a brush biopsy of the nasal mucosa and electron microscopy to assess ciliary ultrastructure, with DNA testing for mutations. These patients characteristically have a low exhaled nasal nitric oxide level, and this can be used as a screening test.

8.8 A

Aspergillus is a ubiquitous fungus that can colonise the airways. It may also occur as a ball of fungus (aspergilloma) within a lung cavity. Allergic aspergillosis is characterised by an intensive IgE-mediated inflammatory response to aspergillus in patients with asthma, giving rise to mucus plugging, fleeting X-ray shadows and proximal bronchiectasis.

8.9 E

Necrobacillosis is caused by infection of the pharynx with *Fusobacterium necrophorum*, which causes local venulitis followed by a septicaemic illness with multiple lung abscesses, often with empyema and septic arthritis.

8.10 D

Cilia are responsible for the normal rotation of structures in embryonic life. Failure of ciliary function in primary ciliary dyskinesia results in random rotation, with about 50% of patients having dextrocardia and situs inversus. This is termed Kartagener's syndrome.

9

Cystic fibrosis

Introduction

Cystic fibrosis is the most common life-limiting inherited disease among white people. **It affects about 1 in 2500 live births** in the UK and is inherited in an autosomal recessive manner. About 10 000 people in the UK have cystic fibrosis and **1 in 25 of the population is a carrier** of the disease.

The basic defect

Cystic fibrosis is caused by mutations of a large gene on the long arm of chromosome 7 that codes for a 1480-amino-acid protein, named **cystic fibrosis transmembrane conductance regulator (CFTR)**. The most common mutation, in which deletion of three base pairs of the gene results in the loss of phenylalanine ('delta F') at position 508 of the protein, is traditionally designated ΔF508 (F508del). This causes misfolding of the mutant CFTR, which is then degraded in the endoplasmic reticulum such that no CFTR protein reaches the cell membrane. CFTR functions as a cyclic adenosine monophosphate (cAMP)-dependent **chloride channel** in the apical membrane of epithelial cells, and the primary physiological defect in cystic fibrosis is reduced chloride conductance at epithelial membranes, most notably in the respiratory, gastrointestinal, pancreatic, hepatobiliary and reproductive tracts. Other ion channels, such as epithelial sodium channels (ENaCs) and calcium-activated chloride channels (CaCCs), also play an important role in membrane physiology (Fig. 9.1). Although CFTR's main function is as a chloride channel, it has other regulatory roles too, including inhibition of sodium transport through ENaCs, inhibition of CaCCs, regulation of intracellular vesicle transport and regulation of bicarbonate–chloride exchange. In sweat ducts, failure of reabsorption of chloride ions results in elevated concentrations of chloride and sodium in the sweat, a characteristic feature of the disease and the basis for the sweat test used in diagnosis.

The traditional treatments of cystic fibrosis have focused on managing the consequences of the disease, such as lung infection, inflammation and thick mucus secretions. However, there is now a new era in treatment with the development of **small-molecule drugs**, which can overcome the effects of certain mutations (e.g. **ivacaftor** for the G551D mutation) and the potential for **gene therapy** to correct the overall genetic defect.

More than 1900 mutations of the CFTR gene have now been identified, which are divided into five major classes according to their effect on CFTR function:

- Class I defects (e.g. G542X) account for about 10% of mutations and disrupt synthesis of CFTR. These include nonsense and frame-shift mutations that lead to premature termination codons (PTCs) with a lack of protein production.
- Class II defects (e.g. ΔF508) account for about 70% of mutations and result in misfolded CFTR, which is then degraded in the endoplasmic reticulum such that no functioning CFTR reaches the cell membrane.
- Class III defects (e.g. G551D) result in CFTR that reaches the apical cell membrane but is not activated. About 5% of patients have a G551D mutation. Ivacaftor is a small-molecule drug that potentiates CFTR function in the apical membrane in the G551D mutation by increasing the amount of time the chloride channel remains open. It was introduced to clinical practice in 2013 as a tablet treatment and it dramatically improves clinical disease, typically reducing sweat chloride levels by about 50 mmol/l, with a 10% improvement in forced expiratory volume in 1 second (FEV_1) and weight gain.

Respiratory Medicine Lecture Notes, Ninth Edition. Stephen J. Bourke and Graham P. Burns.
© 2015 John Wiley & Sons, Ltd. Published 2015 by John Wiley & Sons, Ltd.
Companion Website: www.lecturenoteseries.com/Respiratory

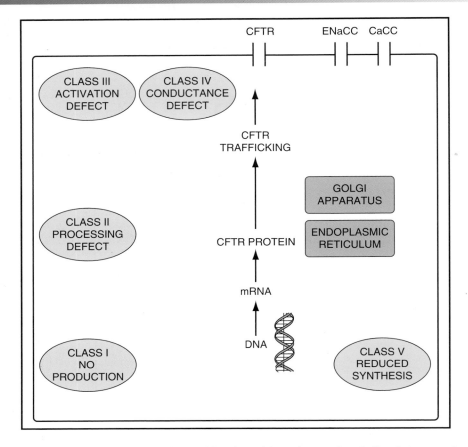

Figure 9.1 The cystic fibrosis gene codes for a 1480-amino-acid protein named cystic fibrosis transmembrane conductance regulator (CFTR) that is trafficked through the cell via the endoplasmic reticulum and Golgi apparatus and inserted into the apical membrane, where it functions as a cAMP-dependent chloride channel. Class I mutations disrupt synthesis of CFTR. These include nonsense and frameshift mutations, which lead to premature termination codons (PTCs) and lack of protein production. Class II mutations result in misfolded CFTR, whcih is then degraded in the endoplasmic reticulum. In class III mutations, CFTR reaches the apical membrane but is not activated. Class IV mutations result in reduced CFTR conductance. In class V mutations, there is reduced synthesis of normal CFTR and therefore reduced CFTR function at the cell membrane. CFTR has additional regulatory effects on epithelial sodium channels (ENaCs) and on calcium-activated chloride channels (CaCCs). Small-molecule therapies are now becoming available, which overcome some of the molecular defects. Ivacaftor is a potentiator that improves CFTR function at the cell surface in patients with class III mutations (e.g. G551D). Lumacaftor is a corrector that improves the trafficking of mutant CFTR through the cell in patients with the ΔF508 mutation. Ataluren allows ribosomes to read through PTCs in some class I mutations.

- Class IV defects (e.g. R117H) result in impaired chloride conductance.
- Class V defects (e.g. A455E) result in reduced amounts of functioning CFTR.

Generally, mutations in classes I–III result in no CFTR function at the cell membrane. This is typically associated with more severe clinical disease. In class IV and V mutations, the mutant CFTR may have some degree of function, which may be associated with less severe clinical disease. However, many other factors influence the clinical phenotype.

Lungs

In the bronchial mucosa, reduced chloride secretion and increased sodium reabsorption result in **secretions of abnormal viscosity**, with reduced water content of the airway surface liquid and reduced depth of the periciliary fluid, which disrupts mucociliary clearance. The **high salt content** of the airway surface fluid **inactivates defensins**, which are naturally occurring antimicrobial peptides on the epithelial surface. There is some evidence that the CFTR also plays a role in the normal uptake and processing of *Pseudomonas aeruginosa* from the respiratory tract. Patients with cystic fibrosis also have abnormal mucus glycoproteins, which act as binding sites such that **bacteria adhere to the mucosa** and proliferate. Thus, the gene defect results in dysfunction of CFTR and predisposes to severe chronic lung infection by a variety of mechanisms at the cellular level. The inflammatory response is unable to clear the infection and a vicious cycle of **infection** and **inflammation** develops, progressing to lung damage, **bronchiectasis**, **respiratory failure** and **death**.

Gastrointestinal tract

In the **pancreas**, the abnormal ion transport results in the plugging and obstruction of ductules, with progressive destruction of the gland. The pancreatic enzymes (e.g. lipase) fail to reach the small intestine and this results in **malabsorption** of fats, with steatorrhoea and failure to gain weight. Progressive destruction of the endocrine pancreas may cause **diabetes**. Abnormalities of bile secretion and absorption cause an increased incidence of **gallstones** and **biliary cirrhosis**. Sludging and desiccation of intestinal contents probably account for the occurrence of **meconium ileus** (neonatal intestinal obstruction) in about 10% of babies with cystic fibrosis and for the development of **distal intestinal obstruction syndrome** (meconium ileus equivalent) in older children and adults.

Clinical features

Fig. 9.2 summarises the clinical features of cystic fibrosis.

Infants and young children

About 10% of children with cystic fibrosis present at birth with **meconium ileus**, a form of intestinal obstruction caused by inspissated viscid faecal material resulting from lack of pancreatic enzymes and from reduced intestinal water secretion. More than half of children affected by cystic fibrosis have obvious malabsorption by the age of 6 months, with **failure to thrive** associated with abdominal distension and copious offensive stools from **steatorrhoea** as a result of malabsorbed fat. **Rectal prolapse** occasionally occurs. Recurrent **respiratory infections** rapidly become a prominent feature, with cough, sputum production and wheeze. Newborn screening programmes are now established and allow the early diagnosis of cystic fibrosis, before the onset of symptoms and complications.

Older children and adults

Respiratory disease

Persistent cough and purulent sputum characterise the development of **bronchiectasis**. Progressive lung damage is associated with the development of digital clubbing and progressive **airway obstruction**, sometimes associated with wheeze. Serial measurements of FEV_1 give an indication of the severity and progression of the disease. Some patients show a significant asthmatic component, with reversible airway obstruction, and some develop colonisation of the bronchi by *Aspergillus fumigatus* and may show features of allergic bronchopulmonary aspergillosis (see Chapter 8). Initially, the typical organisms isolated in sputum cultures are **Staphylococcus aureus**, *Haemophilus influenzae* and *Streptococcus pneumoniae*. By the teenage years, many have become infected with mucoid strains of **Pseudomonas aeruginosa** (Fig. 9.3). There are many different strains of *Pseudomonas aeruginosa*, some of which have increased virulence and are transmissible from patient to patient.

Burkholderia cepacia complex is a group of Gram-negative plant pathogens that cause onion rot. It was initially thought that these organisms were not pathogenic to humans, but in the 1980s it became apparent that patients with cystic fibrosis were vulnerable to them and that infection could spread from patient to patient in an epidemic way, particularly among children in close social contact, such as in holiday camps. The clinical course of patients with *Burkholderia cepacia* complex infection is very variable, but some show an accelerated rate of decline in lung function and some develop a fulminant necrotising pneumonia, the so-called **cepacia syndrome** (Fig 9.4). It is now recognised that there are many different strains of this bacterium, but *Burkholderia cenocepacia* genomovar III is associated with the worst prognosis. *Burkholderia multivorans* is the most common strain and has a high level of resistance to antibiotics. Because of the potential for transmission of infection between patients with cystic fibrosis, it is now standard practice to segregate

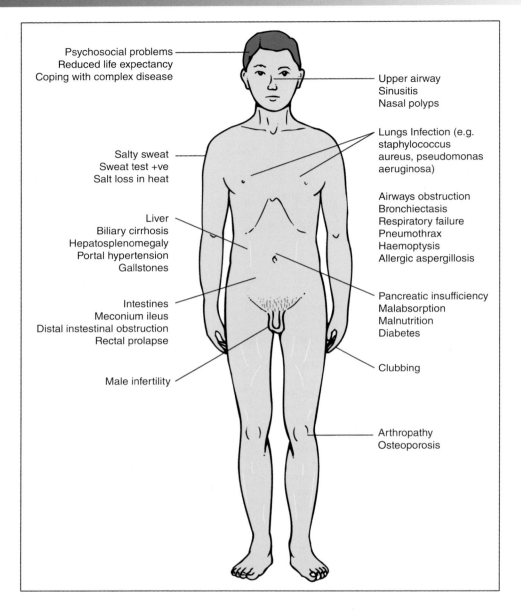

Psychosocial problems
Reduced life expectancy
Coping with complex disease

Upper airway
Sinusitis
Nasal polyps

Salty sweat
Sweat test +ve
Salt loss in heat

Lungs Infection (e.g.
staphylococcus
aureus, pseudomonas
aeruginosa)

Airways obstruction
Bronchiectasis
Respiratory failure
Pneumothrax
Haemoptysis
Allergic aspergillosis

Liver
Biliary cirrhosis
Hepatosplenomegaly
Portal hypertension
Gallstones

Intestines
Meconium ileus
Distal instestinal obstruction
Rectal prolapse

Pancreatic insufficiency
Malabsorption
Malnutrition
Diabetes

Clubbing

Male infertility

Arthropathy
Osteoporosis

Figure 9.2 Clinical features of cystic fibrosis. Cystic fibrosis is a multisystem disease resulting from mutations of the gene that codes for CFTR, which functions as a chloride channel on epithelial membranes. Failure of chloride conductance results in abnormal secretions and organ damage in the respiratory, pancreatic, hepatobiliary, gastrointestinal and reproductive tracts.

patients with different infections such that they attend different clinics and wards, and social contact between patients with cystic fibrosis is discouraged. Nontuberculous mycobacteria (e.g. *Mycobacterium abscessus*) can also colonise and infect the lungs in cystic fibrosis. It is particularly difficult to treat and can also spread between patients.

As the cycle of infection and inflammation progresses, lung damage worsens with deteriorating airway obstruction, destruction of lung parenchyma, impairment of gas exchange and the development of **hypoxaemia**, **hypercapnia** and **cor pulmonale**. The persistent pulmonary inflammation provokes hypertrophy of the bronchial arteries and **haemoptysis**

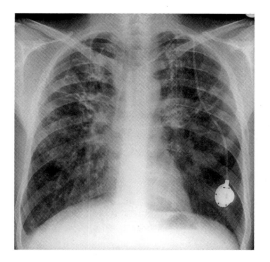

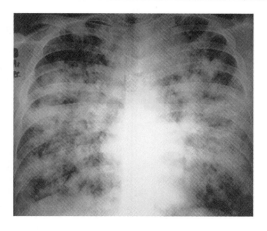

Figure 9.3 Chest X-ray of this 37-year-old man with cystic fibrosis shows hyperinflation, peribronchial thickening, cystic bronchiectasis and perihilar fibrosis. A Portacath central venous system is in place, with the access port situated subcutaneously in the left lower chest. He had chronic *Pseudomonas aeruginosa* infection and received about three courses of intravenous ceftazidime and tobramycin at home each year. His FEV$_1$ was 1.5 l (42% of predicted) and his general condition and lung function had remained stable over 5 years on treatment including long-term nebulised colistin, nebulised dornase alpha (DNase), physiotherapy and nutritional supplements.

Figure 9.4 Chest X-ray of this 23-year-old man with cystic fibrosis shows the typical appearance of 'cepacia syndrome' with fulminant bilateral necrotising pneumonia. He had acquired *Burkholderia cenocepacia* infection 7 years previously during an outbreak of infection among patients with cystic fibrosis attending a holiday camp. His lung function showed an accelerated rate of decline in the years after infection and he then developed a severe exacerbation that failed to respond to treatment and progressed to a fatal fulminant pneumonia over a 2-week period. Patients with cystic fibrosis are advised not to have contact with one other in order to avoid transmission of infections.

becomes common. Occasionally, when severe bleeding occurs, therapeutic embolisation of the bronchial arteries may be required. **Pneumothorax** occurs in about 5–10% of patients with advanced disease and may require prompt tube drainage. Pleurodesis may be required for recurrent pneumothoraces, but this should be performed with care so as not to compromise future potential lung transplantation.

Gastrointestinal disease

About 85% of patients with cystic fibrosis have **pancreatic insufficiency** with **malabsorption of fat** because of lack of lipase. Unless these patients receive adequate pancreatic enzyme supplements, they develop steatorrhoea with frequent bulky offensive stools and failure to gain weight. Progressive destruction of the endocrine pancreas is manifested by an increasing incidence of **diabetes** as these patients get older. A variety of **hepatobiliary abnormalities** occur, including fatty liver, gallstones and focal biliary fibrosis, and about 5% of patients develop

multinodular cirrhosis with hepatosplenomegaly, portal hypertension, oesophageal varices and liver failure. **Distal intestinal obstruction syndrome** (meconium ileus equivalent) (Fig. 9.5) results from inspissated fatty semisolid faecal material obstructing the terminal ileum. A number of factors contribute to the development of this complication, including malabsorption of fat, disordered intestinal motility and dehydrated intestinal contents resulting from defective intestinal chloride transport. The clinical features vary depending on the severity of the obstruction. Typically, the patient suffers recurrent episodes of colicky abdominal pain and constipation, and there is often a palpable mass in the right iliac fossa. In severe cases, complete intestinal obstruction may develop with abdominal distension, vomiting and multiple fluid levels in distended small bowel on an erect X-ray of abdomen. It is treated by a balanced intestinal lavage solution (e.g. Klean-Prep), which is taken orally or by nasogastric tube. The radiocontrast Gastrografin (sodium diatrizoate) may also be used as it has detergent properties that allow it to penetrate the inspissated fatty material and its hypertonicity then draws fluid into the faecal bolus.

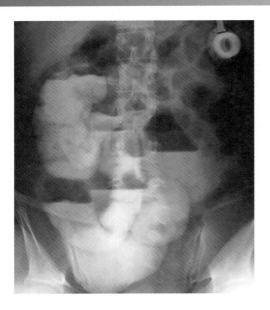

Figure 9.5 This 31-year-old woman with cystic fibrosis was admitted to hospital complaining of abdominal distension, colicky pain and constipation. A mass of inspissated faecal material was palpable in the right iliac fossa. Erect abdominal X-ray (after taking Gastrografin) shows distended loops of small bowel, containing multiple fluid levels. A diagnosis of meconium ileus equivalent (distal intestinal obstruction syndrome) was made and she was treated with Gastrografin (orally and by enema), N-acetylcysteine (orally) and intravenous fluids, followed by flushing of the bowel using balanced intestinal lavage solution.

Other measures include rehydration, stool softeners (e.g. lactulose) and N-acetylcysteine, which probably acts by cleaving disulphide bonds in the mucoprotein faecal bolus. Prevention of recurrence requires adequate pancreatic enzyme supplements, avoidance of dehydration and, sometimes, use of laxatives.

Other complications

Nearly all **male patients are infertile** because of congenital bilateral absence of the vas deferens. The exact mechanism by which this complication occurs is not known, but it has been suggested that it may result from resorption of the vas deferens after it has become plugged with viscid secretions in foetal life. Techniques such as microsurgical sperm aspiration from the epididymis or testes, with in vitro fertilisation by intracytoplasmic sperm injection, can facilitate parenthood for men. Women have near normal fertility, although some abnormalities of cervical

mucus are present. **Pregnancy** places additional burdens on the mother's health and is sometimes associated with deterioration in the disease due to increased nutritional stress and impaired bronchial clearance. However, with the improving prognosis, many women with cystic fibrosis are now successfully undertaking pregnancy. It is important for the mother to maintain all aspects of her own treatment as she focuses on the care of the baby.

Upper airway involvement causes troublesome **sinusitis** and **nasal polyps**. Cystic fibrosis **arthropathy** probably results from the deposition in joints of antigen–antibody complexes produced by the immune response to bacterial lung infections. Vasculitic **rashes** may also occur. In hot weather, patients with cystic fibrosis are at risk of developing **heat prostration** as a result of excess loss of salt in sweat.

As cystic fibrosis patients are now living longer, a number of other complications are being described, including **osteoporosis** and **amyloidosis**. Patients with cystic fibrosis face major **social and emotional stresses** relating to their reduced life expectancy, outlook for employment, ability to form relationships and undertake marriage and general capacity to cope with a complex disease and its treatment.

Diagnosis

The diagnosis of cystic fibrosis is based upon the demonstration of **elevated sweat chloride** concentrations on a sweat test, in association with **characteristic clinical features** such as recurrent respiratory infections and evidence of pancreatic insufficiency. The diagnosis is usually confirmed by the demonstration of **two known cystic fibrosis mutations** (e.g. ΔF508/G542X) on DNA analysis. It is possible to detect abnormal chloride conductance directly by measuring the potential difference of the nasal mucosa, although this is a specialist research technique.

Sweat testing

In cystic fibrosis, the ion-transport defect results in a failure to reabsorb chloride ions from the sweat, so that elevated sweat chloride and sodium concentrations are a characteristic feature of the disease. Sweating is induced by **pilocarpine iontophoresis** and the sweat is collected and analysed for sodium and chloride. Pilocarpine is placed on the skin of the forearm and a small electrical current is passed across it to enhance its penetration of the skin and stimulation of the sweat ducts. Meticulous technique is required to avoid evaporation of secretions or contamination. A sweat flow rate of at least 100 µl/min is required for accurate analysis and sweat chloride levels above 60 mmol/l on repeated tests are highly suggestive of cystic fibrosis. Sweat chloride values of 30–60 mmol/l are considered intermediate and may be associated with atypical cystic fibrosis, while levels below 30 mmol/l make a diagnosis of cystic fibrosis unlikely.

DNA analysis

The discovery of the cystic fibrosis gene in 1989 led to the development of **genotyping as an aid to diagnosis**. Genotyping can also be used to detect **carrier status** and can be applied to chorionic villus biopsy material for **antenatal diagnosis**. However, there are more than 1900 mutations of the cystic fibrosis gene currently identified and routine analysis assesses only the most common mutations, so that it can be difficult to exclude cystic fibrosis resulting from rare mutations. Some variants in the cystic fibrosis gene may not be disease-causing. DNA analysis has established the diagnosis in some individuals with only mild clinical features, and this has extended our knowledge of the clinical spectrum of the disease to include some rare older, less severely affected patients. Affected individuals have two gene mutations, one inherited from each of their parents. Carriers of the disease have only one abnormal gene and do not show any evidence of the disease.

Atypical cystic fibrosis

As more mutations of the CFTR gene are identified, the clinical spectrum of the disease has been extended to include **atypical** or **nonclassic** cystic fibrosis. The vast majority of patients with two mutations of the CFTR gene develop **classic cystic fibrosis**, characterised by the development of pancreatic malabsorption and recurrent respiratory infections in early childhood, with progressive severe lung disease over the years. About 5–10% of patients have a **late diagnosis** of cystic fibrosis in later childhood or adulthood, having been misdiagnosed as having other diseases, such as asthma, bronchitis or bronchiectasis. Sometimes, these patients have had less severe lung disease and may have had normal pancreatic function. It is recommended that all children and adults up to the age of 40 years presenting with bronchiectasis have sweat tests and CFTR gene analysis. The diagnosis of cystic fibrosis should also be considered in older patients with bronchiectasis who have persistent *Pseudomonas aeruginosa* or

Staphylococcal aureus infections, progressive disease or additional features such as malabsorption, pancreatitis, nasal polyps or male infertility. Although diagnosed late, these patients have classic cystic fibrosis and have often already developed severe lung disease by the time of diagnosis, with the risk of progressive disease over time. In contrast, a small number of patients are now being identified who have truly atypical or nonclassic disease associated with CFTR gene dysfunction. Sometimes, these patients present with isolated manifestations such as **male infertility** due to congenital bilateral absence of the vas deferens, **nasal polyps**, recurrent **pancreatitis**, **sclerosing cholangitis**, neonatal hypertrypsinogenaemia or excessive **skin wrinkling** in water. These patients often have intermediate sweat chloride levels of 30–59 mmol/l and, rare, class IV or V mutations with some residual CFTR function, which may protect them from more severe lung disease. These patients need careful assessment and follow-up in specialist cystic fibrosis centres.

Newborn screening

Early diagnosis of cystic fibrosis allows specific treatment to be commenced rapidly, and this is associated with an improved prognosis. Infants with cystic fibrosis have elevated serum **immunoreactive trypsin activity**. This can be measured on a single dried blood spot obtained on a Guthrie card as part of the newborn screening programme for diseases such as phenylketonuria and hypothyroidism.

Treatment

Cystic fibrosis is a complex multisystem disease and skills from several disciplines are needed in treating it. The optimal use of currently available treatments and the introduction of new treatments are best achieved by concentrating the care of cystic fibrosis patients in regional **specialist centres** with comprehensive multidisciplinary teams. The basic elements of treatment comprise clearance of bronchial secretions by **physiotherapy**, treatment of pulmonary infection by **antibiotics** and correction of nutritional deficits by the use of **pancreatic enzyme supplements** and **dietary support**. Patients and their families require continuous encouragement and support in coping with this complex disease. The Cystic Fibrosis Trust in the UK and the Cystic Fibrosis Foundation in the United States act as a focus of **information and support** and coordinate fund raising for research.

Chest physiotherapy

The viscid purulent sputum results in airway obstruction, and clearance of airway secretions by chest physiotherapy is important at all stages of the disease. A variety of techniques can be used, including **postural drainage** (using gravity-assisted positions to aid drainage), chest **percussion** and **positive-expiratory-pressure devices** to aid dislodgement and expectoration of sputum from the peripheral airways. As patients mature, it is important that they learn to perform bronchial clearance themselves. The 'active cycle of breathing' technique is often effective and popular with adult patients. This involves a **cycle of breathing control**, thoracic expansion exercises and the **forced expiratory technique** ('huffing'), which releases secretions from peripheral bronchi. Some patients benefit from using oscillating positive-expiratory-pressure devices (e.g. flutter, Acapella devices). Exercise is an excellent adjunct to physiotherapy but should not replace it.

Antibiotics

Children with cystic fibrosis should be **immunised** against pertussis and measles as part of the childhood vaccination programme, and should receive annual influenza vaccination thereafter. They should avoid contact with people with respiratory infections and avoid inhalation of cigarette smoke. A variety of antibiotic strategies are used. *Staphylococcus aureus* is a major pathogen in the disease from early childhood, and long-term continuous **flucloxacillin** is often used to suppress this infection. Further oral antibiotics are given during exacerbations, in accordance with sputum cultures and sensitivity testing. Common pathogens include *Haemophilus influenzae* and *Streptococcus pneumoniae*, which are usually sensitive to **amoxicillin**.

Infection with *Pseudomonas aeruginosa* becomes an increasing problem as children get older, and an important strategy in antibiotic therapy is to postpone for as long as possible the colonisation of the airways by this organism. Frequent sputum cultures are performed and intensive antipseudomonal antibiotic therapy is given when the organism is first isolated. This often comprises an **initial prolonged course of oral ciprofloxacin** and **nebulised colistin or tobramycin**. If this does not eradicate infection then **intravenous antipseudomonal antibiotics** are recommended. Eventually, chronic infection with *Pseudomonas aeruginosa* becomes established. Attempts at suppressing the effects of this infection involve long-term use of **nebulised antibiotics** such as colistin, tobramycin or aztreonam. Colistin and tobramycin are now also available in inhaler form, which may be more convenient for patients to take. Additional courses of intravenous antipseudomonal antibiotics can be given during infective exacerbations or when there is a decline in lung function. Usually, an aminoglycoside (e.g. gentamicin, tobramycin) is given in combination with a third-generation cephalosporin (e.g. ceftazidime) or a modified penicillin (e.g. piperacillin). Treatment is usually given for 14 days and high doses are required to achieve adequate penetration of antibiotics into scarred bronchial mucosa, because patients with cystic fibrosis have increased renal clearance of antibiotics.

Intravenous antibiotic treatment is often given **at home** by the patient after training. Where venous access is difficult, a totally implanted central venous device can be inserted (e.g. Portacath). This comprises a central venous cannula connected to a subcutaneous port that is accessed by inserting a special non-cutting needle through the skin and the diaphragm of the subcutaneous chamber.

Burkholderia cepacia complex organisms are usually resistant to many of the commonly used antipseudomonal antibiotics, such as colistin, ciprofloxacin and aminoglycosides, but are often sensitive to ceftazidime or meropenem.

Bronchodilator medication

Some patients with cystic fibrosis have a reversible component to their airway obstruction and benefit from bronchodilator drugs (e.g. salbutamol, terbutaline) and inhaled steroids (e.g. beclometasone, budesonide, fluticasone).

Mucolytic medication

The sputum of patients with cystic fibrosis contains high levels of DNA, which is derived from the nuclei of decaying neutrophils. This makes the sputum very viscid and difficult to expectorate. Recombinant human **deoxyribonuclease** (**Dnase**/dornase alfa) is a genetically engineered enzyme that cleaves DNA. This treatment is administered by nebulisation and improves the lung function and reduces the number of exacerbations in some patients. Nebulised **7% hypertonic saline** improves mucociliary clearance by drawing water into the dehydrated periciliary layer. It sometimes provokes bronchoconstriction, such that pretreatment with a bronchodilator (e.g. salbutamol, terbutaline) is needed. **Mannitol**, administered via a dry-powder inhaler, is an osmotic agent that also increases the water content of the airway surface liquid with improved mucociliary clearance.

Anti-inflammatory medication

The inflammatory response is unable to eradicate infection and contributes to the progressive lung damage. Corticosteroid drugs (e.g. **prednisolone**) may have a beneficial effect but their use is limited by adverse effects. High-dose **ibuprofen** may also be useful in reducing lung injury, by inhibiting the migration and activation of neutrophils. **Macrolide antibiotics** (e.g. azithromycin) have been shown to improve lung function in patients with cystic fibrosis. This seems to be due to an anti-inflammatory effect via suppression of inflammatory cytokines, reducing neutrophil function and impairing biofilm formation around *Pseudomonas aeruginosa*.

Nutrition

Pancreatic enzyme supplements (e.g. Creon, Pancrease, Nutrizym) are taken with each meal and with snacks containing fat. Enteric-coated preparations protect the lipase from inactivation by gastric acid, and use of antacid medication (e.g. omeprazole, lansoprazole) may improve effectiveness. The dose of enzyme is adjusted according to the dietary intake in order to optimise weight gain and growth and control steatorrhoea. Use of high doses of pancreatic enzymes has been associated with the development of strictures of the ascending colon – so-called 'fibrosing colonopathy' – in a small number of children, so that it is recommended that the dose of lipase should not exceed 10 000 U/kg/day. Supplements of **fat-soluble vitamins** (A, D, E) are routinely given.

Patients with cystic fibrosis suffer from nutritional deficiencies as a result of malabsorption and the increased energy requirements resulting from increased energy expenditure due to chronic lung infection. Most patients with cystic fibrosis require 120–150% of the recommended daily calorie intake for individuals without cystic fibrosis, so that healthy eating for a patient with cystic fibrosis includes **high-energy foods** and frequent snacks between main meals. **Dietary supplements** (e.g. Fortisip, Scandishake) are useful when factors such as anorexia limit intake. In advanced disease, **nocturnal enteral feeding** of high-energy formulas, via nasogastric tube or gastrostomy, may be required.

Advanced disease

The clinical course of cystic fibrosis is very variable, but an FEV_1 of less than 30% of the predicted value, for example, is associated with a 50% 2-year mortality rate. An awareness of the stage of the disease and the likely prognosis assists in planned management.

Oxygen saturation should be measured by oximetry at each clinic visit in patients with advanced disease, and when hypoxaemia develops, domiciliary **oxygen** may alleviate the complications of respiratory failure. **Lung transplantation** is the main option to consider for patients with advanced disease, but there is a lack of donor organs and about 30% of patients on a transplant waiting list die before donor lungs become available (see Chapter 19). Each year, about 110 patients die from cystic firbosis in the UK and about 440 in the United States. The median age at death is 28 years (range 5–72 years). Death in childhood is now rare. It is important that patients receive high-quality **palliative care**, which often runs concurrently with active treatment of their disease, particularly in those on a transplant waiting list. Death is usually peaceful after a short coma and results from ventilatory failure.

Prognosis

The prognosis of patients with cystic fibrosis has improved dramatically over the years. In the 1950s, survival beyond 10 years was unusual. Now the median survival is about 44 years, and it is predicted to be at least 50 years for children now being born with the disease. There are about 10 000 patients with cystic fibrosis in the UK today, and more than 50% are adults (aged 16 or over). Patients entering adulthood with cystic fibrosis face a number of problems, particularly relating to their chronic lung disease and reduced life expectancy (e.g. life insurance, choice of career, relationships, marriage, pregnancy, fertility). The improved survival of patients with cystic fibrosis has been attributed to a combination of factors, including improved management of meconium ileus in neonates, earlier diagnosis, better dietary management, better pancreatic enzyme supplementation and meticulous attention to physiotherapy and antibiotic treatments in specialist centres. Although cystic fibrosis typically produces severe progressive lung disease, there is a wide **clinical spectrum of severity**. Some 'milder mutations' are associated with residual chloride conductance and less severe clinical disease, but there is generally a poor correlation between specific gene mutations and clinical manifestations. Environmental factors, therapeutic regimens and additional 'modifier genes' that influence cytokine responses, for example, are important. Some patients are well and lead relatively normal lives long into adulthood, and there is a need to adapt treatment to the stage and severity of the disease. With improved survival, treatments need to be planned with care over decades so as to avoid adverse effects (e.g. aminoglycoside nephrotoxicity, antibiotic allergy and resistance) and prevent long-term complications of the disease (e.g. osteoporosis, diabetic complications)

Prospective treatments

Ongoing refinements of conventional care in specialist centres continue to improve survival rates. New formulations of **inhaled antibiotics** (e.g. inhaled ciprofloxacin, nebulised aztreonam) may help control of airway infection. The identification of the cystic fibrosis gene in 1989 revolutionised our understanding of the detailed molecular biology of this disease and offers the prospect of developing treatments directed against the basic underlying defects. Perhaps the most exciting approach is the direct replacement of the defective gene by **gene therapy**. The cystic fibrosis gene has been cloned and given to patients in experimental trials using liposomes or inactivated viruses as gene-transfer agents to introduce it into epithelial cells. Expression of the gene can be detected by measuring transepithelial potential differences. Gene transfer and expression have been achieved and clinical trials are now underway to establish the clinical effectiveness and role of gene therapy.

Substantial progress is being made in **pharmacological treatments** that address the molecular biology processes of CFTR transcription from DNA, trafficking through the cell and activation and regulation at the apical membrane. **Ivacaftor** is the first of a group of drugs known as **small-molecule therapies**; it is a CFTR **potentiator** that improves CFTR function in the cell membrane in patients with the **class III mutation, G551D**. It was introduced to clinical practice in 2013 as a tablet treatment and it dramatically improves clinical disease, typically reducing sweat chloride levels by about 50 mmol/l, with a 10% improvement in FEV_1 and weight gain. **Lumacaftor** is a CFTR **corrector** that improves the trafficking of mutant CFTR through the cell and increases the quantity of CFTR expressed at the cell surface. A combination of lumacaftor and ivacaftor has been shown to improve CFTR function in patients with the main $\Delta F508$ mutation, and clinical trials are in progress. **Ataluren** is a small-molecule drug that induces ribosomes to read through PTCs during mRNA translation in patients with class I mutations (e.g. G542X, W1282X). Recent clinical trials have shown a small clinical improvement in some patients receiving ataluren, although this did not reach statistical significance. A further approach is to attempt to correct the ion-channel defect by **stimulating alternative chloride channels** (e.g. CaCCs) or **inhibiting sodium channels** (e.g. ENaCs). Amiloride and benzamil inhibit ENaC but have not yet shown clinical benefit. Attempts at modifying the inflammatory response involve the assessment of the role of some currently available (e.g. ibuprofen, azithromycin) and some novel (e.g. glutathione, anti-elastases, lipoxins) **anti-inflammatory agents**. Improvements in the field of **lung transplantation** (e.g. extending the donor pool by use of reconditioned lungs) offer the best hope for patients in the advanced stages of the disease. Advances in many different areas of scientific research are being brought into clinical practice in order to improve the outlook for patients with cystic fibrosis.

 KEY POINTS

- Cystic fibrosis is a multisystem disease resulting from mutations of a gene that codes for a chloride channel on epithelial membranes.
- In the lungs, viscid secretions predispose to infection and inflammation with progressive bronchiectasis.
- *Staphylococcus aureus*, *Pseudomonas aeruginosa* and *Burkholderia cepacia* complex are the main pathogens.
- Antibiotics, chest physiotherapy, nutritional support and anti-inflammatory drugs are key elements in treatment.
- Lung transplantation is the main option to consider for patients with advanced lung disease.

 FURTHER READING

Alton EWF, Boyd AC, Cheng SH, et al. A randomized, double-blind, placebo-controlled phase IIB clinical trial of repeated application of gene therapy in patients with cystic fibrosis. *Thorax* 2013; **68**: 1075–7.

Boeck K, Wilschanski M, Castellani C, et al. Cystic fibrosis: terminology and diagnostic algorithms. *Thorax* 2006; **61**: 627–35.

Bott J, Blumenthal S, Buxton M, et al. Guidelines for the physiotherapy management of the adult, medical, spontaneously breathing patient. *Thorax* 2009; **64**(Suppl. 1): 1–51.

Bourke SJ, Doe SJ, Gascoigne AD, et al. An integrated model of provision of palliative care to patients with cystic fibrosis. *Palliative Medicine* 2009; **23**: 512–17.

Bryant JM, Grogono DM, Greaves D, et al. Whole-genome sequencing to identify transmission of *Mycobacterium abscessus* between patients with cystic fibrosis: a retrospective cohort study. *Lancet* 2013; **381**: 1551–60.

Cystic Fibrosis Foundation (USA) Web site (www.cff.org, last accessed 29 December 2014).

Cystic Fibrosis Trust (UK). UK Cystic Fibrosis Registry annual data report 2012. (http://cysticfibrosis.org.uk/about-cf/publications/cf-registry-reports, last accessed 29 December 2014).

Davis PB. Cystic fibrosis since 1938. *Am J Respir Crit Care Med* 2006; **173**: 475–82.

Dodge JA, Lewis PA, Stanton M, et al. Cystic fibrosis mortality and survival in the UK: 1947–2003. *Eur Respir J* 2007; **29**: 522–6.

Flume PA, O'Sullivan BP, Robinson KA, et al. Cystic fibrosis pulmonary guidelines. *Am J Resp Crit Care Med* 2007; **176**: 957–69.

Hoffman LR, Ramsey BW. Cystic fibrosis therapeutics: the road ahead. *Chest* 2013; **143**: 207–13.

Lane MA, Doe SJ. A new era in the treatment of cystic fibrosis. *Clin Med* 2014; **14**: 76–8.

Ramsey BW, Davies J, McElvaney NG, et al. A CFTR potentiator in patients with cystic fibrosis and the G551D mutation. *N Engl J Med* 2011; **365**: 1663–72.

Multiple choice questions

9.1 **A newborn baby is diagnosed as having cystic fibrosis. His parents ask about the risk of future children of theirs having cystic fibrosis. Their risk is approximately:**
  A 10%
  B 25%
  C 50%
  D 75%
  E 90%

9.2 **The most common bacterium causing lung infection in an adult with cystic fibrosis is:**
  A *Burkhoderia cepacia* complex
  B Meticillin-resistant *Staphylococcus aureus*
  C *Pseudomonas aeruginosa*
  D *Achromobacter xylosoxidans*
  E *Mycobacterium abscessus*

9.3 **A 16-year-old boy with cystic fibrosis and chronic *Pseudomonas aeruginosa* infection attends the clinic because of an increase in his cough and sputum. There is a mild reduction in his FEV_1. He is undertaking exams. It is decided that he should have a course of tablet antibiotics at home. The most appropriate choice is:**
  A co-amoxiclav
  B colistin
  C ciprofloxacin
  D tobramycin
  E amoxicillin

9.4 **Men with cystic fibrosis usually:**
  A have normal fertility
  B are infertile due to absence of the vas deferens
  C are infertile because of failure to produce sperm in the testes
  D have reduced fertility due to ciliary dysfunction
  E have reduced fertility because of testosterone deficiency

9.5 **In a child with cystic fibrosis, diarrhoea and failure to thrive typically occur because of:**
  A diabetes
  B antibiotic-associated diarrhoea
  C liver disease
  D pancreatic dysfunction
  E deficiency of vitamins A, D and E

9.6 **Ivacaftor is a small-molecule therapy that improves the function of CFTR in patients with:**
  A G551D mutation
  B ΔF508 (F508del) mutation
  C premature termination codons
  D all CFTR mutations
  E class I mutations

9.7 **Lumacaftor is a small-molecule therapy that acts by:**
  A allowing read-through of premature termination codons
  B improving CFTR function at the cell membrane
  C replacing the mutated gene
  D improving trafficking of the mutant CFTR through the cell
  E improving the function of the epithelial sodium channel (ENaC)

9.8 **Nebulised DNase (dornase alpha) is:**
  A a form of gene-replacement therapy
  B a small-molecule therapy
  C an inhaled antibiotic
  D a mucolytic
  E a potentiator of CFTR

9.9 **At present, the median age of survival for patients with cystic fibrosis in the UK is:**
  A 16 years
  B 20 years
  C 28 years
  D 35 years
  E 44 years

9.10 **A sweat chloride of 70 mmol/l means that a patient is:**
  A unlikely to have cystic fibrosis
  B likely to have cystic fibrosis
  C likely to have nonclassic (atypical) cystic fibrosis
  D likely to have a class III mutation (e.g. G551D)
  E likely to have cystic fibrosis with normal pancreatic function

Multiple choice answers

9.1 B

Cystic fibrosis is an autosomal recessive disease. The baby with cystic fibrosis has two mutations of the cystic fibrosis gene, having inherited one abnormal gene from each of his parents. Each of his parents is thus a carrier of cystic fibrosis. The risk of a child of carrier parents having the disease is 1 : 4 (25%).

9.2 C

Patients with cystic fibrosis are particularly vulnerable to *Pseudomonas aeruginosa* infection, which is the most common infection in adults.

9.3 C

The only oral antibiotic with activity against *Pseudomonas aeruginosa* is ciprofloxacin. Co-amoxiclav and amoxicillin are not active against it. Colistin and tobramycin can be given intravenously or by nebulisation, but are not available in an oral formulation.

9.4 B

Nearly all men with cystic fibrosis are infertile because of congenital bilateral absence of the vas deferens, resulting in azoospermia (no sperm in the ejaculate). However, normal sperm are usually produced by the testes, such that these men can achieve biological fatherhood by assisted reproduction techniques involving aspiration of sperm from the testes and in vitro fertilisation. Women with cystic fibrosis have essentially normal fertility.

9.5 D

Approximately 85% of children with cystic fibrosis have pancreatic insufficiency such that there is a lack of pancreatic enzymes, resulting in malabsorption of fat, which causes diarrhoea and failure to thrive.

9.6 A

G551D is a class III mutation in which the CFTR protein reaches the apical cell membrane but is not activated. Ivacaftor is a small-molecule treatment that enhances CFTR function in this mutation by increasing the amount of time for which the chloride channel remains open.

9.7 D

Lumacaftor is a small-molecule therapy that acts as a 'corrector', allowing mutant CFTR to traffic through the cell. In the ΔF508 mutation, the mutant CFTR fails to fold correctly and is destroyed in the endoplasmic reticulum. Lumacaftor shows some effect in overcoming this trafficking defect.

9.8 D

The sputum of patients with cystic fibrosis contains high levels of DNA, derived from decaying neutrophils. DNase cleaves DNA and reduces the viscosity of the sputum.

9.9 E

The median age of survival for patients with cystic fibrosis is constantly improving. It is currently 44 years.

9.10 B

Sweat chloride levels >60 mmol/l are highly suggestive of cystic fibrosis. Levels <30 mmol/l make a diagnosis of cystic fibrosis unlikely. Levels between 30 and 60 mmol/l are intermediate and may be associated with non-classic (atypical) cystic fibrosis.

10

Asthma

Definition

Asthma is a disease characterised by **airway inflammation** with **increased airway responsiveness**, resulting in **airway obstruction**. The cardinal feature of the airway obstruction in asthma is **variability**. This can occur spontaneously over short periods of time or in response to treatment; in the latter case, it is referred to as **reversibility**. Patients experience **symptoms** such as wheeze, cough and dyspnoea.

Asthma is not a static uniform disease state but rather a **dynamic and heterogeneous clinical syndrome** that has a number of **different patterns** and may progress through different stages, so that not all features are necessarily present in a particular patient at a particular point in time. For example, many patients with well-controlled asthma are asymptomatic, with apparently normal lung function, between attacks (although more detailed investigation may well reveal evidence of airway inflammation and increased airway responsiveness). By contrast, in some patients with chronic asthma, the disease may have progressed to a state of irreversible airway obstruction.

Some patients with smoking-related chronic obstructive pulmonary disease (COPD), bronchiectasis or cystic fibrosis may demonstrate airway obstruction with some degree of reversibility, but it is important to appreciate that these diseases are different from asthma, with distinct aetiologies, pathologies, natural histories and responses to treatment.

Prevalence

Asthma has been recognised since ancient times, and it is now estimated that 235 million people worldwide have the disease. The reported prevalence of asthma greatly depends on the criteria used to define it and is confused by changes in diagnostic habit (**labeling shift**). Patients now diagnosed as having asthma might, in the past, have been labelled as having 'wheezy bronchitis', for example, particularly in the case of children. Notwithstanding issues of labelling, there is a general consensus, based on studies using objective measurement, that the **prevalence of asthma increased greatly over the latter half of the 20th century**. In the developed world at least, prevalence is thought to have plateaued since the turn of the millennium. Nevertheless, the UK still has some of the highest rates in Europe, and 5.4 million are currently in receipt of treatment for asthma. There is considerable interest in the reasons for the increased prevalence over time, but no firm consensus on the environmental factors that underlie it.

Aetiology

Asthma is multifactorial in origin, arising from a complex interaction of **genetic** and **environmental** factors. It seems likely that airway inflammation occurs when genetically susceptible individuals are exposed to certain environmental factors, but the exact processes underlying asthma may vary from patient to patient. In many cases, the most important environmental factors are probably the intensity, timing and mode of exposure to **aeroallergens** that stimulate the production of IgE. However, it is often not possible in an individual case to identify a specific allergen that can be regarded as the 'cause' of the asthma, let alone one for which exposure avoidance would bring about resolution or even an improvement of symptoms.

Genetic susceptibility

There is strong evidence of a hereditary contribution to the aetiology of asthma. It has long been known

Respiratory Medicine Lecture Notes, Ninth Edition. Stephen J. Bourke and Graham P. Burns.
© 2015 John Wiley & Sons, Ltd. Published 2015 by John Wiley & Sons, Ltd.
Companion Website: www.lecturenoteseries.com/Respiratory

that asthma and atopy run in **families**. First-degree relatives of asthmatics have a significantly higher prevalence of asthma than relatives of nonasthmatic patients. It is important to appreciate, however, that families share environments as well as sharing genes, and that environmental factors are necessary for the expression of a genetic predisposition. **Atopy** is a constitutional tendency to produce significant amounts of IgE on exposure to small amounts of common antigens. Atopic individuals demonstrate positive reactions to antigens on skin-prick tests and have a high prevalence of asthma, allergic rhinitis, urticaria and eczema. Several potential gene linkages to asthma and atopy (e.g. chromosome 11q13 location) have been suggested, but it is clear that the genetic contribution to asthma is complex, possibly involving **polygenic inheritance** (several genes contributing to the asthmatic tendency in an individual) and **genetic heterogeneity** (different combinations of genes causing the asthmatic tendency in different individuals). The ADAM33 gene on chromosome 20p13, which is a disintegrin and metalloprotease gene, has been identified as being involved in the structural airway components of asthma, such as airway remodelling, which relates to the development of chronic persistent asthma with irreversible (fixed) airway obstruction and excess decline in forced expiratory volume in 1 second (FEV1) over time.

Environmental factors

The importance of environmental factors in the aetiology of asthma has been particularly evident in studies of populations that have **migrated from one country to another**. For example, children from the Pacific atoll of Tokelau were found develop asthma with similar prevalence to native New Zealand children when they were evacuated to New Zealand following a typhoon that devastated the local economy, whereas children remaining in Tokelau had a significantly lesser prevalence. Similarly, movement of people from East to West Germany in the 1990s was associated with an increased incidence of asthma and atopy. There may be very many aspects of the environment that are important, but a change to a **modern, urban, economically developed society seems to be particularly associated with the occurrence of asthma**.

Indoor environment

People spend at least 75% of their time indoors, and overall exposure to air pollutants and allergens is determined more by concentrations indoors than outdoors. The indoor environment is particularly important in the case of young children, because allergen exposure early in life may be especially important in determining sensitisation. **House dust mites** (*Dermatophagoides pteronyssinus*) are found in high concentrations in carpets, soft furnishings and bedding. Exposure to high levels in early life is associated with an increased likelihood of sensitisation to them by 3–7 years of age. In the Manchester Asthma and Allergy Study, intense environmental manipulation commenced in the pre-natal period, early in pregnancy, and focused mainly on house dust mite avoidance. It showed some reduction in respiratory symptoms in the first year of life. However, there was subsequently a paradoxical effect of increased allergy but better lung function. **Pet-derived allergens** are widespread in homes where dogs, cats or budgerigars are kept. Epidemiological studies suggest that close contact with a cat or dog in early life may reduce subsequent prevalence of asthma and allergy, perhaps via the provocation of immune tolerance. In general, studies on domestic allergen avoidance are inconsistent and there is no clear strategy that can be recommended. Passive exposure to **cigarette smoke** in the home has an adverse effect on asthma and other respiratory diseases in children in particular.

Outdoor environment

Although there is a widespread view among the general public that the increasing prevalence of asthma is attributable to atmospheric pollution from motor vehicles, the balance of evidence suggests that any such influence on the *initiation* of asthma is small. Nevertheless, interactions between atmospheric pollutants, aeroallergens and climatic conditions play an important, although complex and incompletely understood, part in *triggering exacerbations* of pre-existing asthma. **Climatic conditions** such as high pressure and humidity with calm still air can result in an accumulation of airborne pollutants (e.g. particulates, ozone) and of allergens (e.g. pollens, fungal spores). Several epidemics of acute asthma have been associated with thunderstorms, which have particularly affected patients with pre-existing atopic asthma. Warm dry weather may cause a rapid rise in pollen concentrations and in levels of ozone (O_3), nitrogen dioxide and sulphur dioxide, due to atmospheric stability; gusts of wind at the start of a thunderstorm lift allergens into the air, while rain disrupts pollen grains into a number of smaller allergenic particles. Under these circumstances, atopic individuals with pre-existing asthma or hay fever are particularly vulnerable to the resultant allergen challenge.

Occupational environment

Many agents encountered in the workplace may induce **occupational asthma** (e.g. isocyanates, epoxy resins, persulphates, hard wood dusts; see Chapter 14).

Pathogenesis and pathology

A series of factors combine to produce increasing airway inflammation and airway responsiveness, and when these features reach a sufficient level, bronchoconstriction and asthma symptoms are triggered. In a sensitised atopic asthmatic, the inhalation of an allergen typically results in a two-phase response, consisting of an **early asthmatic reaction**, reaching its maximum at about 20 minutes, and a **late asthmatic reaction**, developing about 6–12 hours later. These atopic asthmatics have high levels of specific IgE, which binds to receptors on inflammatory cells, most notably mast cells. Interaction of the IgE antibody and inhaled antigen results in the activation of these inflammatory cells and release of preformed mediators, such as histamine, prostaglandins and leukotrienes, which cause contraction of the smooth muscle of the airways, producing bronchoconstriction. The inflammatory response in asthma is highly complex, involving the full **spectrum of inflammatory cells**, including mast cells, eosinophils, B- and T-lymphocytes and neutrophils, which release an **array of mediators and cytokines**. These mediators regulate the response of other inflammatory cells and have a number of effects resulting in **contraction of airway smooth muscle, increased vascular permeability** leading to increased airway wall oedema and stimulation of airway **mucus secretion**.

T-helper lymphocytes play an important role in the regulation of the inflammatory response. These cells may be divided into two main subsets on the basis of the profile of cytokines that they produce. **Th2 cells** produce proinflammatory interleukins and **upregulate** the specific form of airway inflammation of asthma by enhancing IgE synthesis and eosinophil and mast-cell function. In contrast, **Th1 cells** produce cytokines that **downregulate the atopic response**. In those who are genetically susceptible to developing asthma, antigen presentation to T-helper cells leads to a Th2 response. Infection with respiratory syncytial virus augments a Th2 response, whereas some other microbial antigens lead to a Th1 response.

It has been suggested that exposure to allergens and infections in early childhood is important in determining the pattern of immune response that modulates the genetic susceptibility to developing asthma. In affluent countries, declining family size, improved household amenities and higher standards of cleanliness seem to be associated with an increased incidence of asthma. The **hygiene hypothesis** suggests that allergic diseases may be prevented by certain infections in early childhood. Thus, for example, children with older siblings are more likely to be exposed to childhood infections and have a lower incidence of asthma.

The wall of the airway in asthma is thickened by oedema, cellular infiltration, increased smooth-muscle mass and glands (Fig. 10.1). With increasing severity and chronicity of the disease, **remodelling of the airway** occurs, leading to fibrosis of the airway wall, fixed narrowing of the airway and a reduced response to bronchodilator medication.

Mucus plugging of the lumen of the airway is a prominent feature of acute severe asthma. Although, in clinical practice, patients with asthma are sometimes classified as having atopic asthma (occurring in relation to inhalation of environmental antigens in a susceptible person) or non-atopic asthma (occurring without any definable relationship to an environmental antigen), the pathological features of the airway inflammation are identical. It is likely that the inflammatory cascade of asthma can be initiated by a variety of different factors in different patients.

Clinical features

The typical symptoms of asthma are **wheeze, dyspnoea, cough** and a sensation of 'chest tightness'. These symptoms can first occur at any age and may be episodic or persistent. In mild asthma, the patient may be asymptomatic between episodes but experience symptoms of asthma during viral respiratory tract infections or after exposure to certain allergens or other triggers. Sometimes, the clinical pattern is of more persistent symptoms, with chronic wheeze and dyspnoea. The variable nature of symptoms is a characteristic feature of asthma. Typically, there is a diurnal pattern, with symptoms and peak expiratory flow (PEF) measurements being worse early in the morning: so-called **morning dips**. Symptoms such as cough and wheeze may wake a patient from sleep in the early hours. A history of **nocturnal wakening** should be sought to support a new diagnosis of asthma. In an asthma review, the symptom may not be

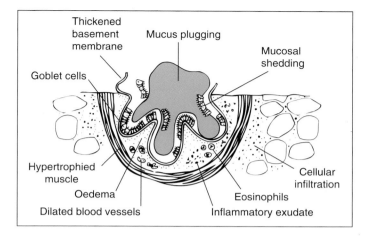

Figure 10.1 The pathogenesis and pathology of asthma. Asthma is characterised by a complex pattern of airway inflammation as a result of an interaction of genetic and environmental factors. Eosinophils, mast cells, neutrophils and B- and T-cells are all involved in the cellular infiltration. Mediators and cytokines regulate the inflammatory response and result in contraction of airway smooth muscle, increased permeability of blood vessels and mucus secretion. In chronic asthma, airway remodelling results in structural changes and fixed airway obstruction.

volunteered by a patient; it needs to be asked about, as it is a strong indicator of poor asthma control.

In some, asthmatic symptoms can be provoked by exercise (**exercise-induced asthma**). This is different from normal exertional dyspnoea; it is the excess ventilation associated with exercise leading to measurable bronchoconstriction. Cough can sometimes be the predominant or only symptom, and the lack of wheeze or dyspnoea may lead to a delay in making the diagnosis: so-called **cough-variant asthma**. Work in recent years has identified a condition termed **eosinophilic bronchitis**. This is also a condition of airway inflammation, although the presence and activation of inflammatory cells is limited to the superficial layers of the airway walls, rather than penetrating further to involve the airway smooth muscle. It usually presents as a chronic cough, perhaps displaying an asthmatic type of diurnal variability, although lung function is essentially normal. This feature may be the semantic divide that separates it from asthma, although clearly the two conditions are very closely related. As with asthma, inhaled corticosteroids are often a very effective treatment.

When assessing a patient presenting with breathlessness, many of these clinical features can be vital clues to the diagnosis of asthma. A careful clinical history is therefore often the principal tool in diagnosis and should include the following:

- **Family history.** There is a significantly increased prevalence of asthma in relatives of patients with asthma or other atopic diseases (eczema, hay fever, allergic rhinitis).
- **Home environment.** Smoking, or exposure to passive smoking in the home environment, is an adverse factor. Indoor allergens, particularly cat dander, may be important in perpetuating asthma symptoms.
- **Occupational history.** It is important to identify whether the patient's asthma could have been caused by exposure to asthmagenic agents at work, by enquiring about current and previous jobs, the tasks performed and materials used. Do symptoms improve away from work at weekends or on holidays? Are symptoms worse on return to work, particularly the evening or night after work? (See Chapter 14.)
- **Trigger factors.** Are there any factors that precipitate symptoms, such as:
  - exercise;
  - cold air;
  - viral respiratory infections;
  - allergen exposure (e.g. feather pillows, cat dander);
  - seasonal factors (e.g. grass pollen); or
  - drugs (e.g. β-blockers, aspirin)?
- **Response to treatment.** Enquiry about the effectiveness of previous treatment with bronchodilator drugs or prednisolone yields clues to the reversibility of the disease and is particularly important in detecting asthma in older patients, who may have been erroneously labelled as having COPD.

The characteristic features **on examination** of patients with asthma are diffuse bilateral **wheeze**, a **prolonged expiratory phase** to respiration and **lower costal margin paradox** (see Chapter 2), but there are often no signs detectable between episodes. There may be features of associated diseases, such as allergic rhinitis, nasal polyps and eczema. It is essential to be alert for atypical features, such as unilateral wheeze, which suggests local bronchial obstruction by a foreign body (e.g. inhaled peanut) in a child or a carcinoma in an adult, for example. It is also important to ensure that there are no signs of cardiac or other respiratory diseases. During acute attacks of asthma, features such as tachycardia, tachypnoea, cyanosis, use of accessory muscles of respiration and features of anxiety and general distress indicate a severe episode. Chronic severe childhood asthma may cause chest deformity, with the lower rib cage being pulled inwards (Harrison's sulcii).

Diagnosis

Asthma is under-diagnosed and under-treated. It creates substantial burden to individuals and families and often restricts individuals' activities for a lifetime.

Although diagnosing asthma is straightforward when the patient presents with classic symptoms and evidence of variable or reversible airway obstruction, there are many pitfalls, and errors in diagnosis are common. **Failure to diagnose** asthma results in the patient being deprived of appropriate asthma treatment; for example, a child with cough might receive recurrent courses of antibiotics for 'chest infections', when in fact they are suffering from asthma. Conversely, **incorrect diagnosis** of asthma might expose the patient to the risks of inappropriate treatment (e.g. recurrent courses of prednisolone) and delay appropriate management of other lung disease, such as an inhaled foreign body in a child or tracheal tumour in an adult producing **wheeze-simulating asthma**. On the one hand, it is necessary to be alert to less well recognised presentations of asthma, such as cough without wheeze, and on the other, it is important to be prepared to review the evidence for asthma if the response to treatment is poor or if unusual features emerge (e.g. could this child have cystic fibrosis?). Evidence establishing the diagnosis of asthma and excluding other diseases often emerges over time, and it is sometimes wise to use interim terms such as '**suspected asthma**' while gathering evidence of variable or reversible airway obstruction, which will allow a **firm diagnosis** of asthma to be established. Doubt may arise where it is difficult to obtain accurate peak flow or spirometry measurements, as in the case of young children. Even when the diagnosis of asthma is established, the diagnostic process should be taken further: **could this be occupational asthma?** Is there evidence of additional lung disease, such as bronchiectasis or allergic bronchopulmonary aspergillosis? The doctor needs to exercise good clinical skills in applying two critical questions: **Could this patient's symptoms be caused by asthma?** and **Does this patient really have asthma?**

Investigations

In a straightforward case, a careful history and clinical assessment may strongly suggest the diagnosis of asthma. If so, a trial of asthma treatment may be a

---

Table 10.1 Diagnosing asthma. 'All that wheezes is not asthma and not all asthma wheezes'

Underdiagnosis: Could this patient's symptoms be caused by asthma?

Overdiagnosis: Does this patient really have asthma?

- Recognise **symptoms** suggestive of asthma (e.g. wheeze, cough, recurrent 'chest infections')
- Establish evidence of **airways obstruction** (e.g. ↓ peak flow, ↓ FEV1, ↓ FEV1/VC ratio)
- Assess **variability, reversibility, provocability** of airway obstruction: serial peak flow chart (e.g. morning dipping; response to bronchodilator and steroid trial; exercise-induced fall in peak flow)
- **Monitor** progress and **review diagnosis** (e.g. has 'wheezy bronchitis' of childhood evolved into established asthma or was it a result of viral bronchiolitis?)
- Consider **additional diagnoses** (e.g. occupational asthma, allergic bronchopulmonary aspergillosis)
- Exclude alternative diagnoses (e.g. cystic fibrosis, COPD, carcinoma, inhaled foreign body)

COPD, chronic obstructive pulmonary disease; FEV1, forced expiratory volume in 1 second; VC, vital capacity.

reasonable next step. (Be prepared to be wrong; if there is not a clear response to treatment, reconsider the diagnosis). In most cases, however, given the likely need for treatment over many years, it is important to try to gain objective support for the diagnosis.

Lung function tests

Confirmation of the diagnosis hinges on the demonstration of airflow obstruction that changes over short periods of time, either spontaneously (**variability**) or in response to treatment (**reversibility**).

Spirometry allows clearer confirmation of airflow obstruction than the peak expiratory flow rate (PEFR), and in that sense is preferable. A reduced FEV/vital capacity (VC) ratio (usually taken to be <0.7) confirms airway obstruction. However, the variability of asthma means that in some individuals (especially with relatively mild disease), spirometry may be normal between attacks.

- **Reversibility.** If airway obstruction is detected by spirometry, the next step is to assess its reversibility to bronchodilator drugs. Typically, the patient is given 200 µg salbutamol and spirometry is repeated 15–20 minutes later. An alternative approach is to employ a 6-week trial of inhaled corticosteroid (e.g. 200 µg of beclometasone) or a 2-week trial of oral steroid (e.g. 30 mg/day of prednisolone). In either case, a >400 ml improvement in FEV_1 strongly suggests a diagnosis of asthma. Smaller improvements are more difficult to interpret and certainly do not exclude the diagnosis. In chronic severe asthma, for example, the response to such treatments may become blunted over time. The diminution of response does not alter the diagnosis, however: it remains asthma.
- **Variability.** Variability in spirometry (irrespective of treatment) may be observed over a number of visits to the clinic. However, **PEFR** has the advantage of being measurable by a cheap, portable device that can be taken away from the clinic by the patient, allowing multiple measurements to be made and giving the potential to record variability in relation to time of day or environment (in the case of asthma triggered by an occupational exposure, for example). The patient needs to be taught how to use the device and record measurements in a **peak flow diary**. A characteristic pattern in asthma is **morning dips**, in which peak flow values are lowest in the morning and improve throughout the day. This diurnal variability is most marked in active, poorly controlled asthma. PEFR variability

is calculated as the difference between the highest and lowest recording, expressed as a percentage of the highest. A 20% or greater variability is highly suggestive of asthma.

Total lung capacity (TLC) is usually increased in asthma, as a manifestation of **hyperinflation**. **Residual volume** is also elevated, indicating **gas trapping**. In contrast to patients with COPD (see Chapter 11), the airway obstruction of asthma is not associated with any impairment of gas diffusion, so that the transfer factor for carbon monoxide (T_Lco) is characteristically normal and the transfer coefficient (Kco) is often slightly elevated (see Chapter 3 for explanation). During an acute severe attack of asthma, **hypoxia** develops, usually in association with increased ventilation and a reduced Pco_2. An elevated (or even normal) Pco_2 in acute severe asthma is a sign of a critically ill patient who is becoming fatigued and failing to maintain ventilation (see later in this chapter).

Airway responsiveness is a measure of the general '**irritability' of the airways**: the degree to which **bronchoconstriction develops in response to physical or chemical stimuli**.

- **Exercise testing.** One of the most useful ways of demonstrating increased airway responsiveness or hyperreactivity is to measure peak flow or spirometry before and after 5–10 minutes of vigorous exercise. A post-exercise fall in FEV_1 or peak flow of 20% is highly suggestive of asthma, as normal subjects usually show a degree of bronchodilatation, rather than bronchoconstriction, during exercise. An **exercise provocation test** is most useful if a patient with suspected asthma has normal peak flow or spirometry when seen in the clinic, such that reversibility testing may be of little use and a 'provocation' test is more useful. The response is greater if exercise is performed in cold air.
- **Methacholine (or histamine) provocation tests.** The degree of airway responsiveness can be measured precisely in the laboratory. Under careful supervision, the patient inhales increasing doses of nebulised methacholine or histamine, starting at a very low dose, and serial spirometry is performed. By plotting the percentage fall in FEV_1, the concentration (C) or dose (D) of the chemical provoking (P) a 20% fall in FEV_1 can be calculated and expressed as a figure (e.g. PD_{20} methacholine 200 µg or PC_{20} histamine 4 mg/ml). Methacholine and histamine provocation tests are not usually required for the diagnosis of asthma in routine practice but are very useful for assessing changes

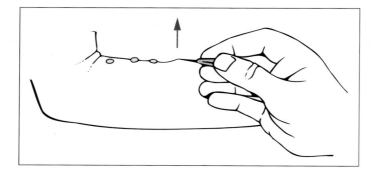

Figure 10.2 Skin-prick test. Drops of antigen extracts and antigen-free control solution are placed on the flexor surface of the forearm. Each drop is pricked with a fine needle. The needle is held parallel to the skin surface and advanced slightly and a tiny fold of skin is lifted briefly, as shown. Deep stabs and bleeding should be avoided. Weal and flare are measured after 10–20 minutes.

in airway responsiveness in relation to exposure to environmental or occupational allergens (see Chapter 14) and in research studies.

Tests for hypersensitivity

Skin-prick tests (Fig. 10.2) may be performed to identify atopy and detect particular sensitivity to a specific antigen, with a view to exclusion of exposure where possible (e.g. cat allergens). A drop of antigen extract is placed on the flexor surface of the forearm and the tip of a small stylet is pressed into the superficial epidermis through the drop. A positive reaction manifests as a weal with a surrounding erythematous flare at about 15 minutes. Reaction to allergens should be compared with the reaction to a drop of histamine and to a drop of control solution containing no antigens. Total **IgE level** is often elevated in patients with atopic asthma, and they sometimes have a mild peripheral blood **eosinophilia**.

Radioallergosorbent testing (RAST) is a means of measuring the level of circulating IgE specifically directed towards a particular antigen.

Some asthmatics develop an allergic reaction to *Aspergillus fumigatus*, a ubiquitous fungus that can colonise the airways. The asthma in these patients is typically severe and persistent, requiring systemic steroid treatment. There is often associated severe airway inflammation and mucus plugging, resulting in bronchiectasis (see Chapter 8). In addition to a positive skin-prick test to *Aspergillus*, these patients often have significant eosinophilia and **precipitating antibodies to *Aspergillus*** in their serum. Very rarely, asthma occurs as part of an eosinophilic vasculitis such as Churg–Strauss syndrome (see Chapter 15), in which case very high levels of blood eosinophilia occur.

General investigations

Further general investigations may be necessary to exclude other cardiorespiratory diseases. **Chest X-ray** is essential in older patients who have smoked, to exclude bronchial carcinoma, for example, and may be needed in children if there are any clinical features to suggest other diseases, such as cystic fibrosis or bronchiectasis. **Bronchoscopy** is occasionally necessary to assess for vocal cord dysfunction, inhaled foreign bodies, bronchial carcinoma or rarer causes of bronchial obstruction, such as carcinoid tumours.

Exhaled nitric oxide (NO) levels are increased in patients with asthma. This is a marker of airway inflammation that can be measured noninvasively. The equipment required is smaller and less expensive than it used to be, but the test hasn't fully established itself as part of routine clinical practice.

Management

Patient education

Asthma is frustrating, frightening and much misunderstood. Successful management of asthma requires that the patient, or their parents if the patient is a child, understand the nature of the condition. The complexity of this explanation will of course vary with the background knowledge and character of the patient, but it is a necessary foundation to an understanding of (and, ultimately, adherence to) treatment. When asthma has only recently developed, for example, the patient may be entirely focused on finding the once-and-for-all cure. Such a patient will not be receptive to the idea of finely tuning lifelong therapy to merely control the disease unless the practicality of the hoped for cure is discussed carefully. Time spent in discussion is very worthwhile. It is particularly important at the time of diagnosis, but education is an ongoing process and should play some part in most consultations.

At clinical review, when attempting to assess the degree of symptom activity, general questions such as 'How's your asthma?' are ineffective and should be avoided. They produce a reply rarely more informative than, 'Fine, doctor'. Specifics, such as the Royal College of Physicians' '3 Questions', are needed to gain a more accurate picture of asthma control:

1 In the last month/week, have you had difficulty sleeping due to your asthma (including cough symptoms)?
2 Have you had your usual asthma symptoms (e.g. cough, wheeze, chest tightness, shortness of breath) during the day?
3 Has your asthma interfered with your usual daily activities (e.g. school, work, housework)?

The patient who reported that their asthma was 'fine', when asked if they wake at night, might, after a brief pause to ensure they have heard you correctly, say, 'Of course I do, doctor; I've got asthma!' This highlights another important issue that needs to be tackled. Many patients (indeed, many doctors) have inappropriately low expectations of what can be achieved with appropriate use of modern inhaled medications. Although we are still some way from a cure, many people with asthma, particularly the young, should be able to achieve something close to complete, if not complete, alleviation of day-to-day symptoms: '**total control**'. Time in consultation often needs to be spent raising expectations of what can be achieved. Many keen sports men and women have given up their sport in the belief that serious competition, or even enjoyment of the activity, is entirely precluded by asthma. This hardly ever needs be the case. Clinical consultation, then, is as much about redefining goals as about the practicalities of treatment regimens.

The practicalities must be addressed, however. Good asthma control for most patients does not depend on the latest, expensive, high-tech treatment; it depends on getting the basics right. Unfortunately, it is the basics that are so often neglected. Good inhaler technique is critical but disappointingly rare.

The fault almost always lies with the clinician, not the patient. An inhaler should never be prescribed unless time is taken to coach (and then check) technique.

Most patients with asthma should be able to **monitor and manage** their own condition to a considerable degree, and to recognise when medical advice is needed, in much the same way that patients with diabetes monitor their blood sugar levels and adjust insulin therapy.

The amount of information given to each patient must be varied in accordance with their needs and, indeed, wishes, but all patients should know about features that indicate when their asthma is deteriorating and what action to take in such circumstances. Healthcare professionals should be aware that it is often those patients least interested in learning about their disease who are at greatest risk and that features such as depression, anxiety, denial of disease and nonadherence with treatment are strongly associated with asthma deaths. Particular effort is required to identify and target resources for such patients. Information conveyed in discussion with the patient should be supplemented by written information. Many organisations, such as the British Lung Foundation and the National Asthma Campaign in the UK, provide excellent literature for patient use. But a preprinted leaflet may sometimes seem to be about 'someone else's asthma'. A few carefully selected notes, including a **personalised asthma plan** *handwritten* in front of the patient, can be a very powerful communication tool. Advice so conveyed is often highly valued by the patient, as it is seen as being about them and their asthma.

Avoidance of precipitating factors

Most patients with atopic asthma react to many different antigens, so that environmental control measures are generally not particularly helpful. The level of **house dust mites** can be reduced by encasing mattresses in occlusive covers and frequently washing blankets and duvets, but the improvement in asthma control, even in those known to be sensitised, is usually disappointing. Avoidance of exposure to **pet allergens** from dogs or cats is more feasible, but the result of these interventions is often not dramatic, either. Similarly, it is difficult to avoid exposure to **outdoor allergens**, although some patients benefit from precautions such as increasing asthma treatment or remaining indoors with closed windows when pollen counts are high.

Desensitisation (immunotherapy) is a highly specialised technique in which repeated injections of an allergen are given to a sensitised subject in an attempt to produce 'blocking antibody' of IgG type that prevents allergen binding to specific IgE on the patient's mast cells. It is most commonly used in the treatment of well-documented life-threatening anaphylactic reactions to insect stings and there is no evidence of its benefit in asthma, while there are major concerns about the risk of anaphylaxis.

Avoidance of irritants such as **cigarette smoke** is advisable. Avoidance of **β-blocker** drugs is important for all patients with asthma, and patients who are sensitive to **aspirin** should avoid all aspirin-containing products and nonsteroidal anti-inflammatory drugs. **Viral infections** often precipitate attacks of asthma, so it is advisable for patients to monitor symptoms (or even peak flow measurements) carefully during such infections and to intensify asthma treatment as required. Because influenza infection may precipitate severe exacerbations of asthma, annual **influenza vaccination** is recommended.

Exercise is a particular factor precipitating asthma. Bronchoconstriction may develop within minutes of onset of vigorous activity. This response usually resolves within 30 minutes and there then follows a refractory period of about 2 hours when further bronchoconstriction is more difficult to provoke. A warm-up period before the main 'event' may help. It is important to remember that exercise-induced asthma is indeed asthma. It responds as asthma does to all the standard therapies. Good overall asthma control is therefore probably more important than a 'quick fix' before the event.

Drug treatment

Short-acting bronchodilator drugs ('relievers') are used to relieve symptoms of bronchoconstriction. **Inhaled corticosteroids ('preventers')** treat the underlying chronic inflammatory process in asthma and are used either alone or in combination with a **long-acting bronchodilator** as maintenance therapy. Most patients with chronic asthma should be able to live perfectly normal lives on a combination of these treatments. The need for oral **prednisolone ('rescue medication')** should be rare, although recognising when it is required is an important part of good asthma management.

Bronchodilators

Short-acting β_2-agonists

Short-acting β2-agonists (e.g. salbutamol, terbutaline) stimulate β-adrenoceptors in the smooth muscle of the airway, producing smooth-muscle relaxation and **bronchodilatation**. They have an onset of action within 15 minutes and a duration of action of 4–6 hours. Side effects include tremor and palpitations, but these are uncommon unless very high doses are used. The principal safety issue with bronchodilators (both long- and short-acting) is not a matter of side effects but of over-reliance at the expense of appropriate use of inhaled corticosteroids. The prompt relief they offer is seductive, but they do nothing to control the underlying disease process: inflammation. Such symptomatic relief can disguise the severity of asthma and delay its treatment. Anyone needing more than three doses of short-acting β_2-agonists per week should have their maintenance therapy increased. An increasing need for bronchodilator medication is a warning of declining control and should be a prompt to action. As a group, patients consuming more than 10–12 puffs of β_2-agonists per day have a recognised increased risk of fatal asthma.

Long-acting β_2-agonists

Long-acting β2-agonists (LABAs) (e.g. salmeterol, formoterol) have a duration of action of more than 12 hours, giving them a convenient twice-daily dosing regimen (which coincides nicely with the usual regimen employed for inhaled corticosteroids). Not long after their introduction, there was concern about an increase in asthma deaths associated with their use. This, however, seems to have been a result of a concomitant reduction in the use of corticosteroids, rather than a direct pharmacological effect of the drugs themselves. Their use is only recommended as an adjunct to inhaled corticosteroids, so that control of the airway inflammation is not neglected.

Combination inhalers, which combine a LABA and an inhaled corticosteroid, are a mainstay in asthma management. They enjoy the benefits of simplicity and convenience (factors associated with better adherence to treatment). They are also a way of ensuring that the improved symptom control brought about by the use of the LABA does not result in a neglect of the inhaled corticosteroid. The particulate combination inhaler Symbicort contains formoterol as its LABA. Formoterol has a 12-hour duration of action but also benefits from an onset of action as brisk as that seen with the short-acting β_2-agonists. **S**ymbicort can therefore be used as both a **M**aintenance **a**nd **R**eliever **T**herapy (**SMART**). The rationale for the so-called SMART regimen is that it automatically delivers an increase in corticosteroid treatment at times when declining control would naturally lead to increasing reliever usage. In selected patients, this has proved to be a useful strategy, but careful patient education about the specific issues related to this regimen is needed. A similar combination, Fostair, now also has a license for maintenance and reliever therapy (MART) use. A third combination, Relvar, contains the inhaled corticosteroid fluticasone furoate and the LABA vilanterol, both of which offer once-daily dosing.

Antimuscarinic bronchodilators

Antimuscarinic bronchodilators (e.g. ipratropium or the long-acting tiotropium) produce bronchodilatation by blocking the bronchoconstrictor effect of vagal nerve stimulation on bronchial smooth muscle. They take about 1 hour to reach their maximum effect and have a duration of action of about 4–6 hours in the case of ipratropium and >24 hours in the case of tiotropium. Side effects are uncommon, but nebulised anticholinergic drugs may be deposited in the eyes, aggravating glaucoma. In most patients with asthma, they are less effective than β_2-agonists; inhaled preparations are therefore not first-choice bronchodilators but can be a useful addition after standard therapy has been deployed in chronic asthma management. Nebulised ipratropium provides a useful adjunct to salbutamol in the treatment of acute severe asthma (see later in this chapter).

Theophyllines

Oral theophyllines increase cyclic adenosine monophosphate (cAMP) stimulation of β-adrenoceptors by **inhibiting the metabolism of cAMP** by the enzyme phosphodiesterase. The additional bronchodilatation beyond that achieved by inhaled bronchodilators is not great, and achieving it requires bringing blood levels close to the toxic range. Hepatic clearance of theophyllines is reduced by drugs such as ciprofloxacin and erythromycin, and toxicity can occur if these medications are prescribed without adjustment in the dose of theophylline. At lower doses, theophylline has a small synergistic anti-inflammatory effect with steroids, which may be useful in some circumstances; however, its place in management is limited. It sits as one of the 'last resorts' when trying to avoid long-term oral steroids. Aminophylline (an intravenous form of theophylline) does not usually result in any additional bronchodilatation compared with standard treatment with nebulised bronchodilators and systemic steroids, and its use is very limited today. It is reserved for patients with near-fatal or life-threatening asthma who show a poor response to initial therapy. The dose must be carefully adjusted according to patient blood levels in order to avoid serious toxicity, such as convulsions and cardiac arrhythmias.

Magnesium

Magnesium sulphate (1.2–2.0 g as an intravenous infusion over 20 minutes) acts as a smooth-muscle relaxant. It is safe and may be useful in treating patients with acute severe asthma who have not had a satisfactory initial response to nebulised salbutamol.

Anti-inflammatory drugs

Inhaled corticosteroids

Inhaled corticosteroids (e.g. beclometasone, budesonide, fluticasone propionate, fluticasone furoate, mometasone, ciclesonide) are the mainstay of asthma treatment because they **counteract airway inflammation**, the key underlying process in asthma. It is essential that the patient understands that this is a **preventative treatment** that needs to be taken regularly and that, in contrast to the short-acting β_2-agonists, these drugs provide no immediate relief of symptoms. Without proper patient education, the drugs may be neglected on the mistaken assumption that 'they're not working'. **Adherence** may be improved when using a twice-daily regime if the patient's 'preventative' steroid inhaler is left at their bedside or by their toothbrush and taken regularly every night and morning. The dose is adjusted to give optimal control and varies greatly from patient to patient.

The **potency** of the various available inhaled steroids differs; the same anti-inflammatory effect can be achieved with one drug at half the dose required with another. Clinical guidelines, in specifying steroid dosage, therefore refer to 'beclometasone equivalent'. This variation does *not* imply superiority of one steroid over another. The critical comparator is not potency but the efficacy-to-side effect profile. In this regard, there is no great difference between any of the available products. In choosing an inhaled steroid, it is probably as wise to choose on the basis of the inhaler device in which the drug is available. A device that the patient can use is likely to be the most effective. Many adult patients with relatively mild asthma achieve good control with a dosage of about 400 μg/day beclometasone, but some with chronic severe asthma may require up to 2000 μg/day. In adult patients, '**low-dose**' (below the equivalent of about 800 μg/day beclometasone) inhaled steroids are not usually associated with any significant adverse effects, apart from oropharyngeal candidiasis or hoarseness of the voice, which can be reduced by using a spacer device in the case of metered-dose inhalers (MDIs) or by using a dry-powder device and gargling the throat with water after inhalation. With '**high-dose**' inhaled steroids (above about

800 µg/day beclometasone), biochemical evidence of suppression of adrenal function and increased bone turnover are detectable in some patients. The clinical significance of such systemic effects needs to be considered in the context of the dangers of uncontrolled asthma and alternative therapies such as oral prednisolone. The dosage of inhaled steroids should be reviewed regularly to ensure that the patient is taking as much as is necessary to control their asthma ('step up') but, equally, as little as is necessary ('step down') to minimise the risk of adverse effects with long-term usage. Patients taking high-dose inhaled corticosteroid should carry a steroid treatment card advising of the risk of adrenal suppression.

Sodium cromoglycate

Sodium cromoglycate was once a commonly used nonsteroid preventative. It no longer has a recommended role in treatment guidelines.

Oral steroid treatment

'Rescue' courses of oral steroids may be needed to control exacerbations of asthma. Typically, these consist of 30–40 mg/day of prednisolone for about 7 days in an adult. Treatment is continued until asthma control has been achieved. Most patients should be taught to start their own short course of oral prednisolone in accordance with a predetermined action plan (e.g. when peak flow falls below 60% of the patient's best value). Patients should understand the potential adverse effects of long-term use of prednisolone and the difference between this and infrequent short courses, which, if truly infrequent, are safe. A very small number of patients require **long-term systemic prednisolone** to control severe asthma. These patients should be attending a hospital specialist and it should have been clearly established that their asthma cannot be controlled by other measures. The dosage of steroids needs to be kept as low as possible. All other effective therapies, particularly inhaled steroids, should be continued at full dose. In these circumstances, the patient should be given a **steroid treatment card** documenting the dosage of steroids used, advised about adverse effects and warned not to stop the use of steroids suddenly, because of the risk of adrenal insufficiency. Booster doses may be required during illnesses and patients may be particularly susceptible to infections such as chickenpox. Other **adverse effects** include peptic ulceration, myopathy, osteoporosis, growth suppression, depression, psychosis, cataracts and cushingoid features. Patients receiving long-term oral prednisolone should be considered for preventative treatment of osteoporosis, such as smoking cessation, exercise, hormone replacement therapy, adequate dietary calcium intake and bisphosphonate treatment, where appropriate.

Leukotriene receptor antagonists

Leukotriene receptor antagonists (e.g. montelukast, zafirlukast) block the effects of cysteinyl leukotrienes: metabolites of arachidonic acid with bronchoconstrictor and proinflammatory actions. Leukotriene antagonists are a modality of anti-inflammatory therapy in asthma, given orally in tablet form. Some patients report a clear improvement in symptoms, although in many the response is disappointing. Their place is as add-on therapy (only to be used after inhaled steroids and a long-acting bronchodilator), but in this role they are a reasonable option. If no benefit can be discerned after 1 month, however, they should be stopped.

Anti-IgE treatment

Omalizumab is a monoclonal antibody that binds to IgE. As such, it is reserved for patients with severe, IgE-mediated (allergic) asthma who are not controlled by high-dose inhaled corticosteroid and LABA medication. It must be given under the direction of a specialist. It is administered by subcutaneous injection every 2–4 weeks, with the dose depending on the baseline IgE level. Its impact on carefully selected patients who were once dependent on continuous oral steroids can be dramatic. It has revolutionized the treatment of severe allergic asthma.

Bronchial thermoplasty

Bronchial thermoplasty is a novel, still rather experimental, technique in which heat is applied directly to the central airways via bronchoscopy. Thermal 'damage' to smooth muscle reduces its quantity and functionality, and in one major study led to improved lung function and reduced need for reliever medication over a 22-week follow-up. More evidence of both safety and efficacy will be required before the technique can be established as a component of clinical practice.

Stepwise approach to the treatment of asthma

The British Thoracic Society guidelines on the management of asthma recommend a stepwise approach to treatment according to the severity of the asthma (Fig. 10.3). The **aim of treatment** is to control the disease. **Control** is defined as:

- no daytime symptoms;
- no nighttime wakening due to asthma;

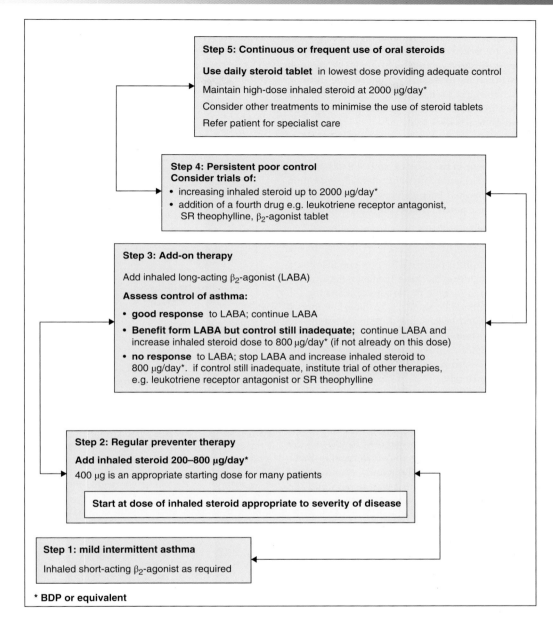

Step 5: Continuous or frequent use of oral steroids

Use daily steroid tablet in lowest dose providing adequate control

Maintain high-dose inhaled steroid at 2000 μg/day*

Consider other treatments to minimise the use of steroid tablets

Refer patient for specialist care

Step 4: Persistent poor control
Consider trials of:

• increasing inhaled steroid up to 2000 μg/day*
• addition of a fourth drug e.g. leukotriene receptor antagonist,
  SR theophylline, β₂-agonist tablet

Step 3: Add-on therapy

Add inhaled long-acting β₂-agonist (LABA)

Assess control of asthma:

• **good response** to LABA; continue LABA
• **Benefit form LABA but control still inadequate;** continue LABA and
  increase inhaled steroid dose to 800 μg/day* (if not already on this dose)
• **no response** to LABA; stop LABA and increase inhaled steroid to
  800 μg/day*. if control still inadequate, institute trial of other therapies,
  e.g. leukotriene receptor antagonist or SR theophylline

Step 2: Regular preventer therapy

Add inhaled steroid 200–800 μg/day*
400 μg is an appropriate starting dose for many patients

Start at dose of inhaled steroid appropriate to severity of disease

Step 1: mild intermittent asthma

Inhaled short-acting β₂-agonist as required

* BDP or equivalent

Figure 10.3 Summary of the stepwise management of asthma in adults. (Reproduced with permission from British Thoracic Society/Scottish Intercollegiate Guidelines Network. *British Guideline on the Management of Asthma 2012* (www.brit-thoracic.org.uk).

• no need for reliever medication;
• no exacerbations;
• no limitations on activity, including exercise;
• normal lung function (in practical terms, FEV_1 and/or PEF >80% predicted or best); and
• minimal or no side effects.

Patients should start treatment at the step most appropriate to the initial severity of their asthma and treatment should be adjusted as appropriate thereafter. For the majority of patients, asthma is controlled by a combination of a regular inhaled steroid and occasional use of an inhaled bronchodilator drug as required. Bronchodilator drugs are primarily intended to provide symptom relief, whereas inhaled steroids are targeted at the underlying inflammatory process in the airways. Treatment should be **'stepped up' as much as necessary** to control the asthma; when control has been achieved, treatment may be **'stepped down'** so that the patient is on **no more treatment than is necessary**.

Asthma is a dynamic condition, changing over time, and ongoing management requires a continuous assessment of the level of control that has been achieved and a continuous adjustment of medication to find the optimal balance between control of the asthma and the potential adverse effects of treatment.

Inhaler devices

The inhaled route is preferred for bronchodilator and corticosteroid drugs because it allows these drugs to be delivered directly to the airway, reducing the risk of systemic adverse effects. A large number of different inhaler devices and drug formulations are available. Current evidence suggests that there is no major difference in the clinical effectiveness of the various devices, **provided the patient is able to use them appropriately**.

Metered-dose inhalers

Pressurised MDIs (Fig. 10.4) use hydrofluoroalkane (HFA) as a propellant. It is essential to instruct the patient in the correct use of the inhaler and to check they are using it correctly frequently. About 10% of the drug is delivered to the lower airways and the remainder is mainly deposited in the oropharynx and swallowed. It is absorbed into the blood, but is mostly metabolised by first-pass metabolism in the liver. MDIs delivering corticosteroids should not be used without a spacer device.

Spacer devices

Poor inhaler technique is a significant problem in the use of MDIs. Large-volume spacer devices (e.g. Volumatic, Nebuhaler, Aerochamber) (Fig. 10.5)

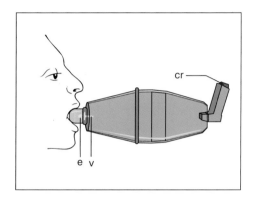

Figure 10.5 Example of a spacer device for use with MDIs. This allows the patient to inhale after discharge of the aerosol. The Volumatic (Allen and Hanbury) is a large-volumed device designed to allow free dispersal of the discharged material, so that a high proportion of it forms particles small enough to be inhaled. It also allows large doses of aerosol to be inhaled relatively efficiently (see text). cr, canister of pressurised aerosol; e, expiratory port; v, valve (closes on expiration).

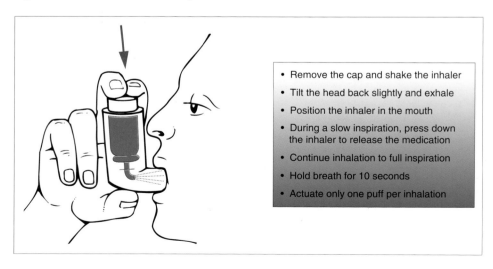

- Remove the cap and shake the inhaler
- Tilt the head back slightly and exhale
- Position the inhaler in the mouth
- During a slow inspiration, press down the inhaler to release the medication
- Continue inhalation to full inspiration
- Hold breath for 10 seconds
- Actuate only one puff per inhalation

Figure 10.4 Pressurised metered-dose inhaler.

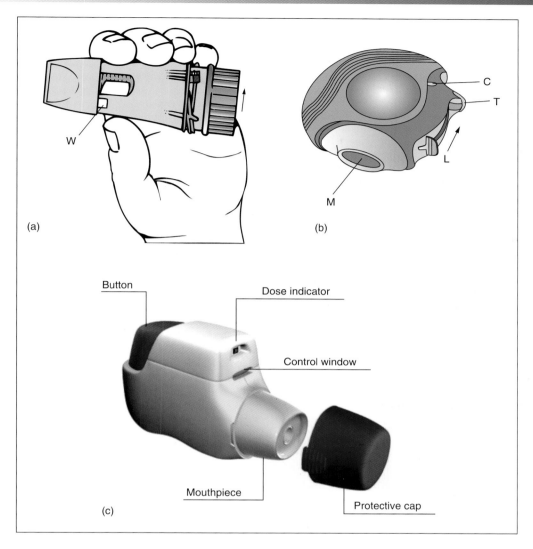

(a)

(b)

Button

Dose indicator

Control window

Mouthpiece

Protective cap

(c)

Figure 10.6 Examples of dry-powder inhalers. (a) Turbohaler. The inhaler is shown with the cover removed, the mouthpiece to the left. Up to 200 doses of the powdered drug are stored in a reservoir, through which the air channel passes. A dose of the dry powder is rotated into the air channel by turning the distal section (arrow). The number of doses remaining is indicated in a small window (W). (b) Accuhaler. The inhaler is opened by pushing the thumb grip (T) right around until it clicks. The inhaler is shown open. Sliding the lever (L) around as far as it will go pierces an individual blister and places a dose of the drug in the mouthpiece (M). There is a counter (C) indicating how many doses are left. (c) Genuair. When the button is pressed and released, the control window changes to green, indicating the drug is ready to be inhaled. Inhalation changes the control window to red and locks the inhaler out, preventing further inhalation until the button is pressed again.

overcome this to some extent and improve deposition of the drugs in the lower airway to about 20%, on average. A canister of pressurised aerosol is inserted into one end of the spacer device and the patient breathes through the other end via a one-way valve, which closes on expiration. This **reduces the need for coordination of inspiration and actuation of the inhaler**. Distancing the inhaler from the mouth ('spacing') results in a fine aerosol of small particles, **improving delivery of the drug to the lower**

airways. Spacer devices should be cleaned monthly by washing in detergent and air-drying. They should be replaced at least every 12 months.

Breath-actuated aerosol inhalers

Breath-actuated inhalers (e.g. Autohaler, Easi-breathe) avoid the need for the patient to coordinate actuation of the inhaler and breathing: the valve on the inhaler is actuated as the patient breathes in, delivering the drug only during inspiration.

Dry-powder devices

In dry-powder devices (e.g. Turbohaler, Accuhaler, Genuair, Ellipta) (Fig. 10.6), the β-agonist or steroid drug is formulated as a dry powder, without a propellant. Inspiratory airflow releases the powder from the device (it is **breath-actuated**), reducing the need to coordinate inspiration and inhaler actuation. Some patients find dry-powder devices easier to use, but they require an adequate inspiratory flow rate to achieve drug delivery.

Nebulisers

In this form of inhaled therapy (Fig. 10.7), oxygen or compressed air is directed through a narrow hole, creating a local negative pressure (Venturi effect) that draws the drug solution into the air stream from a reservoir chamber. The droplets are then impacted against a small sphere: small particles are carried as an aerosol, whereas larger particles hit the side wall of the chamber and fall back into the reservoir solution. The aerosol is administered by mask or via a mouthpiece. Nebulisers are a convenient means of giving **high doses of bronchodilator drugs in acute attacks of asthma** where coordination of inhaler administration may be difficult due to patient distress. They may also be used to deliver inhaled steroids (e.g. budesonide) in very young children, although it is important to realise that properly used dry-powder devices (e.g. Turbohaler), MDIs and spacer devices deliver a greater percentage of the administered dose to the lower airway and are therefore the devices of choice for routine long-term treatment.

The danger of patients having nebulisers at home lies in the fact that they may come to over-rely on the temporary alleviation of symptoms these devices offer, to the detriment of regular anti-inflammatory therapy. It might also lead to a delay in their seeking urgent medical advice during acute severe asthma attacks.

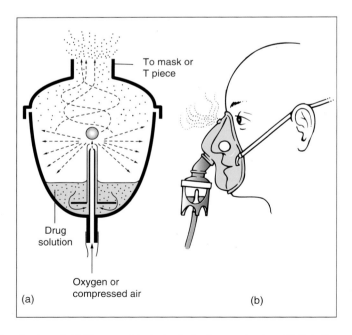

Figure 10.7 Nebuliser treatment. (a) Diagram of typical nebulisation mechanism. (b) Nebuliser mask for administration of high-dose bronchodilator (see text).

Acute severe asthma

Some patients with asthma are particularly suscepti- ble to recurrent sudden attacks of severe asthma, but any patient with asthma may develop an acute attack under certain circumstances (e.g. viral infection, allergen exposure). It is crucial that all patients with asthma know how to recognise the features of a severe attack and know what action to take. Most of the people who die of acute asthma do so because the severity of the attack was underestimated and not treated adequately or promptly. It is important there- fore that doctors and patients recognise the features of worsening asthma control and a severe attack.

Signs of acute severe asthma

Any one of:

- PEF 33–50% of best or predicted;
- respiratory rate ≥25/min;
- heart rate ≥110 bpm; and/or
- inability to complete sentences in one breath.

Life-threatening asthma

Any one of the following in a patient with acute severe asthma:

- **Clinical signs.**
  - altered conscious level
  - exhaustion
  - arrhythmia
  - hypotension
  - cyanosis
  - silent chest
  - poor respiratory effort
- **Measurements.**
  - PEF <33% of best or predicted
  - O_2 saturation <92%
  - $P_aO_2 < 8$ kPa
  - normal P_aCO_2

Near-fatal asthma

- Raised P_aCO_2 and/or need for mechanical ventila- tion with raised inflation pressures.

Immediate management

- **Oxygen.** The highest concentration available should be used. Masks delivering 24% or 28% are not appropriate. Aim for a saturation >94%.
- **High-dose nebulised β-agonist**. For example, salbutamol 5 mg or terbutaline 10 mg. This may

be repeated after 15–30 minutes if the patient's condition is not improving. Multiple doses from an inhaler should be given with a spacer device if a nebulizer is not available.

- **High-dose systemic steroid.** For example, pred- nisolone 40–50 mg daily orally or hydrocortisone 100 mg 6-hourly intravenously, given immediately.

If response to this initial therapy is poor, add the following:

- **Nebulised ipratropium.** Add ipratropium 0.5 mg to the nebulised β-agonist. Use 4–6-hourly
- **Intravenous magnesium sulphate.** 1.2–2.0 g infu- sion over 20 minutes.
- **Intravenous bronchodilators.** Intravenous aminophylline is unlikely to result in any addi- tional bronchodilatation compared with standard care. Side effects such as arrhythmias may also be problematical. Some patients with near-fatal or life-threatening asthma may gain additional benefit from intravenous aminophylline, but such patients have been difficult to identify in trials and are probably rare. Aminophylline should only be used after consultation with senior medical staff.
- **Intravenous β$_2$-agonists.** These are sometimes used (salbutamol or terbutaline 250 μg over 10 minutes, then infusion of 5 g/min), but they should be reserved for those patients in whom nebulised therapy cannot be used reliably.

Investigations

- Arterial blood gases, urea and electrolyte concen- trations, electrocardiogram in older patients, chest X-ray.

Monitoring treatment

Continued vigilance is required. The patient's con- dition may deteriorate some hours after an initial improvement (e.g. during the night after admission). Measure and record PEF 15–30 minutes after starting treatment and at least 4 times daily thereafter, accord- ing to the response. Monitor respiratory rate, pulse, patient's general condition and oxygen saturation frequently. Deterioration in these signs should prompt consideration of admission to the intensive therapy unit (ITU). Acute severe asthma usually acts as a powerful stimulus to ventilation, resulting in a reduced PCO_2. By the time of admission, however, the patient may have had progressive symptoms over a few days, with very little sleep. Fatigue and exhaustion are often present. Even a normal PCO_2 (let alone an elevated value) in the context of acute severe asthma is therefore an ominous sign. Transfer of the patient to an ITU may be advisable, so that their condition can be monitored more closely. Intermittent positive-pressure ventilation is only rarely necessary but is used when the patient shows signs of exhaustion (rising Pco_2), failure to maintain oxygenation or deterioration in vital signs.

Management during recovery in hospital and following discharge

The opportunity should be taken to improve the patient's understanding of asthma and its management and to provide written guidance on future management. Ways of improving the patient's response to worsening asthma should be identified. Most crises resulting in hospital admission are probably preventable. The importance of peak flow measurement in determining treatment changes should be explained. Possible precipitating factors should be identified. Inhaler technique should be checked and performance recorded. If necessary, alternative inhaler devices should be used. No single physiological marker defines safety for discharge but patients should be stable on medical therapy that they can continue at home (this usually means they have managed overnight without the need for nebulised bronchodilators). Follow up with the general practitioner within 2 working days of discharge and with a specialist within a month.

Respiratory emergencies Asthma

- **Oxygen.** High flow. Aim for a saturation >94%.
- **Nebulised β-agonist.** Salbutamol 5 mg or terbutaline 10 mg. This may be repeated after 15–30 minutes if the patient's condition is not improving. Continue 4–6-hourly or more frequently, as required.
- **High-dose systemic steroid.** For example, prednisolone 40–50 mg orally or hydrocortisone 100 mg 6-hourly intravenously immediately.

If response to initial therapy is not adequate, add the following:

- **Nebulised ipratropium.** 0.5 mg 6-hourly
- **Intravenous magnesium sulphate.** 1.2–2.0 g infusion over 20 minutes.
- **Closely monitor** clinical condition, PEF and arterial blood gases. If there is poor response to treatment, fatigue or failure to achieve adequate oxygenation or if Pco_2 is within normal range, discuss with ITU.

 KEY POINTS

- Asthma is a dynamic heterogenous clinical syndrome, characterised by chronic airway inflammation, airway hyperresponsiveness and airway obstruction.
- Asthma is multifactorial in origin, arising from a complex interaction of genetic and environmental factors.
- The clinical diagnosis of asthma should be supported by evidence of variable or reversible airway obstruction on spirometry or peak flow measurements.
- Most patients with asthma can be managed perfectly well by proper attention to detail with the basic therapies (regular inhaled corticosteroids and an inhaled bronchodilator).
- Instruction in the correct use of an appropriate inhaler device is crucial in the treatment of asthma.
- Most patients (and many doctors) have inappropriately low expectations of disease control. Aim for 'total control'.

 FURTHER READING

Asthma UK Web site (www.asthma.org.uk, last accessed 29 December 2014).

British Thoracic Society/Scottish Intercollegiate Guidelines Network. *British Guideline on the Management of Asthma 2009*. London: British Thoracic Society, 2009 (http://sign.ac.uk/guidelines/fulltext /101/, last accessed 29 December 2014).

Carlsen KH, Delgado L, DelGiacco S. Diagnosis, prevention and treatment of exercise-related asthma, respiratory and allergic disorders in sports. *Eur Respir Mon* 2005; **10**: 1–105.

Chu EK, Drazen JM. Asthma: one hundred years of treatment and onward. *Am J Respir Crit Care Med* 2005; **171**: 1202–8.

Dolovich MB, Ahrens RC, Hess DR, et al. Device selection and outcomes of aerosol therapy: evidence based guidelines of the American College of Chest Physicians/American College of Asthma, Allergy and Immunology. *Chest* 2005; **127**: 335–71.

Global Initiative for Asthma (GINA) Web site (www. ginasthma.org, last accessed 29 December 2014).

Holgate ST, Yang Y, Haitchi HM, et al. The genetics of asthma. *Proc Am Thorac Soc* 2006; **3**: 440–3.

Masoli M, Fabian D, Holt S, Beasley R. The global burden of asthma: executive summary of GINA Dissemination Committee report. *Allergy* 2004; **59**: 469–78.

Multiple choice questions and answers

10.1 Most patients with asthma:

A are overoptimistic in their expectations of what can be achieved with treatment

B are fastidious about treatment compliance

C can manage simple inhalers well

D need more than just the basics (inhaled corticosteroids and short-acting bronchodilators) to maintain good control

E are capable of managing the disease themselves

10.2 In a patient presenting with breathlessness, a diagnosis of asthma is most strongly supported by:

A breathlessness on exertion

B a family history of hay fever

C FEV1/VC < 0.7 at the time of clinic visit

D nocturnal wakening due to cough

E asymmetry of chest expansion on examination

10.3 The following are features of a life-threatening attack of asthma:

A PEF 33–50% of best or predicted

B respiratory rate > 25/min

C O_2 saturation < 92%

D respiratory rate > 25/min

E heart rate >110 bpm

10.4 In chronic asthma management, current protocols and treatment specify:

A use of reliever medication only once per day suggests good control

B inhaled corticosteroids do not improve symptoms

C long-acting bronchodilators should never be used without inhaled corticosteroids

D omalizumab is a new effective oral medication for severe disease

E leukotriene receptor antagonists are effective in most patients

10.5 Common triggers for asthma do not include:

A cigarette smoke

B influenza vaccine

C beta blockers

D aspirin

E cold air

10.6 Options at step 4 of asthma management include:

A nebulised salbutamol

B theophylline

C aspirin

D leukotriene receptor antagonist

E oral (tablet) salbutamol

10.7 In relation to lung function tests, signs typical of asthma include:

A reduced FEV1

B reduced Kco

C reduced total lung capacity (TLC)

D reduced variability in peak expiratory flow rate (PEFR)

E reduced residual volume (RV)

10.8 The BTS definition of good asthma control includes:

A waking up due to asthma no more than twice per week

B < 2 exacerbations per year

C daytime symptoms twice per week

D PEFR variability of 20%

E modest exercise limitation no more than twice per week

10.9 In a new diagnosis of asthma:

A start with p.r.n. (as required) salbutamol first and assess response

B start with the simplest inhalers: pressurised metered dose inhalers (pMDIs)

C an elevation in total IgE is important to confirm the diagnosis

D a peak flow diary is needed to confirm the diagnosis before treatment is started

E warn the patient that asthma has no cure and may well lead to lifelong limitation of activity

10.10 First-line management of acute severe asthma includes

A controlled oxygen

B nebulised salbutamol

C nebulised ipratropium

D high-dose inhaled steroids

E intravenous magnesium

Multiple choice answers

10.1 E

Patients often have inappropriately low expectations of what can be achieved with treatment. Adherence to treatment is a major issue in any chronic disease; the additional complexity of inhaled medication (as opposed to oral) only adds to this. Inhaler technique is generally very poor. This is usually the prescribing clinician's fault, not the patient's. Most people can be managed perfectly well at step 2 of the BTS guidelines, provided attention is paid to the detail. Self-monitoring and management are essential to good control in this variable condition. Education is key.

10.2 D

Any cause of breathlessness tends to be worse on exertion. While hay fever may be linked with asthma, the association between a family history and a personal diagnosis of asthma is a little weak. FEV1/VC < 0.7 confirms airway obstruction, but variability is required for a diagnosis of asthma. Nocturnal symptoms of cough or breathlessness suggest diurnal variability consistent with asthma. Asymmetry of chest expansion on examination suggests the diagnosis is something else.

10.3 C

All are features of acute severe asthma, but only C is a feature of a life-threatening attack

10.4 C

The need for reliever medication more than 3 times per week implies inadequate control. Of course, corticosteroids improve symptoms; they just don't do it instantly. Omalizumab is given by injection. LTRA can be very effective in some patients, but only a minority.

10.5 B

Influenza vaccine is recommended.

10.6 B, D, E

The other option at step 4 is to increase the dose of inhaled corticosteroid – up to 2000 mcg per day. Aspirin can be dangerous in some asthmatic patients.

10.7 A

Kco is typically increased (see text). TLC is usually increased as a manifestation of hyperinflation, PEFR displays increased variability (a cardinal feature of asthma). Gas trapping with early small airway closure leads to an increase in residual volume.

10.8 None

Good asthma control includes: no daytime symptoms, no nighttime wakening due to asthma, no need for reliever medication, no exacerbations, normal lung function, no limitation of exercise.

10.9 None

Although p.r.n salbutamol is a step 1 drug, in a new diagnosis of asthma the patient should be commenced at the treatment step judged by the clinician to be the most appropriate – treatment can be later stepped up or down. pMDIs may be the oldest inhalers but they are certainly not the simplest to use. A diagnosis is confirmed by a good history and demonstration of variability (or reversibility) of airflow obstruction (e.g. spirometry). A peak flow diary takes time, and treatment may be needed more urgently. Well controlled asthma should mean no disability.

10.10 B

High-flow (not controlled-rate) oxygen should be used. Systemic (not inhaled) steroids are used. Nebulised ipratropium and IV magnesium are used if response to first-line treatment is poor.

11

Chronic obstructive pulmonary disease

Introduction

Chronic obstructive pulmonary disease (COPD) is a major cause of morbidity and mortality worldwide. It not only shortens life but has a devastating impact on quality of life. In the UK, an estimated 3 million people have COPD, yet more than 2 million of these remain undiagnosed. There are 110 000 admissions to hospital with exacerbations of COPD and 30 000 people die of the disease each year. Mortality has fallen in men but continues to rise in women, reflecting smoking patterns over the second half of the twentieth century. As the worldwide epidemic of smoking spreads, with increasing smoking rates in China, Africa and Asia, it is predicted that COPD will become the third most common cause of death worldwide by 2020. There is an urgent need to improve awareness, prevention and treatment of this disease.

Definitions

Chronic obstructive pulmonary disease

COPD is defined as a chronic, slowly progressive disorder characterised by **airflow obstruction** that does not change markedly over several months. Although there is some overlap in the features of COPD and asthma, they are separate disorders with different aetiologies, pathologies, natural histories and responses to treatment. In asthma, airway inflammation and hyperreactivity are the key factors giving rise to bronchial muscle contraction and manifestly variable airway obstruction. In COPD, structural and histological changes give rise to the various facets of the condition: chronic bronchitis, emphysema and airway obstruction.

Chronic bronchitis

Chronic bronchitis is a hypersecretory disorder defined as the presence of **cough productive of sputum on most days for at least 3 months of 2 successive years** in a patient in whom other causes of a chronic cough have been excluded (e.g. tuberculosis, bronchiectasis). The diagnosis is made on the basis of symptoms. The airways of patients with chronic bronchitis show mucous gland hypertrophy and an increased number of goblet cells. Although chronic bronchitis and obstructive lung disease result from inhaling cigarette smoke, they do not show a clear relationship to each other and are distinct components of the spectrum of COPD. Mucus hypersecretion is mainly caused by changes in the central airways, whereas progressive airway obstruction arises principally from damage to the peripheral airways and alveoli.

Emphysema

Emphysema is defined in terms of its pathological features that consist of **dilatation of the terminal air spaces of the lung distal to the terminal bronchiole with destruction of their walls**. The reduced surface area for gas transfer is marked by a reduction in the transfer factor for carbon monoxide and transfer coefficient, physiological hallmarks of emphysema (Chapter 3). High-resolution computed tomography (CT) scans can demonstrate the parenchymal lung destruction of emphysema. Two main patterns of

Respiratory Medicine Lecture Notes, Ninth Edition. Stephen J. Bourke and Graham P. Burns.
© 2015 John Wiley & Sons, Ltd. Published 2015 by John Wiley & Sons, Ltd.
Companion Website: www.lecturenoteseries.com/Respiratory

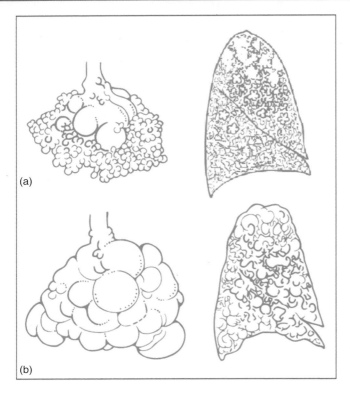

(a)

(b)

Figure 11.1 Emphysema. Diagrammatic view of lobule and whole lung section in (a) centrilobular and (b) panacinar emphysema.

emphysema are recognised (Fig. 11.1): **centriacinar (centrilobular) emphysema** involves damage around the respiratory bronchioles with preservation of the more distal alveolar ducts and alveoli. Characteristically, it affects the upper lobes and upper parts of the lower lobes of the lung. **Panacinar (panlobular) emphysema** results in distension and destruction of the whole of the acinus, and particularly affects the lower half of the lungs. Although both types of emphysema are related to smoking and may be present together, it is possible that they may arise by different mechanisms. Panacinar emphysema is the characteristic feature of patients with α_1-anti-trypsin enzyme deficiency.

Airway obstruction

Airway obstruction is an increased resistance to airflow caused by diffuse airway narrowing (see Chapter 3). The term denotes a disturbance of physiology made manifest by a **reduced forced expiratory volume in 1 second/vital capacity (FEV_1/VC) ratio**. From a practical perspective, an FEV_1/VC ratio less than 0.7 is deemed to denote airway obstruction, although in truth the normal value of this ratio varies with age (see later in this chapter). A number of factors contribute to airway obstruction in

COPD: destruction of alveoli by emphysema (leading to loss of elastic recoil and a loss of outward traction on the small airways, leaving them prone to collapse on expiration; Figs. 11.1 and 11.2), airway inflammation with thickening of the airway wall (different to that seen in asthma and usually the result of tobacco smoke) and accumulation of mucous secretions (obstructing the airway lumen).

Aetiology

Worldwide, a number of factors may be important in the development of COPD. In the developing world, the smoke from biomass fuel used for indoor cooking is a major cause, while in the developed world, **tobacco smoking** is far and away the most important. Even in the developing world, smoking is of increasing importance. The total dose of tobacco inhaled is critical and depends on factors such as **age at starting** smoking, **depth of inhalation** and total **number of cigarettes** smoked (one pack-year is defined as the equivalent of one pack (20 cigarettes) per day for 1 year). Although nearly all patients with COPD have smoked heavily, only about 15% of smokers develop COPD, indicating that genetic susceptibility plays a

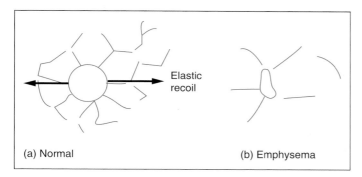

(a) Normal   (b) Emphysema

Elastic recoil

Figure 11.2 Emphysema consists of dilatation of the terminal air spaces of the lungs, distal to the terminal bronchiole, with destruction of their walls. (a) Small peripheral airways lack cartilage and depend on the support of the surrounding alveoli to maintain their patency. (b) Alveolar destruction in emphysema results in a loss of elastic recoil and a loss of outward traction on the small airways such that they collapse on expiration, contributing to the observed airway obstruction.

part. There is a higher prevalence of COPD in **men** than in women, in patients of **lower socioeconomic status** and in **urban** rather than rural areas.

There is evidence that COPD may be aggravated by **air pollution**, but the role of pollution in the aetiology of COPD appears to be small when compared with that of cigarette smoking. Some dusty occupational environments are associated with the development of chronic bronchitis and COPD, such as those involving exposure to coal dust, cotton dust and grain (see Chapter 14). However, the contribution of occupation to the development of COPD is again small when compared with the dominant effect of cigarette smoking.

A variety of **factors in early childhood** have an important influence on the development of obstructive airway disease in adulthood, by determining the maximum lung function achieved in adolescence and possibly also the subsequent rate of decline in lung function. Such factors include **passive exposure** to **cigarette smoke**, either transplacentally **in utero** or environmentally in the **home**. Some studies suggest that the presence of **airway responsiveness** predicts an accelerated rate of decline in lung function in smokers. The **genetic factors** that contribute to the differences between individuals in their susceptibility to developing COPD if they smoke are poorly defined, except in the case of the inherited **deficiency of antiprotease enzymes**. It is thought that emphysema develops as a consequence of destruction of lung tissue by proteolytic digestion resulting from an imbalance between proteases and antiproteases and between oxidants and antioxidants. Genetic deficiency of the principal antiprotease, α_1-antitrypsin, is associated with the development of severe emphysema at a young age. This deficiency accounts for fewer than 1% of all cases of COPD, but it is possible that other, unidentified proteases may be important.

Clinical features and progression

COPD has a wide spectrum of severity. The characteristic clinical manifestation of the **emphysema and airway obstruction** of COPD is **breathlessness**, which responds only partially to treatment and **progresses** gradually but relentlessly over the years. Wheeze is not the prominent feature it tends to be in asthma. Because of the large pulmonary reserve, patients with a sedentary lifestyle often do not notice breathlessness until a great deal of lung function has been permanently lost. Many people are in their 50s at the time of diagnosis and may have been smoking since their teens. Fig. 11.3 illustrates the insidious progressive way in which lung function is lost in COPD. It also demonstrates the benefits of smoking cessation (see later in this chapter).

Chronic **cough** and **sputum** production are the clinical manifestations of the mucus hypersecretion of chronic bronchitis. **Infective exacerbations** of bronchitis are common and are characterised by an increased cough with purulent sputum. Non-typeable unencapsulated strains of *Haemophilus influenzae* often colonise the normal upper respiratory tract. In chronic bronchitis, disruption of the mucociliary defence mechanism facilitates spread of infection to the bronchial tree, where infection may provoke inflammation and a self-perpetuating vicious circle of inflammation and infection, further compromising pulmonary clearance mechanisms and aggravating airway obstruction. Extension of infection into the lung parenchyma, if it occurs, gives rise to **bronchopneumonia** (see Chapter 6).

Two main clinical patterns of disturbance may be discerned in patients with advanced COPD, which differ mainly in the extent to which ventilatory drive is

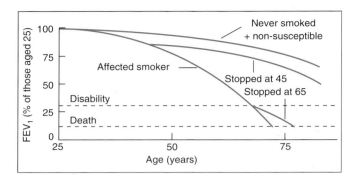

Figure 11.3 Change in FEV$_1$ with age: effect of smoking and stopping smoking. Nonsmokers show a small progressive decline in function with age. Many smokers are unaffected by smoking and show the same decline as nonsmokers. Some smokers are affected, however, and show a steeper decline. By the time disability is noted, ventilatory function is seriously reduced, to about one-third of predicted normal values. Those affected by smoking can be detected by measurement of FEV$_1$ many years before they become disabled. Stopping smoking slows the rate of decline. (From Fletcher C, Peto R. The natural history of chronic airflow obstruction. *BMJ* 1977; **1**: 1645.)

preserved in the face of increasing airway obstruction: **'pink puffers'** and **'blue bloaters'** (Fig. 11.4). These represent two extremes of a spectrum, and most patients do not fit either pattern completely, but have some features of both. 'Pink puffers' have well-preserved ventilatory drive even in the presence of severe airway obstruction. Dyspnoea is usually intense, but Pco_2 is often maintained in the normal range at rest until the terminal stages of the disease. 'Blue bloaters' have poor ventilatory drive and easily drift into respiratory failure with hypercapnia, hypoxaemia and right heart failure, particularly during exacerbations.

Investigations

There is no single diagnostic test for COPD. Diagnosis relies on clinical judgment based on a combination of history, physical examination and confirmation of the presence of airflow obstruction using spirometry.

Lung function tests

Spirometry is the most accurate measure of airflow obstruction and is therefore crucial in the diagnosis of COPD. In the context of COPD, the diagnosis of airflow obstruction and the assessment of severity are based on **post-bronchodilator spirometry**.

The FEV$_1$/VC ratio declines naturally with age and airway obstruction should more correctly be defined by the lower limit of the normal range for the patient's age, but for convenience an FEV$_1$/VC ratio

< 0.7 is generally taken to define airway obstruction irrespective of age. Once airway obstruction has been determined to be present (by this ratio), its severity is usually classified by comparing FEV$_1$ to the predicted value. Descriptors such as **mild** (FEV$_1$ >80% predicted), **moderate** (FEV$_1$ 50–79% predicted), **severe** (FEV$_1$ 30–49% predicted) and **very severe** (FEV$_1$ <30% predicted) are broadly accepted and used, although they are, of course, intrinsically arbitrary.

Spirometry can also be used to assess the degree of reversibility of the airway obstruction to bronchodilators or corticosteroids, but this is a complex area. There is considerable variability in the change in FEV$_1$ in response to the same stimulus from day to day and the overall clinical usefulness of inhaled corticosteroids is generally not predicted by the response to a reversibility test (see the section on Management later in this chapter). Nevertheless, the performance of reversibility tests can be very useful in identifying an unsuspected case of asthma. Asthma and COPD are different conditions with different treatment algorithms, so diagnostic accuracy matters. The two conditions can coexist; when they do, treatment strategies must deal with both.

Total lung capacity (TLC) and **residual volume** are often elevated, signifying hyperinflation and gas trapping. **Transfer factor for carbon monoxide** and **transfer coefficient** are typically reduced in emphysema.

Oximetry is useful in measuring oxygen saturation noninvasively, but a sample of **arterial blood** is necessary to assess Po_2 and Pco_2 levels.

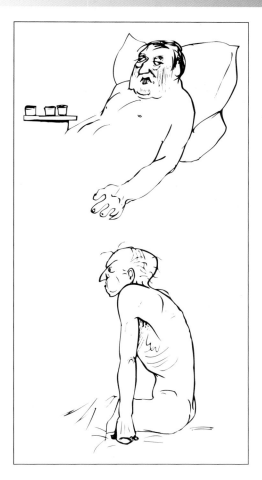

Figure 11.4 'Blue bloater' (top) and 'pink puffer' (bottom). (Original drawings reproduced by kind permission of Dr R.A.L. Brewis. From Brewis, *Lecture Notes on Respiratory Disease*, 1st edn. Oxford: Blackwell Science, 1975)

Lung function tests are discussed in more detail in Chapter 3.

Radiology

The **chest X-ray** typically shows hyperinflation of the chest, with flattened, low hemidiaphragms, a long narrow cardiac shadow and an increased retrosternal airspace on the lateral film (Fig. 11.5). The chest X-ray is also an important investigation in excluding additional diagnoses (e.g. lung cancer) and in detecting complications of COPD (e.g. pneumothorax, bronchopneumonia). **High-resolution CT scans** (Fig. 11.6) can demonstrate the extent of emphysema and the presence of bullae but are not required for the routine care of patients with COPD.

A multisystem disease

It is common for patients with COPD to have a number of other medical conditions, termed **comorbidities**. Some of these are the result of a common aetiological factor (e.g. smoking and ischaemic heart disease), some are a direct consequence of the lung condition itself. COPD can lead to a number of different pathophysiological changes outside the lung, including simple mechanistic effects (e.g. pulmonary hypertension due to hypoxia) and **inflammatory overspill**, wherein inflammatory mediators from the lung are transported to other organs (see later in this chatper). The nonrespiratory aspects of a patient's condition are important to obtaining a full appreciation of the impact of the disease process on them.

Hypoxia within the lungs leads to pulmonary vasoconstriction. This puts a strain on the right side of the heart, leading to right ventricular hypertrophy (right axis deviation, dominant R wave in V_1) on electrocardiography (ECG) and ultimately to a dilated ventricle with tricuspid regurgitation on echocardiography (echo). Right heart failure caused by lung disease is known as cor pulmonale. Some patients with chronic hypoxaemia develop polycythaemia with elevated haemoglobin levels.

Severe COPD can result in **cachexia** and **loss of muscle mass**. This is probably multifactorial, including the effects of breathlessness on both appetite and activity and an increase in circulating inflammatory mediators (e.g. IL-6, TNF-α). The result is further impairment of mobility and increased restriction on the patient's ability to function socially. A low **body mass index** (BMI) should be managed with nutritional support. Conversely, if an obese patient can be encouraged to lose weight, the impact on symptoms can be enormous.

Inflammatory overspill is also thought to play a part in the development of a number of other comorbidities, including **osteoporosis, cardiac failure** and **diabetes**.

There are a number of tools which can give us a general impression of the impact of the disease on a patient's life. Breathlessness can be quantified using the Medical Research Council dyspnoea scale:

- **Grade 1.** Breathless only on strenuous exertion.
- **Grade 2.** Breathless when walking up a slight hill.
- **Grade 3.** More breathless than contemporaries when walking on level ground.
- **Grade 4.** Breathless on walking about 100 m.
- **Grade 5.** Breathless on dressing or undressing.

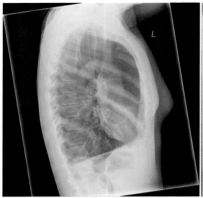
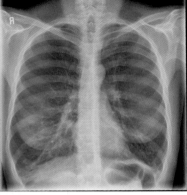

Figure 11.5 The chest X-ray in COPD typically shows hyperinflation of the chest, with flattened, low hemidiaphragms, a long narrow cardiac shadow and an increased retrosternal airspace on the lateral film.

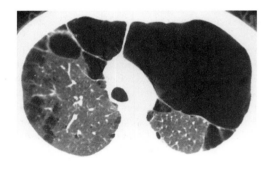

Figure 11.6 This 42-year-old man had smoked 20 cigarettes a day since the age of 14. He presented with a 5-year history of progressive breathlessness and could walk only 100 m. He had severe airway obstruction, with an FEV_1 of 0.5 l and a transfer factor for carbon monoxide and transfer coefficient reduced to 30% of predicted values. High-resolution CT shows extensive emphysematous bullae with dilated distal airspaces, cysts and destruction of alveolar architecture. Levels of α_1-antitrypsin were unrecordable.

A number of questionnaires are available for assessment of the overall function, quality of life and impact of the disease, such as the COPD Assessment Test (CAT). The BODE index (body mass index, airflow obstruction, dyspnoea and exercise capacity) can be calculated to give an indication of prognosis.

Depression and anxiety are very common accompaniments to COPD, reported in up to 50% of patients. Breathlessness is not just unpleasant, but at times is very frightening. It is not surprising, therefore, that frequent but unpredictable attacks of breathlessness may ultimately lead to a persistently anxious state. The general debility and potential for social isolation that COPD can bring are obvious risk factors for depression. Despite their prevalence, these debilitating conditions are usually entirely overlooked by doctors. Screening (e.g. Hospital Anxiety and Depression Scale, HADS) is necessary to identify cases. Active screening is, of course, only worthwhile if there is a therapeutic option available. This has been a stumbling block in the past. **Cognitive behavioural therapy (CBT)** is proven to reduce both anxiety and depression, but its effectiveness in the context of chronic lung disease has been less certain. Access to therapy has also been a problem, with a shortage of trained psychologists even in many developed healthcare economies. A study is now underway to assess the impact of CBT on anxiety in the context of COPD and to determine whether clinicians armed with only basic CBT skills can make a difference.

Management

For years, COPD was dogged by a rather negative profile. Like asthma, it is characterised by airway obstruction, but unlike asthma, that obstruction is generally regarded as 'nonreversible'. In imprecise minds, 'nonreversible' is too easily confused with 'nontreatable'. COPD was the disease for which 'little could be done', and, indeed, little was done. Over the latter half of the 20th century, as medicine had a positive impact on many diseases that afflicted the developed world, the age-adjusted death rate for coronary heart disease (CHD), for example, fell by almost 60% – a testament to what medicine and good public health measures can achieve. Over the same period, the age-adjusted death rate for COPD rose by 163%. The reasons for this stark divergence in fortunes are manifold, but it is noteworthy that, where CHD was a disease that affected the affluent in society, COPD was perhaps a disease of the 'disenfranchised'. The socioeconomic influence on COPD persists. Not only is there a higher prevalence of COPD in those of **lower socioeconomic status**, this group also has the highest rate of underdiagnosis. COPD accounts for a considerable part of the **reduced life expectancy** in areas of deprivation compared with the UK as a whole.

In the past decade, there has been a revolution in our approach to COPD.

With the development of new treatments, and indeed a fresh look at some of the old, we have managed to move beyond the old nihilistic mindset. In COPD, we now recognise that it is possible to have a very positive impact on a great number of clinically important outcomes, including breathlessness, cough, sputum, exacerbation rate, hospital admission rate, disability, exercise endurance, quality of life, anxiety, depression, rate of disease progression and even mortality. The interventions that achieve these outcomes still do not have a great short-term impact on FEV_1, but in the face of such evidence it would be difficult to continue to view COPD as an 'untreatable' condition.

In managing patients with COPD, we now have a number of tools at our disposal, including pharmacological, physical and psychological interventions. The application of each needs to be considered carefully for every patient and integrated into an overall comprehensive individualised management plan.

The first consideration in any patient still smoking has to be **smoking cessation**. If this can be achieved, it will have a far greater impact on long-term prognosis than any other intervention.

Smoking cessation

Fig. 11.3 illustrates the decline in lung function seen in smokers with COPD. Many patients are well down the slippery slope before the diagnosis is established. The graph also demonstrates the effect of smoking cessation on disease progression. Although it is clear that the lung function lost is never regained (emphysema is permanent damage), smoking cessation changes the course of the disease. Indeed, despite the vast sums of money spent on drug development, smoking cessation remains the only proven **disease-modifying** intervention for COPD. If smoking cessation occurs early enough in the course of the disease then the rate of decline in FEV_1 returns (approximately) to what it would have been had the patient never smoked – a natural age-related decline. Clearly, the earlier smoking cessation can

be achieved, the better the preservation of lung function. Although lung function never returns to normal, it is clear that the patient will be far better off than if they had continued to smoke. Year on year, they will experience fewer symptoms and a better quality of life, as well, of course, as living longer. Smoking cessation therefore remains one of the most important components of management. Doctors need to do more than just pay lip service to smoking cessation. All patients still smoking, regardless of age, should be encouraged to stop, and offered help to do so, at every opportunity. The risks of lung cancer and heart disease are important issues to discuss, of course, but many patients are well aware of this increased 'risk' and have already rationalised the issue in their own mind. What many COPD patients are not aware of is the startling decline in quality of life that awaits them (not a risk: a certainty) if they continue to smoke. A description of the practical implications of declining lung function (a transition from mild breathlessness to being entirely housebound) can have a powerful impact on a patient's determination to quit. Without a firm commitment by the individual, smoking-cessations aids will achieve little. When used in conjunction with willpower, pharmacotherapy can improve quit rates.

Pharmacotherapy for smoking cessation

Small doses of nicotine produce predominantly stimulant effects, such as arousal, whereas larger doses produce mainly depressant effects, such as relaxation and relief of stress. **Nicotine withdrawal** can cause irritability, restlessness, anxiety, insomnia and a craving for cigarettes. Nicotine replacement therapy approximately doubles the success rates of attempts at smoking cessation and smokers should be encouraged to use it to avoid withdrawal symptoms. Typically, a heavy smoker is given **transdermal nicotine patches** 21 mg/day for 4 weeks, reducing to 14 mg/day for 2 weeks and then 7 mg/day for 2 weeks. Most withdrawal symptoms have resolved within that period of time. The patch is applied to the skin each morning and delivers a constant dose over 16–24 hours, but the onset of action is quite slow. Patients who experience marked cravings for cigarettes may benefit from using nicotine **chewing gum**, **lozenges**, **inhalators** or **nasal sprays**, which provide more rapid peak blood levels from absorption of the nicotine through the buccal or nasal mucosa. Nicotine replacement therapy is safe, but is not recommended in pregnancy. Addiction to nicotine replacement therapy can occur in a few patients who use it in the long term, but most patients can be weaned off treatment over a few weeks.

Bupropion (amfebutamone) is an antidepressant drug that significantly improves the success of attempts at smoking cessation, although its mode of action is uncertain. It has some significant side effects, most notably a 1 in 1000 risk of epileptic seizures, such that it is contraindicated in patients with convulsive disorders, central nervous system disease, bulimia or anorexia nervosa and in patients experiencing symptoms of withdrawal from alcohol or benzodiazepines.

Varenicline is a nicotinic receptor partial agonist. As such, it both reduces cravings for and decreases the pleasurable effects of cigarettes, and through these mechanisms it can assist some patients in quitting smoking. Side effects include nausea (common), headache, difficulty sleeping and abnormal dreams.

Electronic cigarettes (e-cigarettes) are battery-powered devices designed to resemble a cigarette. They generally use a heating element, known as an atomizer, which vaporizes a liquid solution containing nicotine and a mixture of other chemicals (e.g. propylene glycol, vegetable glycerin, flavourings). The vapour is inhaled in a manner that mimics cigarette smoking. They remain controversial. Whilst some doctors (quite rightly) argue that they are significantly safer than smoking cigarettes, they are not without problems. They are made by the tobacco companies, who, of course, have no incentive to reduce nicotine addiction: the devices generally deliver a large dose of nicotine (accounting for their popularity) and so only reinforce nicotine addiction. Only by breaking addiction to nicotine does an individual have any prospect of remaining a sustained quitter long-term. At present, they remain entirely unregulated, so there is no control at all on what other chemicals are inhaled along with the nicotine. Regulation would restrict the use of chemicals to a prescribed 'safe list', but, even if these are benign in the short term, the long-term effects of inhaling them into the lung are not yet known. It is also difficult to see how the use of flavours such as *bubble gum* can do anything other than attract children to the market and increase nicotine addiction.

Pharmacological treatments in the management of stable COPD

Short-acting bronchodilators

Short-acting β$_2$-agonists, such as salbutamol and terbutaline, relax bronchial smooth muscle by stimulating β-adrenoreceptors. **Short-acting anticholinergic drugs**, such as ipratropium, produce bronchodilatation by blocking the bronchoconstrictor effect of vagal nerve stimulation of the bronchial smooth muscle. Although some bronchodilatation is in fact achievable, it is the impact on breathlessness that is of most relevance. These old, long-established drugs are reasonably effective short-term symptom relievers. β$_2$-agonists remain first-line drugs, particularly in mild COPD.

Long-acting bronchodilators

Tiotropium and **glycopyrronium** are **long-acting muscarinic antagonists (LAMAs)**. They have greater affinity and a slower rate of dissociation from muscarinic receptors than ipratropium. Their duration of action is at least 24 hours, giving them a convenient once-daily dosage. They also outperform the short-acting ipratropium on all important indices, effectively superseding it as a maintenance therapy in chronic stable disease. **Aclidinium** has a shorter duration of action and needs to be delivered twice daily but it has the advantage of having fewer anticholinergic side effects (e.g. dry mouth).

Long-acting β$_2$-agonists (LABAs), such as **salmeterol** and **formoterol** (with a 12-hour duration of action) and **indacaterol** (24 hours), also offer prolonged relief of symptoms and would seem to be a reasonable additional maintenance therapy. However, for a variety of reasons not always associated with clinical efficacy, these agents have generally not become as established in routine clinical practice as the LAMAs.

The latest class of treatment launched is the **dual bronchodilator (LAMA/LABA)** combination. Undoubtedly more efficacious then either agent alone, its place in routine clinical practice will inevitably ultimately be determined by its perceived cost-effectiveness.

Although symptomatic relief of breathlessness is an important aim of treatment, COPD is a multifaceted disease and modern, comprehensive treatment strategies must therefore offer more than just short-term relief from this symptom.

Corticosteroids

In many other areas of medicine, drugs are employed that offer prognostic benefit. Statins, for example, don't improve symptoms in ischaemic heart disease but do have a measurable impact on the frequency of future events. In relation to exacerbations and hospital admissions – the events that blight the lives of COPD patients – inhaled corticosteroids offer a similar prognostic benefit. This effect is greatest when inhaled corticosteroids are combined with a LABA in a **combination inhaler** (e.g. Symbicort, Seretide, Fostair). The combination typically produces a 30% reduction in exacerbation frequency, with a positive knock-on effect in reducing hospital admission rates. These important benefits are seen principally in moderate to severe disease; at the mild end of the spectrum there are usually fewer exacerbations to prevent. The combination inhalers are now licensed for use with the indication of reducing exacerbation frequency in patients with a predicted $FEV_1 < 60\%$. Inhaled corticosteroids alone are not licensed and have no place in the management of COPD.

Long-acting muscarinic antagonists (prognostic issues)

The symptomatic relief of breathlessness offered by LAMAs has already been discussed. In this sense, they are effective in all grades of severity. In addition, as with the inhaled corticosteroid/LABA combination inhalers, in moderate to severe disease LAMAs have a beneficial impact on both exacerbation frequency and hospital admission rate.

Treatment strategy

In relation to inhaled therapies, the treatment strategy differs depending on the severity of the disease. In mild disease (other than smoking cessation support, for which benefit is prognostic), treatment is principally aimed at short-term symptom control. Options such as SABA, LAMA and LAMA/LABA combinations can be tried. They are usually effective; if they are not, it is likely to be evident within the first month and they should be stopped. In moderate and severe disease, the situation is very different. Although symptom control remains important, there is, in addition, evidence of prognostic benefit from certain treatments. Group mean data from very large studies tell us that the use of a LAMA and/or an ICS/LABA combination inhaler will reduce the frequency of both exacerbations and hospital admissions. In contrast to the symptom controllers in mild disease, prognostic treatments should not be stopped if the patient reports no perceived benefit in the first month. This may seem obvious enough, but the approach is quite a radical departure from traditional practice with inhaled therapies, where a 'try it and see' approach has been the norm. The principle of prognostic treatment is, of course, well understood and accepted in other clinical contexts, such as blood pressure control, hypercholesterolaemia and the use of β-blockers post acute coronary syndrome.

Inhaler technique

If you assume that **most people who have inhalers don't use them properly**, you'll not go far wrong! This is not usually the fault of the patient but of the prescriber who failed to spend time teaching and checking inhaler technique. There seems to be a general assumption that getting the inhaler technique 'about right' is good enough. It's not: lung delivery falls sharply if technique is not perfect, and in many cases technique is so poor that lung delivery is likely to be zero. Whenever an inhaler is prescribed, care must be taken to coach (and then test) inhaler technique. This should, of course, be done by someone who understands it themselves. Technique should then be tested every time the patient is reviewed.

Oral medications

Methylxanthines, such as aminophylline and theophylline, have a number of effects, including cyclic adenosine monophosphate (cAMP) stimulation of β-adrenoceptors through inhibition of the metabolism of cAMP by the enzyme phosphodiesterase. Theophylline should only be used after a trial of short- and long-acting bronchodilators. Plasma levels need to be monitored, as the therapeutic window is narrow. The dose should be reduced if a macrolide or fluroquinolone antibiotic is prescribed. A large-scale study is now underway in the UK to determine whether regular low-dose theophylline can reduce exacerbation frequency.

The newer long-acting **PDE-4 inhibitor** roflumilast has some benefit in reducing exacerbation frequency in patients at the severe end of the spectrum with the chronic bronchitis phenotype. It is licensed for use in Europe but not in the United States.

Mucolytics are drugs that increase the expectoration of sputum by reducing its viscosity. They were once 'blacklisted' in the UK, deemed not to work. The rationale for this belief stemmed from the fact that they did not improve FEV_1. A reappraisal of the earlier studies led to a significant change in opinion. Although mucolytics do not have an impact on FEV_1, they can improve cough symptoms and may reduce the frequency of exacerbations in some patients with COPD who have a chronic productive cough.

Psychological treatment

Anxiety and depression are common in COPD of all grades of severity and not just confined to severe disease. **CBT** should be the first-line therapy (see earlier in this chapter).

Pulmonary rehabilitation

Pulmonary rehabilitation is a multidisciplinary programme of care for patients with COPD that is individually tailored and designed to optimise physical and social performance and autonomy. Typically, a pulmonary rehabilitation programme involves the skills of doctors, respiratory nurse specialists, physiotherapists, dieticians, social workers and occupational therapists. Many patients with COPD are in a vicious cycle of breathlessness, reduced physical activity and deconditioning of skeletal muscles, with resultant loss of social contact and autonomy. Pulmonary rehabilitation can break this vicious cycle and can **reduce dyspnoea and improve exercise tolerance and quality of life**. When delivered early after an admission, it can **reduce the chance of future admission**.

The key components of a rehabilitation programme must be adjusted to meet the needs of the individual patient, but typically include the following:

- **Exercise training.** Breathless patients often reduce their level of exercise and lose general fitness and muscle mass. Exercise training (e.g. walking, cycling) can counteract muscle atrophy and improve fitness. Improvement in lower limb function may help walking, and arm training improves performance of day-to-day tasks such as lifting, dressing, washing and brushing one's hair. Typically, an exercise training programme involves three supervised aerobic exercise sessions per week over a period of 8 weeks.
- **Smoking cessation.** Advice, encouragement and support should be offered in achieving and maintaining smoking cessation.
- **Optimisation of drug treatment.** The patient should take a comprehensive treatment regimen, with a good inhaler technique.
- **Education.** An education programme for patients and their families should include advice on how and when to take medications, the benefits of exercise, the importance of smoking cessation and the use of techniques such as breathing control, relaxation and anxiety management. Patients who are vulnerable to exacerbations can be taught to recognise the onset of symptoms and instructed to start a 'rescue pack' (including a course of prednisolone, and an antibiotic if sputum is purulent) and to increase their use of bronchodilator drugs.
- **Breathing control techniques.** These involve pursed-lip breathing, slower deeper respirations and better coordination of breathing patterns. Physiotherapy techniques such as active cycle breathing, chest percussion and forced expiratory techniques may be useful in patients who have difficulty expectorating secretions.
- **Social support.** Patients with advanced disability may have difficulty in performing daily tasks, such as climbing stairs, shopping and washing, and may benefit from assessment by an occupational therapist with regard to home aids such as stair lifts and bath aids. Assessment by a social worker will allow a patient to obtain appropriate allowances (e.g. disability or mobility allowances) from government agencies.
- **Psychological support.** Depression and social isolation are common and can be helped by psychological support focusing on restoring coping skills. Patient self-help groups may be useful. Some patients will require referral for more formal treatment, such as CBT.
- **Nutrition.** Poor nutrition is common in patients with advanced COPD and is associated with poor overall health status and an increased mortality. Patients with COPD are often underweight because of the increased work of breathing, the systemic effects of inflammatory cytokines and a decreased food intake from anorexia and breathlessness. Some patients, however, are overweight, because of reduced activity and overeating. A patient's weight and body mass index should be measured and appropriate dietary advice should be given.

Pulmonary rehabilitation is an enormously valuable intervention, but if the patient does not continue to exercise after completion of the formal programme, the benefits in exercise performance are likely to be lost gradually over the following 6 months. Ideally, patients should be encouraged to continue regular exercise; many such opportunities exist in local sports centres and gyms. Patients also benefit in this context from being on appropriate inhaled medication. The right symptom relievers are proven to both amplify the fitness benefits gained from pulmonary rehabilitation and slow the 'post-programme' decline.

Oxygen therapy in stable disease

'Short of breath' does not imply 'short of oxygen'. It is important to understand that it is quite possible to experience breathlessness from a physiological cause without being hypoxic. In this context, breathing supplemental oxygen will achieve nothing. As a simple analogy, imagine a car breaking down despite having a full tank of petrol: supplying more petrol will do nothing to get the car restarted. Supplemental oxygen in a patient who is not hypoxic is just as pointless. Many breathless patients ask their doctor for oxygen therapy and many well-meaning doctors duly prescribe it. These prescriptions are costly and many are of no benefit to the patient whatsoever.

There are, nevertheless, a number of circumstances in which oxygen therapy can not only improve symptoms but also extend life. Proper (specialist) assessment is required to ensure that the patients who need oxygen therapy receive it and those who do not, do not.

Long-term oxygen therapy

Hypoxia within the lung leads to pulmonary vaso-constriction. The increased vascular resistance puts a strain on the right heart. The right heart struggles for a while, hypertrophies, but eventually fails. Right heart failure caused by lung disease is known as **cor pulmonale**. The first sign is often ankle swelling. This is sometimes (incorrectly) perceived as a minor 'cosmetic' issue to be fixed with a small dose of diuretic. It should be obvious to anyone after a moment's reflection, however, that having half of the heart not working is likely to be serious. It is. Cor pulmonale is a fatal disease. Patients with COPD and chronic hypoxia have a poor prognosis, with a mortality rate of about 50% within 3 years.

The clinical features of hypoxia are nonspecific and it is often overlooked; periodic measurement of oxygen saturation by oximetry is therefore useful in detecting these patients. In the early 1980s, two major studies – the British Medical Research Council (MRC) Study and the American Nocturnal Oxygen Therapy Trial (NOTT) – showed that the administration of oxygen for *at least* 15 hours/day (preferably longer) improved survival in patients with hypoxia. It is important to understand that oxygen therapy has no impact on the progression of COPD (rate of decline of FEV_1); the improvement in survival is via the relaxation of pulmonary vasoconstriction and the alleviation of the strain on the right heart. It is the premature death from a complication of COPD – cor pulmonale – that is prevented.

Prescribing criteria

Long-term home oxygen therapy is indicated for **patients with severe COPD ($FEV_1 < 1.5 l$) and persistent hypoxia ($Po_2 < 7.3 kPa$ (55 mmHg))**. Many patients who are hypoxic during an exacerbation will recover over a few weeks and will not require long-term oxygen. Arterial blood gases should therefore be measured on two occasions, at least 3 weeks apart, during a stable phase before diagnosing persistent hypoxia. Patients with more borderline oxygen levels ($7.3-8.0 kPa$ (55–60 mmHg)) who have elevated haematocrit or already have features of cor pulmonale, such as oedema, are also likely to benefit from long-term oxygen. The oxygen is usually given via nasal cannulae at a flow rate of about 2 l/min, but the dose required and mode of administration should be decided by a specialist in the context of the patient's arterial blood gas measurement.

Oxygen concentrator

Long-term home oxygen therapy is often provided by an oxygen concentrator. This is an electrically powered machine that separates oxygen from the ambient air using a molecular sieve. The machine is installed in the patient's house and plastic tubing relays oxygen to points such as the bedroom and living room. Providing oxygen cylinders to the patient's home for long-term oxygen therapy is impractical and much more expensive than installation of an oxygen concentrator. The patient and their family should be warned not to smoke in the presence of oxygen, because of the risk of causing a fire. It is essential that the patient understands that the main aim of long-term oxygen therapy is to improve prognosis (reduce mortality rate), rather than to alleviate symptoms, and that it is necessary to comply with oxygen therapy for at least 15 hours/day. Patients often have to be reminded of this 15-hour rule, as it runs counter to the instruction ('don't take more than … ') that accompanies most other prescriptions.

When first advised of the need to spend so much of the day 'tied to an oxygen machine', patients are often visibly deflated. They imagine sitting next to a large oxygen cylinder, looking at the clock and waiting for 15 hours to pass. In fact, the treatment can be accommodated far more easily than is first imagined, and time should be spent reassuring the patient on this matter. For a start, oxygen can be applied at night as the patient sleeps (that's 8 hours clocked up with no effort at all). Sufficient tubing around the home allows the patient to continue ordinary domestic activities during the day. A further 7 hours can therefore usually be clocked up without any significant limitation to lifestyle. Remind patients that the 15-hour rule still leaves them 9 hours in the day to be 'out and about'. Most patients find that if they simply use the oxygen whenever they are at home, they can quite easily accumulate a sufficient number of hours with no deleterious effect on quality of life.

Ambulatory oxygen

Ambulatory oxygen may be appropriate for patients who are active enough to leave the home regularly, who demonstrate a fall in oxygen saturation to below 90% on exercise and who show symptomatic benefit from oxygen in terms of walking distance (assessed formally using a 6-minute walk test). It is given using a refillable portable container of liquid oxygen.

Short-burst oxygen

Short-burst oxygen involves breathing oxygen from a cylinder for a few minutes to relieve dyspnoea after exercise. However, the benefit of this form of oxygen therapy is not clearly established. It is most commonly employed as a palliative measure in 'end-stage' disease.

Hypoxia during air travel

Patients with lung disease are vulnerable to developing hypoxia when travelling by plane. Commercial aircraft routinely fly at about 11 400 m (38 000 feet) and are pressurised to a cabin altitude of 2438 m (8000 feet) The reduced partial pressure of oxygen at this altitude is equivalent to breathing 15% oxygen at sea level, and causes the Po_2 of a healthy passenger to fall to between 7.0 and 8.5 kPa (52–64 mmHg). Although this does not usually cause symptoms or problems for most passengers, it can produce critical hypoxia for patients with lung disease. Pre-flight assessment should include an overall assessment of the patient's condition, with particular regard to dyspnoea, exercise capacity, previous flying experience, spirometry and oxygenation. If the oxygen saturation is >95% then in-flight oxygen is not required. If oxygen saturation is <92%, supplementary in-flight oxygen is usually prescribed by nasal cannulae at a rate of 2–4 l/min. If the oxygen saturation is between 92 and 95% then further assessment is recommended. This may include a **hypoxic challenge test**, during which arterial blood gases are measured when the patient has been breathing 15% oxygen for 20 minutes. In-flight oxygen is usually recommended if the Po_2 falls below 7.4 kPa (56 mmHg).

Surgery

A small number of patients with COPD may benefit from surgery. **Lung transplantation** is an option, although lack of donor organs severely limits the utilisation of this procedure (see Chapter 19). **Bullectomy** may be appropriate where a large bulla is compressing surrounding viable lung. **Lung volume-reduction surgery** is an option for selected patients with severe disability. In emphysema, destruction of the alveoli results in a loss of elastic recoil (with collapse of small airways on expiration) and hyperinflation of the lungs

(with flattening of the diaphragm). Volume-reduction surgery aims to resect functionally useless areas of the lungs, thereby reducing the overall volume. This relieves compression of the relatively normal portion, restores elastic recoil (increasing outward traction on the small airways) and re-establishes more normal diaphragmatic and thoracic contours, allowing better respiratory motion during breathing. Patients whose emphysema preferentially affects the upper lobes may be the most suitable for this procedure. In certain patients, lung function, exercise performance and quality of life are improved, but the benefit tends to decline with time.

Emergency treatment

Exacerbations of COPD are characterised by an acute worsening of symptoms, with increased breathlessness, sputum volume and sputum purulence. They may occur spontaneously or as a result of infections. There are associations between COPD admissions and the weather: the strongest relate to cold weather (admissions peak 12 days after a cold snap) and season (worse over the New Year).

Patients can be taught to recognise the onset of an exacerbation and to institute a **self-management plan**, whereby they increase the dose and frequency of bronchodilator medication and start a course of oral prednisolone and an antibiotic, according to a predetermined plan. Mild exacerbations can be **managed at home** but patients with severe exacerbations require **admission to hospital**. Deciding whether a patient can be managed at home requires an overall assessment of the severity of the COPD (e.g. baseline FEV_1, oxygen saturation, exercise capacity), the home circumstances (e.g. family support, able to cope) and key adverse features that indicate a severe exacerbation (e.g. confusion, cyanosis, severe respiratory distress).

Patients admitted to hospital should have a chest X-ray, oximetry, arterial blood gas measurement, an ECG (to exclude comorbidities), full blood count and urea and electrolyte measurements. Culture of sputum is often performed but rarely produces a result in time to influence antibiotic prescribing. Blood cultures should be taken if the patient is pyrexial and a theophylline level should be measured in patients on theophylline therapy.

Bronchodilator therapy is usually given by nebuliser, using a combination of **salbutamol** 2.5–5.0 mg and **ipratropium** 500 mcg with **prednisolone** 30 mg/day for 5 days.

Antibiotics

In some cases, exacerbations of COPD are associated with infections by viruses or bacteria, and antibiotics should be used to treat exacerbations associated with a history of more purulent sputum. Common bacteria include *Haemophilus influenzae*, *Streptococcus pneumoniae* and *Moraxella catarrhalis*. Although **amoxicillin** has a reasonably good spectrum of activity against many of these organisms, 15–20% of *Haemophilus influenzae* and many strains of *Moraxella catarrhalis* are resistant to it, so that other antibiotics such as **co-amoxiclav** (amoxicillin and clavulanic acid), **doxycycline**, **ciprofloxacin** or **clarithromycin** may be needed. In many cases, exacerbations of COPD seem to arise as a result of a spontaneous worsening or are provoked by noninfectious events such as air pollution, smoking or adverse weather conditions. Patients with exacerbations without more purulent sputum do not need antibiotic therapy unless there is consolidation on a chest radiograph or there are clinical signs of pneumonia.

Pneumococcal vaccination and annual **influenza vaccination** are recommended for patients with COPD.

Emergency oxygen

Oxygen is delivered in most emergency situations, with the aim of achieving a near normal saturation (94–98%). However, for some patients, such levels are dangerous and may be life-threatening.

Patients with established respiratory failure who have chronically raised P_{CO_2} (type 2 respiratory failure) become unresponsive to the carbon dioxide stimulus to ventilation and rely increasingly on hypoxaemia to maintain the drive to breathe. If they are given high concentrations of oxygen, they lose the drive to breathe and underventilation results in increasing hypercapnia, acidosis, narcosis, respiratory depression and, ultimately, death. Uncontrolled oxygen therapy poses a risk to this subset of patients. The risk must of course be balanced against the threat of hypoxia. Because of the shape of the oxyhaemoglobin dissociation curve, there is little benefit in increasing a patient's oxygen saturation above about 90% (P_{O_2} above about 8 kPa (60 mmHg)). In patients at risk of hypercapnic respiratory failure (which, unless proven otherwise, includes any patient with an exacerbation of COPD), treatment should be commenced using controlled oxygen (e.g. 28% Venturi mask (Fig. 11.7) in pre-hospital care or 24% Venturi mask in hospital settings), with an initial target saturation of **88–92%** pending urgent blood gas assessment to determine the patient's ventilatory status (pH and P_{CO_2}) (see Chapter 3). In this 'Goldilocks zone' (88–92%), the patient will not die of hypoxia and it is very unlikely there will be any appreciable respiratory depression.

It is essential to document carefully the amount of oxygen being breathed when measuring arterial gases. Avoid measuring gases immediately after the patient has received nebulised drugs using

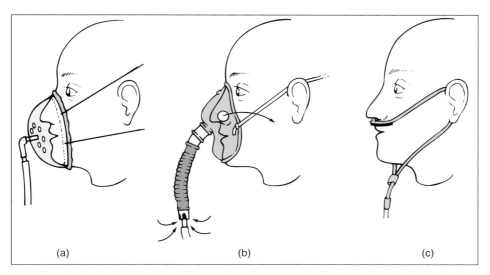

(a)   (b)   (c)

Figure 11.7 Oxygen administration. (a) Simple uncontrolled high-concentration face mask with oxygen supplied directly to the mask space. (b) Fixed-performance Venturi mask delivering a controlled (fixed) dose of low-concentration oxygen. (c) Nasal cannulae delivering an uncontrolled level of oxygen in a convenient continuous manner.

high-flow oxygen. Sometimes there is concern about using high-flow oxygen (e.g. 6–8 l/min) to nebulise bronchodilator drugs in patients with hypercapnia; occasionally, compressed air is used instead. However, nebulising drugs that use air during acute exacerbations of COPD may leave the patient dangerously hypoxic. One option it to deliver concomitant supplemental oxygen via nasal cannulae. Alternatively, it is safe to use oxygen to nebulise the drug, provided the nebulisation time can be strictly limited to 10 minutes. The patient is then not exposed to the risk of either hypoxia or prolonged high-concentration oxygen.

Ventilatory support

Occasionally, acute respiratory acidosis complicates an exacerbation of COPD. This can occur despite the best efforts of doctors (when high-flow oxygen is inappropriately delivered, it may occur *because* of the efforts of doctors). It is crucially important to recognise respiratory acidosis when present, so blood gas analysis is essential to the management of acute exacerbations of COPD in hospital.

After initial management with nebulised bronchodilators and appropriate oxygen therapy, if the pH is below the normal range (<7.35) then **noninvasive ventilation (NIV)** should be employed (unless there is a specific contraindication (rare) or the patient declines it). It should be delivered in a dedicated setting by staff trained in its application, and there should be a clear plan covering what to do in the event of deterioration.

When used in this context, NIV not only reduces the likelihood that the patient will progress to need invasive ventilation but is demonstrated to **reduce inpatient mortality by 50%**. Despite the overwhelming evidence of such a substantial clinical benefit, a number of national audits have demonstrated that NIV is not utilised as often as it should be. This seems to be a result of both a lack of knowledge of the specific indication and a failure to appreciate the magnitude of the benefit. A rather laissez-faire and fatalistic approach is still worryingly common. In the light of current evidence, such an approach is frankly wrong.

Practical application

NIV is delivered via a tight-fitting mask strapped in place over the nose and mouth and connected to a specifically designed ventilating machine. The spontaneous respiratory efforts of the patient are used to trigger the ventilator to deliver additional tidal volume under positive pressure. Lack of familiarity with the technical aspects of NIV may be what deters many doctors from employing this therapy. In most UK hospitals, however, the practical aspects of NIV use are handled by the on-call physiotherapy team or specialist nurses: all the doctor really needs to know is the arterial pH and how to pick up a telephone.

Prior to the advent of NIV, the intravenous respiratory stimulant **doxapram** was used in a similar context. This option may still be useful for those few patients unable to tolerate NIV, but **invasive ventilation** (i.e. endotracheal intubation and ventilation on the intensive therapy unit (ITU)) should be considered.

Admission avoidance and early supported discharge for COPD

Novel ways of managing patients with acute exacerbations of COPD are being developed. In some cases, admission to hospital can be avoided by undertaking an initial assessment in the patient's home, usually by a specialist nurse and according to an agreed protocol, with the back-up of a respiratory specialist and admission to hospital if needed. Easy access to such a reassuring review can often prevent patients from calling an ambulance unnecessarily. Such schemes are being increasingly adopted, although they are perhaps still rather probationary, with, as yet, no proven model firmly established.

For other patients, **early supported discharge** is more appropriate. This involves providing ongoing care in the patient's own home, after initial treatment and stabilisation in hospital. Early supported discharge is now well established. It is safe, effective and very popular with patients.

Both of these models of care are very cost-effective compared with a standard, prolonged hospital admission. Their safety and success are entirely dependent on the expertise and experience of the staff delivering care.

Respiratory emergencies COPD

Tests

Chest X-ray, oximetry, arterial blood gases, ECG, sputum culture, blood count, urea, electrolytes

Treatment

- **Bronchodilators.** For example, nebulised **salbutamol** 2.5–5.0 mg and **ipratropium** 500 mcg; repeat as needed and continue 4–6 hourly.

- **Steroids. Prednisolone** 30 mg/day orally for 5 days.
- **Antibiotics.** For example, **doxycycline** 200 mg followed by 100 mg o.d. orally. Check previous sputum microbiology and consider ciprofloxacin, clarithromycin or co-amoxiclav, if needed.
- **Oxygen.** Aim for O_2 saturation 88–92%, unless and until hypercapnia is excluded on arterial blood gases.
- **Ventilatory support. NIV** if hypercapnic with pH <7.35 or endotracheal ventilation in ITU, if appropriate.

🔑 KEY POINTS

- Smoking-related COPD is a major cause of morbidity and mortality worldwide.
- Spirometry is essential in assessing airway obstruction (FEV_1/VC ratio < 0.7) in COPD.
- Smoking cessation is the most important intervention. It can slow the rate of progression of COPD.
- COPD is an eminently treatable condition.
- Inhaled β_2-agonist and LAMA bronchodilators improve symptoms, exercise capacity and quality of life.
- Combination inhalers and LAMAs can reduce exacerbations and hospitalisations in moderate to severe disease.
- During exacerbations of COPD, patients who remain hypercapnic and acidotic (pH <7.35) despite nebulised bronchodilators, systemic steroids, antibiotics and controlled oxygen therapy should be treated with NIV.
- Pulmonary rehabilitation improves the patient's physical and social performance and quality of life and, if delivered early, can reduce future admissions.
- Long-term oxygen therapy at home improves the prognosis of patients with COPD who have persistent hypoxia (Po_2 < 7.3 kPa (55 mmHg)).

📖 FURTHER READING

British Thoracic Society Standards of Care Committee. Managing passengers with respiratory disease planning air travel. *Thorax* 2002; **57**: 289–304 (2011 update available from https://www.brit-thoracic.org.uk/document-library/clinical-information/air-travel/bts-air-travel-recommendations-2011/, last accessed 29 December 2014).

British Thoracic Society Standards of Care Committee. Non-invasive ventilation in acute respiratory failure. *Thorax* 2002; **57**: 192–211.

British Thoracic Society Standards of Care Committee. Guideline for emergency oxygen use in adult patients. *Thorax* 2008; **63**(Suppl. VI): 1–81.

British Thoracic Society Standards of Care Committee Intermediate Care. Hospital-at-home in chronic obstructive pulmonary disease guideline. *Thorax* 2007; **63**(Suppl. 3): 200–10.

Celli BR, MacNee W. Standards for the diagnosis and treatment of patients with COPD: a summary of the ATS/ERS position paper. *Eur Respir J* 2004; **23**: 932–46.

Department of Health. Home oxygen services (https://www.gov.uk/government/publications/home-oxygen-services, last accessed 29 December 2014).

Fletcher C, Peto R. The natural history of chronic airflow obstruction. *BMJ* 1977; **1**: 1645.

National Institute for Health and Care Excellence (NICE). *Chronic Obstructive Pulmonary Disease: Management of Chronic Obstructive Pulmonary Disease in Adults in Primary and Secondary Care (2010)*. London: NICE, 2010 (http://guidance.nice.org.uk/CG101/Guidance/pdf/English, last accessed 29 December 2014).

Ram FSF, Wedzicha JA, Wright J, Greenstone M. Hospital at home for patients with acute exacerbations of chronic obstructive pulmonary disease: systematic review of evidence. *BMJ* 2004; **329**: 315.

Royal College of Physicians, British Thoracic Society, Intensive Care Society. The Guideline Development Group. *Non-Invasive Ventilation in Chronic Obstructive Pulmonary Disease: Management of Acute Type 2 Respiratory Failure*. Concise Guidance to Good Practice Series No 11. London: Royal College of Physicians, 2008 (https://www.rcplondon.ac.uk/resources/concise-guidelines-non-invasive-ventilation-chronic-obstructive-pulmonary-disease, last accessed 29 December 2014).

Multiple choice questions

11.1 The physiological changes typically seen in COPD are:

A FEV_1 reduced, TLco normal, Kco reduced

B FEV_1/FVC reduced, FEV_1 normal, FVC normal

C FVC reduced, TLC increased, RV increased

D FEV_1/FVC reduced, TLC reduced, RV reduced

E FEV_1/FVC reduced, FEV_1 reduced, TLco normal

11.2 The pathological changes typically seen in COPD are:

A chronic bronchitis, principally affecting the distal airways

B emphysema, resulting in increased elastic recoil of the lung

C airway inflammation, causing airway obstruction

D emphysema, perhaps showing some recovery with smoking cessation

E emphysema independent of airway obstruction

11.3 In relation to oxygen therapy in COPD:

A Long-term oxygen therapy can extend life

B Long-term oxygen therapy can slow the progression of COPD

C Most patients experiencing limiting dyspnoea will benefit from ambulatory oxygen

D Short-burst oxygen therapy is only used in the terminal stages of the disease

E In an acute exacerbation, oxygen should be delivered to achieve a saturation >94%

11.4 In the management of COPD, the following cannot be achieved by some intervention:

A spirometry (FEV_1/VC ratio)

B improved mortality (extension of life)

C disease modification (slowing of the decline in FEV_1)

D frequency of exacerbations

E exercise tolerance

11.5 In relation to epidemiology, current evidence is best reflected by the statement:

A COPD was a disease of the 20th century and the global prevalence is now falling in association with changes in smoking patterns

B COPD affects all socioeconomic groups equally

C most COPD in the industrial world is caused by occupational exposures and air pollution

D in the UK, COPD affects urban more than rural populations

E most smokers develop COPD

11.6 In the aetiology of COPD:

A tobacco smoke is the only cause

B asbestos exposure can be a potent factor

C susceptibility to tobacco smoke follows an autosomal recessive inheritance

D occupation is irrelevant

E air pollution is a major contributory factor

11.7 In the natural history of COPD:

A symptoms are usually evident once modest changes in lung function are present

B the rate of decline in FEV is essentially the same for all smokers

C stopping smoking will allow normalisation of lung function

D if smoking cessation is achieved before the age of 35, there will be no discernible damage

E after smoking cessation, there will be no further decline in lung function

11.8 The following are critical to the diagnosis of COPD:

A (personal) clinical history

B lung function

C family history

D chest X-ray

E CT scan

11.9 In COPD, the following interventions have a disease-modifying effect (slowing the rate of FEV1 decline):

A long-acting muscarinic antagonists

B inhaled corticosteroids

C smoking cessation

D long-term oxygen therapy

E exercise

11.10 In COPD, pulmonary rehabilitation can:

A improve lung function

B increase exercise tolerance

C reduce breathlessness

D reduce the risk of hospitalisation

E improve oxygenation

Multiple choice answers

11.1 C

TLco is reduced, FEV_1 is reduced, FVC is usually also reduced (although not as much as FEV_1)

11.2 C

Chronic bronchitis principally affects the larger airways. Emphysema results in reduced elastic recoil. Airway inflammation, in conjunction with emphysema and chronic bronchitis, contributes to airway obstruction. Emphysema is permanent.

11.3 A

Long-term oxygen therapy can extend life in severe disease associated with hypoxia by slowing the progression of cor pulmonale. It has no effect on the progression of COPD (FEV_1 decline). Many breathless patients are not hypoxic; supplemental oxygen is of no benefit to them. Short-burst oxygen is often used as a 'palliative' measure but is not confined to the terminal stages of the disease. Emergency oxygen should be delivered to achieve a saturation of 88–92% pending arterial blood gas assessment.

11.4 All of them

Bronchodilators work in COPD (but not as dramatically as in asthma). Long-term oxygen therapy extends life. The rate of decline of FEV1 will be slowed by smoking cessation. ICS/LABA combination inhalers and tiotropium reduce exacerbation frequency. Many interventions, including pulmonary rehabilitation, improve exercise tolerance.

11.5 D

The global prevalence if COPD is increasing. COPD affects lower socioeconomic groups more than others – largely due to smoking prevalence. Smoking is the main cause of COPD in the developed world, although only about 15% of smokers will develop the condition.

11.6 None

Tobacco smoke is the most important cause of COPD in the developed world, but in the developing world biomass fuel use may be even more important. Asbestos exposure can cause many chest diseases (Chapter 14) but COPD isn't one of them. Susceptibility runs in families but is generally polygenic. Occupations associated with smoke and dust are associated with increased risk. Air pollution in general plays a small role.

11.7 None

Severe airway obstruction may be present before the patient is 'aware' of symptoms. Lung function decline varies considerably based on susceptibility. Stopping smoking halts the rapid decline in lung function but the damage is done and is permanent. Even after stopping, lung function will continue to decline at (something like) the natural age-related rate. Damage starts when smoking starts – there is nothing magic about the age of 35 (see Figure 11.3).

11.8 A,B

11.9 C

Smoking cessation is the only proven disease modifier.

11.10 B,C,D

If rehab is delivered early after a hospital admission for an exacerbation, it can reduce the risk of readmission.

12

Carcinoma of the lung

Introduction

Lung cancer is the most common cause of cancer death in the world, with more than 1 million deaths occurring annually. In the UK, it kills about 35 000 people each year and it has overtaken breast cancer as the leading cause of cancer deaths in women. It is a lethal disease, with only 25% of patients surviving 1 year and only 7% surviving 5 years from diagnosis. About 90% of lung cancers are caused by smoking, and smoking prevention and smoking cessation are the crucial issues in dealing with this major public health problem.

Aetiology

The epidemic spread of lung cancer in the 20th century came about 20 years after increases in **tobacco-smoking** habits. The commercial manufacture of cigarettes started around 1900 and smoking soon became popular among men. At that time, lung cancer was a very rare disease. By the end of the 1940s, about 70% of men and 40% of women smoked. Doctors then started to become aware of an increasing incidence of lung cancer and noticed that the patients were smokers. By 1950, an epidemic of lung cancer had become apparent and studies, such as those of Doll and Hill in the 1950s, established the causative link between smoking and lung cancer. Doll and Hill studied the smoking habits and causes of death of UK doctors and showed a significant and steadily rising incidence of deaths from lung cancer as the amount of tobacco smoked increased. At that time, 83% of doctors smoked, but thereafter the medical profession was the first to put research into practice, by stopping smoking! In the early 1960s, the Royal College of Physicians of London and the Surgeon General of the United States published their landmark reports documenting the causal relationship between smoking and lung cancer.

The risk of death from bronchial carcinoma increases by a factor roughly equal to the number of cigarettes smoked per day. For example, a man smoking 30 cigarettes/day has over 30 times the risk of dying from lung cancer compared to a man who has never smoked. On stopping smoking, excess risk is approximately halved every 5 years thereafter. Smoking has decreased in popularity such that in the UK today, about 22% of men and 19% of women smoke, compared to 51% of men and 41% of women in 1974. Reflecting these changes, lung cancer mortality rates have fallen by about 20% over the last 40 years in the UK. Although smoking in the UK is declining, it is increasing in developing countries, so that the epidemic of smoking-related mortality and morbidity that has dominated health trends in the Western world in the 20th century may be repeated in the developing world in the 21st.

Breathing other people's tobacco smoke – **passive or environmental smoke** – is also a cause of lung cancer. For example, a woman who has never smoked has an estimated 24% greater risk of developing lung cancer if she lives with a smoker. Genetic factors may be important in determining the way individuals metabolise inhaled carcinogens or in the expression of oncogenes or tumour-suppressor genes, and a **family history** of lung cancer is a risk factor for the development of the disease. There is an increased incidence of lung cancer in patients with **diffuse lung fibrosis** such as idiopathic pulmonary fibrosis, and so-called **scar carcinomas** may occur in areas of focal fibrosis resulting from previous tuberculosis. The male to female ratio for lung cancer is now almost equal, at approximately 1.2 : 1, reflecting past trends in smoking prevalence. Smoking and lung cancer are both associated with **social deprivation**.

Respiratory Medicine Lecture Notes, Ninth Edition. Stephen J. Bourke and Graham P. Burns.
© 2015 John Wiley & Sons, Ltd. Published 2015 by John Wiley & Sons, Ltd.
Companion Website: www.lecturenoteseries.com/Respiratory

Table 12.1 Aetiology of carcinoma of the lung

- Tobacco smoking
- Passive smoking
- Genetic factors
- Ionising radiation (e.g. radon gas)
- Asbestos exposure
- Diffuse lung fibrosis (e.g. fibrosing alveolitis)
- Lack of dietary fruit and vegetables

Some studies suggest that a high dietary intake of fruit and vegetables containing β-carotene reduces the risk of lung cancer. Exposure to **ionising radiation** such as that from radon gas arising from the ground and from building materials in some homes may be important and accounts for a proportion of lung cancers in nonsmokers. Occupational exposure to **asbestos** is associated with an increased risk of lung cancer, with an approximately linear relationship between the dose of asbestos and the occurrence of lung cancer. The interaction between asbestos and smoking is multiplicative.

Table 12.1 summarises the aetiology of lung carcinoma.

Pathology

Although the pathology of lung cancer is complex (Fig. 12.1), for clinical purposes the disease is classified into two groups:

1 **Small-cell carcinoma** (15% of lung cancer).
2 **Non-small-cell carcinoma** (85%), comprising **squamous-cell carcinoma** (40%), **adenocarcinoma** (30%) and **large-cell (undifferentiated) carcinoma** (15%).

Small-cell (oat-cell) carcinoma arises from neuroendocrine cells of the bronchial tree and its endocrine potential is sometimes manifest clinically by ectopic hormone production. This is a highly malignant cancer that grows rapidly and metastasises early. Squamous-cell carcinoma is the most common type of lung cancer and shows the greatest tendency to cavitate. The incidence of adenocarcinomas seems to be rising and is currently about 30%. These tumours often arise in the periphery of the lung, sometimes as 'scar carcinomas', and show the least relationship to smoking. About 13% of lung cancers do not show squamous or glandular differentiation and are classified as large-cell undifferentiated carcinomas.

Diagnosis

Lung cancers arising centrally in the bronchial tree often present with **chest symptoms** (e.g. haemoptysis), whereas peripheral tumours may grow silently without causing local symptoms until late in the course of the disease (Fig. 12.2). Such tumours may be found coincidentally on a **chest X-ray** or present with nonspecific **general symptoms** (e.g. weight loss), with effects of **metastases** (e.g. to brain, bone) or with nonmetastatic **paraneoplastic syndromes**.

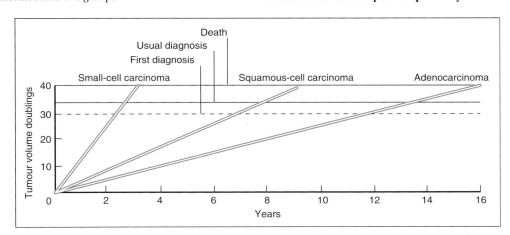

Figure 12.1 Lung cancer growth rates. As a rough approximation, small-cell carcinomas double monthly, squamous-cell carcinomas 3-monthly and certain adenocarcinomas 6-monthly. A tumour typically becomes evident on a chest X-ray when it reaches about 1 cm in diameter, corresponding to about 30 doubling volumes. Symptoms usually arise later than this. By 40 doublings, death will usually have occurred. Diagnosis occurs late in the course of the disease and most of the tumour's life history is subclinical.

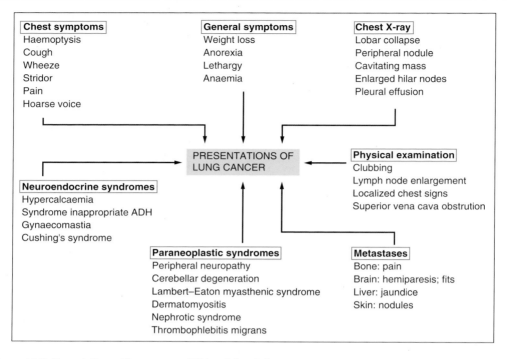

Figure 12.2 Presentations of lung cancer. ADH, antidiuretic hormone.

Paraneoplastic syndromes arise at sites distant from the tumour or its metastases and result from the production of hormones, peptides, antibodies, prostaglandins or cytokines by the tumour. The **syndrome of inappropriate antidiuretic hormone (ADH) secretion** is most common with small-cell cancer and results in a low serum sodium, potassium and urea, a serum osmolarity below 280 mosmol/l and a urine osmolarity greater than 500 mosmol/l. Treatment consists of restriction of fluid intake and drugs such as tolvaptan (a vasopressin receptor antagonist) 15–60 mg/day or demeclocycline (which competes for ADH renal tubular binding sites) 600–1200 mg/day. **Hypercalcaemia** in patients with lung cancer may be indicative of bone metastases, but squamous-cell carcinomas sometimes secrete a parathyroid hormone-related protein that causes nonmetastatic hypercalcaemia. Clearly, some patients will present primarily with chest symptoms, often against a background of pre-existing smoking-related lung disease (e.g. chronic obstructive pulmonary disease, COPD). Equally, a diagnosis of lung cancer must be considered in patients presenting with a variety of medical problems.

Tumours in certain specific locations may cause problems by direct invasion of adjacent structures.

Direct invasion of the mediastinum can cause paralysis of the **phrenic nerve**, manifest by elevation of the hemidiaphragm, or of the **recurrent laryngeal nerve**, particularly on the left side, where it passes around the aortic arch to the superior mediastinum, causing vocal cord palsy with hoarseness and diminished cough reflex. Injection of Teflon or Bioplastique into the paralysed vocal cord under general anaesthesia can improve voice quality by building up the volume of the vocal cord, enabling better apposition. **Obstruction of the superior vena cava** causes venous engorgement of the upper body with facial oedema, headache, distended pulseless jugular veins and enlarged collateral veins over the chest and arms. These symptoms require urgent treatment by chemotherapy in the case of small-cell cancer or radiotherapy in the case of other tumours. Insertion of an expandable metallic wire stent into the strictured vein under radiological guidance can give rapid relief of symptoms in severe cases. A **Pancoast tumour** (Fig. 12.3) is a carcinoma situated in the superior sulcus of the lung, where the subclavian artery forms a groove over the lung apex. Because of its particular anatomical location, a tumour here gives rise to a characteristic syndrome: ipsilateral Horner's syndrome (ptosis, meiosis, enophthalmos, anhydrosis).

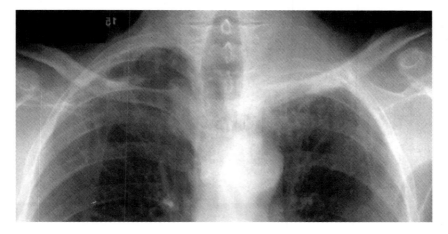

Figure 12.3 Pancoast tumour. This 68-year-old man presented with a 3-month history of left shoulder pain. On examination, he had features of a left Horner's syndrome (ptosis, meiosis, enophthalmos, anhydrosis). The chest X-ray shows a mass at the apex of the left lung eroding the first and second ribs posteriorly. Percutaneous biopsy showed squamous-cell carcinoma. He was treated with palliative radiotherapy.

Anhydrosis is due to stellate ganglion involvement, with pain resulting from erosion of the posterior first and second ribs and wasting of the small muscles of the hand due to brachial plexus invasion. The tumour may invade a vertebral foramen, giving spinal cord compression. These tumours are notoriously difficult to detect on a chest X-ray and the cause of the patient's pain is often misdiagnosed initially.

The chest X-ray plays a pivotal role in the investigation of lung cancer, and a range of abnormalities may be apparent. A peripheral tumour may be seen as a small nodule or mass in the lung. A cavitating mass is characteristic of squamous-cell carcinoma (Fig. 4.8). Central tumours may cause bronchial obstruction, typically giving rise to atelectatic collapse of a lung or lobe of a lung (Fig. 12.4), or to pneumonic consolidation distal to the obstruction. Thus, 'loss of volume' of a lobe (atelectatic collapse) on a chest X-ray in a patient with apparent pneumonia is a sinister feature, suggesting bronchial obstruction by a carcinoma. The chest X-ray may show evidence of spread of the tumour to bone (e.g. rib or vertebral destruction), pleura (e.g. effusion), hilar or mediastinal structures. **Computed tomography (CT) scanning** is the next key investigation in defining the extent and spread of the tumour and in planning the best approach to obtaining histological diagnosis.

Histological–cytological diagnosis should be obtained wherever possible. **Sputum cytology** is positive in about 40% of cases, and is particularly useful in patients unfit for invasive tests. **Bronchoscopy** allows direct visualisation and biopsy of central tumours. Peripheral tumours seen on chest X-ray may not be accessible to bronchoscopy and **percutaneous needle biopsy** of these lesions under radiological guidance is a useful technique (Fig. 12.5). Small peripheral cancers need to be distinguished from rare benign tumours (e.g. hamartomas) and from inflammatory nodules, but it may be advisable to proceed to surgical resection without histological confirmation of the diagnosis if the risk of cancer is high and if the nodule shows a high level of metabolic activity on positron emission tomography (PET) or is enlarging on serial CT scans. Diagnosis may also be achieved by obtaining material from a site of metastasis (e.g. lymph node, skin, pleural effusion).

Studies of **screening for lung cancer with low-dose CT** have been undertaken and show a reduction in the mortality from the disease in selected populations of smokers with early detection and treatment. However, there are concerns about the potential harm from radiation dose and from the investigation and treatment of 'false-positive' benign nodules.

Bronchoscopy

Flexible fibreoptic bronchoscopy is usually performed as an outpatient procedure under sedation (e.g. midazolam) and topical anaesthesia (e.g. lidocaine to the vocal cords and airways). The bronchoscope is usually passed through the nose into the orophayrynx, and then through the vocal cords into the trachea and bronchial tree to the subsegmental

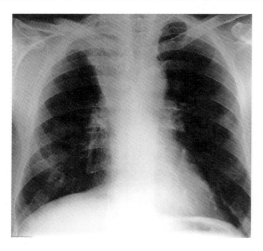

Figure 12.4 Right upper lobe collapse. This 65-year-old smoker presented with haemoptysis. The chest X-ray shows a triangular-shaped opacity in the right upper zone, indicating collapse of the right upper lobe. Bronchoscopy showed a tumour occluding the orifice to the right upper lobe and biopsy showed a large-cell undifferentiated carcinoma. CT showed that the tumour was confined to the right upper lobe without mediastinal invasion or metastases. He was treated by right upper lobectomy. Coincidentally, the X-ray also shows an old un-united fracture of the right clavicle.

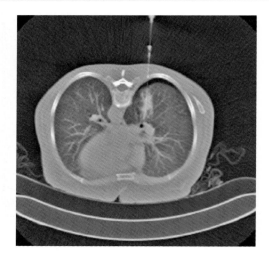

Figure 12.5 This 66-year-old smoker was found to have a mass in the periphery of the lung when an X-ray was performed during an exacerbation of COPD. Percutaneous fine-needle aspiration of the lesion was performed under CT guidance and showed adenocarcinoma on cytology. The procedure caused a small pneumothorax, which resolved spontaneously without the need for intervention.

level. The bronchial tree is illuminated by light transmitted from a light source to the tip of the bronchoscope and the image is transmitted to the eyepiece or displayed on a screen. About two-thirds of lung cancers are visible through the bronchoscope, and therefore bronchoscopy is a key investigation for lung cancer or haemoptysis. A biopsy forceps or cytology brush may be passed through the channel to obtain samples from a tumour, and saline washings can be aspirated for cytology or microbiology tests (Fig. 13.1). Bronchoscopy is a very safe procedure but is contraindicated in patients with uncontrolled angina or recent myocardial infarction. Sedation should be avoided or used with particular caution in patients with respiratory depression. Pulse oximetry is used to monitor oxygen saturation and supplemental oxygen is given. The bronchoscope is carefully cleaned with detergent and immersed in glutaraldehyde to prevent transmission of infection between patients. It is recommended that the bronchoscopist and nurses should wear masks, goggles and gowns in order to prevent contraction of infections (e.g. tuberculosis) from the patient through aerosols generated by coughing.

Endobronchial ultrasound (EBUS) allows needle aspiration to be performed on mediastinal lymph nodes (e.g. subcarinal, paratracheal nodes) and on tumours causing extrinsic compression of bronchi, through ultrasound guidance via a specially designed bronchoscope. It is a very useful technique in the diagnosis and staging of lung cancer. Ultrasound needle biopsy of small supraclavicular nodes is also a useful, minimally invasive method of obtaining cytology. About 50% of patients with mediastinal adenopathy on CT scan will also have small pathological supraclavicular nodes that can be detected and aspirated using ultrasound.

Communicating the diagnosis

Telling patients they have been diagnosed with lung cancer is a difficult clinical skill that needs to be developed through training and experience. Patients want to talk honestly about what is happening to them and to know what is in store for them in the future. Their awareness of the diagnosis often emerges over a number of consultations, and the time that elapses between initial suspicion of tumour and histological confirmation of the diagnosis is often useful in allowing the patient an opportunity to come to terms with the situation. When discussing the diagnosis, it is essential to allow adequate time for questions, to ensure privacy during the interview, to encourage a relative or friend to accompany the patient for support and to have further counselling available from skilled nurses. Some patients may find written information about lung cancer and its treatment useful.

Inevitably, patients will experience such emotions as shock, anger and denial, and the doctor must work through these with them. It is a good idea to try to bring the interview to a conclusion on a relatively positive note by discussing a management plan. Many patients will initially be too shocked to understand the information given and it is often useful to arrange a further interview with either the hospital doctor, a nurse or a general practitioner to answer the patient's questions. Rapid communication between all members of the medical team is crucial in these circumstances.

Treatment

Treatment depends on the histological **cell type**, the **stage** of the disease and the **fitness** of the patient (Fig. 12.6). The management plan is discussed by the **multidisciplinary team** following a review of the patient's radiological, histopathological and clinical details.

Small-cell carcinoma (15%)

Small-cell carcinoma is a highly malignant cancer that has usually disseminated widely by the time of diagnosis, such that systemic treatment in the form of **chemotherapy** is required. On rare occasions, when small-cell carcinoma is diagnosed by surgical resection of a peripheral nodule, adjuvant chemotherapy is given postoperatively. Various combinations of chemotherapeutic agents are available, using drugs such as carboplatin, cisplatin, etoposide, cyclophosphamide, doxorubicin, vincristine, gemcitabine, vinorelbine, irinotecan and taxanes (paclitaxel, docetaxel). Combinations of these drugs (e.g. carboplatin and etoposide) are usually given as a day treatment in pulses at intervals of about 4 weeks for up to six cycles of treatment. Untreated patients with small-cell carcinoma are usually very symptomatic, with a median survival of only 3 months. Combination chemotherapy achieves a symptom-relieving remission of the cancer in about 70% of patients, with reduction in tumour size and prolongation of survival. Small-cell cancer may be staged using the TNM system (based upon the size, location and degree of invasion of the tumour (T), the presence of regional lymph node involvement (N) and distant metastases (M)) but is often described as **limited stage disease** when it can be encompassed within a 'tolerable' radiotherapy port (involving one hemithorax, including ipsilateral mediastinal, subcarinal and supraclavicular nodes or contralateral hilar nodes) or as **extensive stage disease** when it has spread beyond a radiotherapy port (distant metastases or spread beyond one hemithorax). In limited stage disease, chemotherapy improves survival from an average of 3 months without treatment to 12 months with treatment, and 5–10% of patients achieve a 5-year survival. In extensive stage disease, chemotherapy improves survival from an average of 6 weeks to 8 months. **Consolidation radiotherapy** is usually given to the site of the tumour and mediastinal nodes. Cerebral metastases are common, so that prophylactic cranial radiotherapy is also given to patients with limited disease who have responded to chemotherapy. Patients receiving chemotherapy require careful monitoring of their full blood count to avoid problems arising from bone marrow suppression, such as anaemia, haemorrhage or infection. Hair loss occurs with some drugs and patients may choose to wear a wig. Careful attention to anti-emetic medications (e.g. ondansetron, domperidone, metoclopramide) can usually prevent nausea and vomiting.

Non-small-cell carcinoma (85%)

Surgical resection of the tumour offers the best chance of cure in non-small-cell carcinoma but is only possible if the patient is fit for surgery and if the tumour has not already metastasised. **Staging** (Table 12.2) is the assessment of the extent and spread of the disease and is important in determining the potential resectability of the tumour and the prognosis of the patient. The TNM system is the most widely used. The accuracy of staging depends on the degree of assessment; for example, staging at thoracotomy may show more advanced disease than was apparent on CT scanning.

When staging a tumour, the patient's **symptoms** should be carefully reviewed for any indication of metastatic disease (e.g. bone pain). Clinical **examination** may show evidence of tumour spread to lymph nodes or reveal features of distant metastases. **Bronchoscopy** allows direct visualisation of many tumours and may show features of inoperability (e.g. vocal

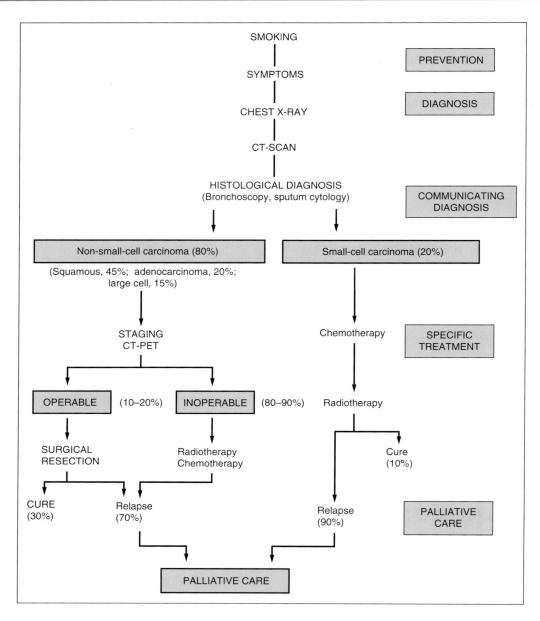

Figure 12.6 The 5-year mortality rate of lung cancer is about 93%, emphasising the fact that the disease is usually disseminated at the time of presentation. Prevention by avoidance of smoking is the most important strategy in the fight against lung cancer. Choice of treatment depends on cell type and stage of disease. About 15% of lung cancers are small-cell carcinomas and are best treated by chemotherapy followed by radiotherapy. There is usually a good response to chemotherapy, but relapse is likely. About 85% are non-small-cell carcinomas and require careful staging and assessment for potential operability. About 10–20% of non-small-cell carcinomas are suitable for surgery but only 30% of patients undergoing resection will be alive in 5 years. A judicious plan of assessment allows careful selection of the best choice of specific anticancer treatment, with either curative or palliative intent. Symptom relief and palliative care are crucial aspects in the overall management, and the communication of information between doctor and patient at all stages of the disease is of paramount importance. CT, computed tomography; PET, positron emission tomography.

Table 12.2 Outline of the main examples of TNM staging of non-small-cell lung cancer

Stage	TNM			Operability	5-year survival (%)
IA	$T_{1a,b}$	N_0	M_0		70%
IB	T_{2a}	N_0	M_0		50%
IIA	$T_{1a,b}$	N_1	M_0	Resectable	
	T_{2a}	N_1	M_0		45%
	T_{2b}	N_0	M_0		
IIB	T_{2b}	N_1	M_0	Resectable	30%
IIB	T_3	N_0	M_0		
IIIA	T_1, T_2	N_2	M_0		
	T_3	N_1	M_0	Not-resectable	<10%
	T_4	N_0, N_1	M_0	(chemo/radiotherapy)	
IIIB	T_4	N_2	M_0		
	Any T	N_3	M_0		
IV	Any T	Any N	M_1		0%

Tumour (T)

T_1 Tumour <3cm without invasion more proximal than a lobar bronchus

T_{1a} Tumour <2cm

T_{1b} Tumour >2cm <3cm

T_2 Tumour>3cm <7 cm, or tumour involving main bronchus (but more than 2 cm away from carina), or invading visceral pleura

T_{2a} Tumour >3cm <5cm

T_{2b} Tumour >5cm <7cm

T_3 Tumour>7cmor invading chest wall, diaphragm, phrenic nerve, mediastinal pleura or within 2 cm of carina or separate tumour nodule in same lobe

T_4 Tumour of any size invading mediastinum, heart, great vessels, trachea, recurrent laryngeal nerve,

oesophagus, vertebrae, carina; separate tumour nodule in different ipsilateral lobe

Nodes (N)

N_0 No node metastasis

N_1 Metastasis in ipsilateral bronchial or hilar nodes

N_2 Metastasis in ipsilateral mediastinal or subcarinal nodes

N_3 Metastasis in contralateral mediastinal, hilar or supraclavicular nodes

Metastasis (M)

M_0 No distant metastasis

M_1 Distant metastasis

Carcinomas that are stage I or IIA are treated by surgical resection with curative intent, if the patient is fit for surgery. Some tumours that are Stage IIb have poor results when surgery is attempted. Sometimes the tumour is up-staged after surgery when histology shows more extensive disease, and adjuvant chemotherapy may be used. Carcinomas that are stage III or IV are not suitable for surgery, but may be suitable for treatment with chemotherapy and radiotherapy with palliative intent.

cord palsy, splaying of the carina by subcarinal lymphadenopathy or extension of the tumour to within 2 cm of the main carina). Elevated liver function tests or bone **biochemistry** is an indication for imaging of the liver by ultrasound or CT scans and of bone by isotope scans. CT scanning is the key investigation in staging lung cancer, particularly in assessing mediastinal invasion by the tumour and involvement of hilar and mediastinal nodes. Enlarged (>1 cm) lymph nodes are suggestive of malignant involvement, but if the tumour otherwise appears operable, **PET** (see Chapter 4) is undertaken to assess active disease in mediastinal nodes and to detect distant metastases. Biopsy of the mediastinal nodes may then be undertaken by **mediastinosopy** or by **endobronchial ultrasound**-guided needle aspiration.

- **Surgery.** Only about 10–20% of non-small-cell carcinomas are suitable for surgical resection, because of the advanced stage of the disease at diagnosis. The decision concerning the **patient's fitness** to undergo resection of the tumour is based principally upon the lung function tests and the patient's general fitness. Unfortunately, these patients often have substantial cardiovascular disease and smoking-related COPD. No single test predicts the feasibility of surgical resection and greater risks may be justified for a tumour that is otherwise curable by resection, but a forced expiratory volume in 1 second (FEV_1) < 50% of predicted or the presence of hypoxaemia (Po_2 < 8 kPa (60 mmHg)) would suggest that the patient is not fit for thoracotomy. Lobectomy has a 30-day mortality of about 3%, compared to 8% for pneumonectomy. Mortality and morbidity increase with age. Surgery typically achieves a 70% 5-year survival in patients with stage IA ($T_1N_0M_0$) disease, a 40% 5-year survival in stage IB ($T_2N_0M_0$) disease and a 25% 5-year survival in stage 2 (T_{1-2},N_1M_0) disease. **Adjuvant chemotherapy** (i.e. post-surgery) can improve survival rates by about 4% at 5 years in selected patients.
- **Radiotherapy.** Radiation treatment is chiefly undertaken for the relief of symptoms. Superior vena caval obstruction (SVCO), lobar collapse from bronchial obstruction, haemoptysis and chest wall pain usually respond well to radiotherapy. Radical radiotherapy, using larger doses, is occasionally used with curative intent for small localised tumours that are not treatable by surgery due to poor patient fitness. This sometimes involves continuous hyperfractionated accelerated radiotherapy (**CHART**), with fractions of radiotherapy being given at 8-hour intervals in a concentrated fashion. **Stereotactic radiotherapy** involves giving

Table 12.3 **World Health Organization performance status scale. Patients with performance status 3 or 4 are usually regarded as not being fit enough to tolerate chemotherapy**

WHO Performance Status

0: Fully active

1: Restricted on strenuous activity but ambulatory and able to do light work

2: Ambulatory for >50% of day, able to self-care but unable to work

3: In bed or chair >50% of day, unable to care for self

4: Confined to bed or chair, unable to self-care

very high-dose radiation to a very precisely targeted area. It is mainly used to treat patients with localised non-small-cell carcinoma who are not fit to undergo surgical resection of the tumour.

- **Chemotherapy.** Chemotherapy can improve the survival and quality of life of some patients with advanced non-small-cell lung cancer. First-line chemotherapy typically consists of cisplatin or carboplatin combined with gemcitabine, paclitaxel or vinorelbine. Docetaxel may be used as second-line therapy when relapse occurs after previous chemotherapy, although a variety of regimens are available. For patients with advanced (stage III or IV) non-small-cell cancer who are fit to undergo chemotherapy (Table 12.3), treatment on average extends survival by about 2 months, improving 1-year survival from 5% to 25%. The role of chemotherapy before (neoadjuvant) and after (adjuvant) surgery is being studied in ongoing clinical trials.

Advances in the understanding of cancer cell biology have led to new treatments. Overexpression of the **epidermal growth factor receptor** (EGFR) is a feature of some non-small-cell lung cancers. Geftinib and erlotinib are oral EGFR inhibitors that have demonstrated antitumour activity in patients with non-small-cell lung cancer who have failed to respond to chemotherapy. The best results have been seen in women with adenocarcinoma who are nonsmokers.

Palliative care

Palliative care focuses on improving the patient's functioning and psychosocial well-being through relief of symptoms. Even when the disease cannot be cured, rapid assessment and diagnosis is important in addressing the patient's symptoms and anxieties. Regular review of patients with lung cancer is essential in providing support and in identifying the nature and origin of symptoms as they arise.

When dealing with a symptom such as pain, specific anticancer treatment (e.g. radiotherapy) is often the most effective method of symptom relief. Where there is persistent pain, analgesics need to be given regularly and prophylactically in advance of its return. Mild pain may be treated by a **non-opioid analgesic** (e.g. a nonsteroidal anti-inflammatory drug (NSAID) or paracetamol). More severe pain may be treated by a combination of a **weak opioid** (e.g. codeine) and a non-opioid (e.g. naproxen) drug. **Strong opioids** should be used immediately for any severe pain. Often, pain control is achieved by use of slow-release morphine tablets 12-hourly, with additional use of morphine solution for any breakthrough pain. Certain types of pain may benefit from the use of **co-analgesics**, such as steroids (e.g. dexamethasone for nerve compression), benzodiazepines (anxiolytic), tricyclic antidepressants or anti-epileptics (e.g. gabapentin or pregabalin for neuropathic pain). Whenever opiates are prescribed, it is necessary to prescribe a laxative (e.g. co-danthramer) to prevent constipation, and an anti-emetic (e.g. metoclopramide) may be required initially.

Anorexia, weight loss, fatigue and general debility are common in the advanced stages of lung cancer. It is important to check for conditions requiring specific treatment, such as anaemia (blood transfusion) or hypercalcaemia (pamidronate). Prednisolone may be useful in boosting appetite, and nutritional supplements may be helpful. Attention needs to be given to the patient's level of social support and help often needs to be given with tasks of daily living. If control of symptoms is not being achieved, help should be sought from a specialist in palliative care.

Other thoracic neoplasms

Alveolar cell carcinoma (lepidic adenocarcinoma)

This is a rare malignant tumour that arises in the alveoli of the lung and spreads along the alveolar and bronchiolar epithelium. Histologically, it resembles adenocarcinoma. Occasionally, this tumour produces large amounts of mucin, causing copious sputum production (bronchorrhoea). On chest X-ray, it may appear as more diffuse shadowing, resembling pneumonic consolidation, rather than as a discrete mass, and it is sometimes multifocal in origin. A transbronchial biopsy of alveolar tissue is often necessary for diagnosis. When the tumour is confined to one lobe, surgical resection is the treatment of choice.

Carcinoid tumour

This rare tumour is less malignant than bronchial carcinomas in that it rarely metastasises and is often slow-growing, although it may invade locally. It is not related to smoking and often affects younger patients. It normally arises in the main bronchi and presents with haemoptysis and wheeze. At bronchoscopy, the tumour often has a smooth rounded appearance, resembling a cherry, and it may bleed profusely on biopsy because of its vascularity. Most such tumours can be cured by surgical resection. Very rarely, a carcinoid tumour of lung metastasises to the liver, where secretion of substances such as 5-hydroxy indoleacetic acid (5-HIAA) produces the carcinoid syndrome of flushing, diarrhoea and wheeze.

Respiratory emergencies Superior vena caval obstruction (SVCO)

- SVCO presents with headache, **distended neck veins** that are nonpulsatile, **oedema of the face** and arms and dilated collateral veins over the chest.
- **Lung cancer** is the most common cause of SVCO. Lymphoma, metastatic carcinoma, mediastinal tumours and thrombosis of central veins can also cause it.
- Urgent diagnosis of the underlying cause is needed to allow specific treatment. Chest X-ray and **urgent CT scan** allow a decision as to the best method of obtaining histological diagnosis.
- A short tapering course of **dexamethasone** (initially 16 mg/day) may be useful in reducing oedema and inflammation around a tumour.
- Insertion of a **metallic stent** into the compressed vein under radiological guidance can provide rapid relief of symptoms.
- Urgent **chemotherapy** for small-cell carcinoma or **radiotherapy** for non-small-cell carcinoma is likely to achieve tumour shrinkage with relief of SVCO.

- **Anticoagulation** is sometimes used to reduce thrombosis, but it carries an increased risk of haemorrhage and is usually only indicated if there is associated thrombosis in the compressed vein.

 KEY POINTS

- Lung cancer is the most common cause of cancer death, causing about 35 000 deaths each year in the UK.
- Cigarette smoking is the main cause of lung cancer.
- Non-small-cell carcinoma accounts for 85% of lung cancer cases. It is suitable for surgical resection in 10–20% of cases.
- Chemotherapy and radiotherapy improve survival and quality of life when surgery is not feasible.
- Small-cell cancer accounts for 15% of lung cancers and is treated by chemotherapy followed by radiotherapy.

 FURTHER READING

Auvinen A, Pershagen G. Indoor radon and deaths from lung cancer. *BMJ* 2009; **338**: 184–5.

Baldwin DR, Hansell DM, Duffy SW, Field JK. Lung cancer screening with low dose computed tomography. *BMJ* 2014; **348**: 9.

British Thoracic Society. Guidelines on the selection of patients with lung cancer for surgery. *Thorax* 2001; **36**: 89–108.

Doll R, Hill AB. The mortality of doctors in relation to their smoking habits. *BMJ* 1954; **i**: 1451–5.

Lababede O, Meziane M, Rice T. Seventh edition of the cancer staging manual and stage grouping of lung cancer. *Chest* 2011; **139**: 183–9.

National Institute for Health and Care Excellence (NICE). *The Diagnosis and Treatment of Lung Cancer. Clinical Guideline 24*. London: NICE, 2005 (http://guidance.nice.org.uk/CG24/Guidance/pdf/English, last accessed 29 December 2014).

Popwell CA, Halmos B, Nana-Sinkam SP. Update in lung cancer and mesothelioma. *Am J Respir Crit Care Med* 2013; **188**: 157–66.

Silvestri GA, Rivera MP. Targeted therapy for the treatment of advanced non-small cell lung cancer: a review of the epidermal growth factor receptor antagonists. *Chest* 2005; **128**: 39.

Simone CB, Wildt B, Haas AR, et al. Stereotactic body radiation therapy for lung cancer. *Chest* 2013; **143**: 1784–90.

Temel JS, Greer JA, Muzikansky A, et al. Early palliative care for patients with metastatic non-small cell lung cancer. *N Engl J Med* 2010; **363**: 733–42.

Multiple choice questions

12.1 The most common type of bronchial carcinoma is:
A squamous cell carcinoma
B small-cell carcinoma
C carcinoid tumour
D adenocarcinoma
E large-cell undifferentiated carcinoma

12.2 A 71-year-old man, who is usually fit and well, is coincidentally found to have a 2 cm mass in the periphery of the right upper lobe on a chest X-ray performed when he undergoes cholecystectomy. He is a smoker. PET/CT scan confirms avid uptake of FDG in a 2 cm mass in the right upper lobe, with no other abnormality. The features suggest a bronchial carcinoma. Confirmation of the cell type is best sought by:
A bronchoscopy
B endobronchial ultrasound-guided needle aspiration
C video-assisted thoracoscopic biopsy
D percutaneous CT-guided needle aspirate
E mediastinoscopy

12.3 A 60-year-old woman who has smoked and has mild COPD presents with swelling of her face and arms, with dilated veins over her chest wall. Chest X-ray shows a widened bulky mediastinal shadow with a 2 cm opacity in the left upper lobe. The clinical features suggest:
A dissection of the thoracic aorta
B nephrotic syndrome
C central venous thrombosis
D superior vena caval obstruction
E thymoma

12.4 A 72-year-old man is diagnosed as having a $T_1N_0M_0$ adenocarcinoma of the left upper lobe of the lung. PET/CT confirms avid uptake of FDG within the tumour, without any other abnormality. He is otherwise fit and well, with an FEV_1 of 3.21 (98% predicted) and a WHO performance status of zero. The best treatment option is:
A left pneumonectomy
B radical radiotherapy

C chemotherapy
D left upper lobectomy
E monitoring of the tumour by serial CT scans until symptoms arise

12.5 A 65-year-old woman is diagnosed as having an extensive stage small-cell carcinoma of the lung with bone metastases. After discussion, she decides upon chemotherapy as the initial treatment option. Her 5-year survival is likely to be approximately:
A 80%
B 60%
C 40%
D 20%
E 0%

12.6 The number of deaths from lung cancer in the UK each year is about:
A 10 000
B 20 000
C 25 000
D 35 000
E 50 000

12.7 A 55-year-old man who has smoked 20 cigarettes/day for 30 years has a single episode of haemoptysis. His chest X-ray is normal and he is now asymptomatic and well. The most appropriate course of action is to:
A proceed directly to bronchosopy
B undertake a CT scan
C arrange annual follow-up chest X-rays
D reassure him and discharge him from further follow-up
E arrange a PET scan

12.8 A 65-year old-woman with an adenocarcinoma of the left upper lobe of the lung and mediastinal lymphadenopathy develops hoarseness of her voice. This is most likely to indicate:
A phrenic nerve palsy
B recurrent laryngeal nerve palsy
C oropharyngeal candidiasis
D superior vena caval obstruction
E a Pancoast tumour

12.9 A patient with small-cell lung cancer develops the syndrome of inappropriate antidiuretic hormone secretion. This is:

A   usually treated by fluid restriction

B   often associated with hypercalcaemia

C   an indication of metastases to the adrenal gland

D   an indication of metastases to the pituitary gland

E   characterised by hypernatraemia

12.10 A 72-year-old man has a 2.5 cm tumour in the periphery of the left upper lobe of his lung. He has chronic low back pain due to degenerative disease of the spine. Transthoracic needle biopsy shows squamous cell carcinoma. CT and PET scans show a high level of metabolic activity in the tumour but no abnormality elsewhere. The staging of this carcinoma is:

A   T1aN0M0

B   T1bN0M0

C   T3N1M0

D   T1aN0M1

E   T2N0M1

Multiple choice answers

12.1 A

Squamous carcinoma is the most common form of lung cancer. Small-cell carcinoma accounts for approximately 20% and non-small-carcinoma for 80% (comprising squamous carcinoma, 45%, adenocarcinoma, 20%, and undifferentiated carcinoma, 15%).

12.2 D

The nodule is peripherally located such that it is not likely to be amenable to biopsy at bronchoscopy or by endobronchial ultrasound. Percutaneous fine-needle aspirate of the nodule under CT scan guidance provides the best method of seeking cytological diagnosis and is less invasive than video-assisted thoracoscopic biopsy. Mediastinoscopy gives access to the mediastinal nodes but not to nodules in the lung.

12.3 D

Obstruction of the superior vena cava causes oedema of the face, neck and arms, with dilatation of collateral veins often visible on the chest wall.

12.4 D

This patient has a stage I adenocarcinoma, which is best treated by surgical resection in the form of a left upper lobectomy. He has adequate lung function and general fitness for lobectomy. Pneumonectomy is not required to resect the tumour. Radiotherapy and chemotherapy are not appropriate, as they offer a much lower chance of cure for stage I carcinoma.

12.5 E

Small-cell carcinoma is a highly malignant cancer. She has extensive stage disease at presentation. Average survival without treatment is approximately 6 weeks, improving to 8 months with chemotherapy, but long-term survival is extremely unlikely.

12.6 D

Lung cancer kills about 35 000 people each year in the UK. It is now the most common cause of cancer death in the world.

12.7 B

Haemoptyis in a smoker is a sinister symptom that requires further investigation even if the patient is now asymptomatic and well. CT scan is much more sensitive than a chest X-ray in detecting early lung cancer. Bronchoscopy may also be needed, but CT scan should be performed first.

12.8 B

On the left side, the recurrent laryngeal nerve passes around the aortic arch, where it may be damaged by cancer that has spread to the mediastinal lymph nodes.

12.9 A

The syndrome of inappropriate antidiuretic hormone secretion is most common with small-cell cancer and results in a low serum sodium, a serum osmolarity below 280 mosml/l and a urine osmolarity greater than 500 mosmol/l. Initial treatment usually consists of fluid restriction.

12.10 B

The TNM staging system for lung cancer is based upon the size, location and degree of invasion of the primary tumour (T), the involvement of lymph nodes (N) and the presence of distant metastases (M). CT and PET scans in this patient do not show evidence of lymph node involvement or metastases (N0M0). A tumour >2 cm and <3 cm is T1b.

13

Interstitial lung disease

Introduction

Clinical presentation

'Interstitial lung disease' and 'diffuse parenchymal lung disease' are imprecise clinical terms used to refer to a diverse range of diseases that result in inflammation and fibrosis of the alveoli, distal airways and septal interstitium of the lung. Patients with these diseases typically present with progressive **breathlessness**, a dry cough, lung **crackles** and diffuse **infiltrates on chest X-ray**. Lung function tests usually show a restrictive defect (reduced total lung capacity (TLC) and vital capacity (VC)), with normal forced expiratory volume in 1 second (FEV_1)/VC ratio, **impaired gas diffusion** (reduced transfer factor) and **hypoxaemia** with hypocapnia (Table 13.1).

Differential diagnosis

At presentation, interstitial lung disease must be distinguished from a number of other diseases, such as infective pneumonia, pulmonary oedema, bronchiectasis and malignancy (e.g. lymphangitis carcinomatosa). The overall context of the disease is important and exclusion of other diseases may require further investigations (e.g. echocardiography) or observance of the response to treatment (e.g. antibiotics, diuretics). Once the clinical features suggest interstitial lung disease, a careful search for potential causes must be undertaken. Particular attention should be paid to any environmental **antigens** (e.g. budgerigar), **toxins** (e.g. paraquat) or **dusts** (e.g. asbestos) that the patient encounters in their **occupational** or **home environments**. **Systemic diseases** (e.g. rheumatoid disease) commonly involve the lung parenchyma and many **drugs** can cause lung fibrosis (e.g. amiodarone, nitrofurantoin, bleomycin) or eosinophilic reactions in the alveoli (e.g. sulphonamides, naproxen).

Investigations

After a detailed clinical assessment, chest X-ray and lung function tests, the next key investigation is high-resolution computed tomography (CT), which gives precise information about the extent and pattern of the disease. In many cases, this allows a diagnosis to be made with reasonable certainty, but it may sometimes be useful to proceed to biopsy of the lung parenchyma in order to study the histological pattern of the disease. Small samples can be obtained by **transbronchial biopsy** of the lung parenchyma through a flexible bronchoscope (Fig. 13.1). Larger samples can be obtained by **surgical biopsy** under general anaesthesia by **video-assisted thoracoscopy**. In many cases, the histological features are characteristic of a particular disease (e.g. granulomas in sarcoidosis or extrinsic allergic alveolitis; tumour cells in lymphangitis carcinomatosa), but in advanced disease the histology may show established lung fibrosis without clues to its aetiology. **Bronchoalveolar lavage** may be performed through the bronchoscope at the same time as transbronchial biopsy. Aliquots of saline are instilled via the bronchoscope, which is held in a wedged position in a subsegmental bronchus, and fluid is then aspirated for cell analysis. A lymphocytic alveolitis is characteristic of sarcoidosis, for example. Some of these diseases are characterised in their early stages by an inflammatory alveolitis, which is responsive to corticosteroids, whereas in the later stages there may be irreversible lung fibrosis. Careful clinical investigation of patients presenting with features of interstitial lung disease aims to move from this imprecise clinical label to a diagnosis of a specific disease process (Fig. 13.2).

Respiratory Medicine Lecture Notes, Ninth Edition. Stephen J. Bourke and Graham P. Burns.
© 2015 John Wiley & Sons, Ltd. Published 2015 by John Wiley & Sons, Ltd.
Companion Website: www.lecturenoteseries.com/Respiratory

Table 13.1 Clinical features of airway disease and interstitial lung disease. Some lung diseases, such as asthma and chronic obstructive pulmonary disease (COPD), affect the airways, and are characterised by wheeze and an obstructive pattern on spirometry (reduced FEV_1/VC ratio). Interstitial lung disease affects the alveoli and lung parenchyma and is characterised by progressive dyspnoea, crackles and a restriction of lung volumes. Gas diffusion measurements (transfer factor for carbon monoxide ($T_L co$) and transfer coefficient (Kco)) are a measure of parenchymal lung function: they are normal or elevated in asthma, but are reduced in emphysema (where there is destruction of the lung parenchyma) and in interstitial lung disease. In emphysema, the chest X-ray typically shows hyperinflated clear lungs, whereas in interstitial lung disease, the chest X-ray typically shows small lungs with reticular infiltrates

	Airway disease	Interstitial disease
Example	COPD, asthma	Lung fibrosis
Risk factors	Smoking	Environmental exposures
Symptoms	Wheeze	Progressive dyspnoea
Signs	Wheeze, hyperinflation	Crackles
Chest X-ray	Hyperinflated clear lungs	Small lungs with reticular infiltrates
FEV_1/VC	Obstructive	Restrictive
Kco, $T_L co$	Reduced in emphysema Elevated in asthma	Reduced
PaO_2	Low	Low
$PaCO_2$	High	Low

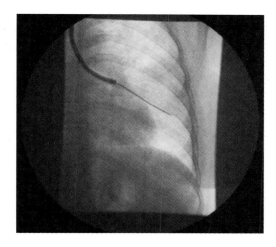

Figure 13.1 Transbronchial lung biopsy. A small specimen of lung parenchyma can be obtained by passing a biopsy forceps through a flexible bronchoscope, usually under radiological guidance, into the lung periphery. A sample of lung tissue is obtained by biopsying between two limbs in a branching small bronchus. There is a small risk of causing haemorrhage or pneumothorax, so the patient's condition and lung function should be adequate to tolerate these complications.

Idiopathic pulmonary fibrosis

Idiopathic pulmonary fibrosis (IPF) is the classic example of a diffuse fibrotic lung disease. About 5000 new cases of IPF are diagnosed each year in the UK, and the incidence seems to be rising. It is a serious disease, with about 50% of patients dying within 3 years of diagnosis. It is more common in men (**male/female ratio 2 : 1**) and in the older age groups (**mean age 70 years**). It presents with the typical features of an interstitial lung disease, as progressive dyspnoea, dry cough, crackles, restrictive defect in lung function and reticulonodular **infiltrates on chest X-ray** (Fig. 13.3). About 60–70% of patients have clubbing. The aetiology is unknown, but it appears to be the result of a failure of repair of lung tissue, whereby epithelial injury culminates in fibrosis rather than a controlled inflammatory and healing process. A possible association with previous exposure to environmental dusts (e.g. metal or wood dust) has been found in some epidemiological studies. Cigarette smoking may be a cofactor for the

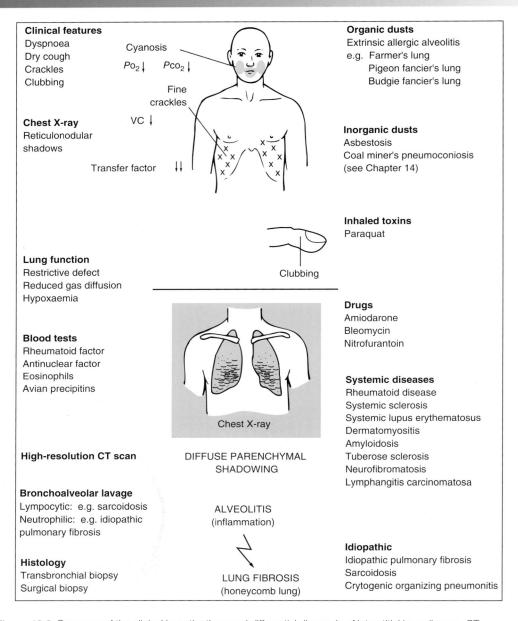

Clinical features
Dyspnoea
Dry cough
Crackles
Clubbing

Cyanosis

$Po_2\downarrow$ $Pco_2\downarrow$

Fine crackles

Chest X-ray
Reticulonodular shadows

VC $\downarrow$

Transfer factor $\downarrow\downarrow$

Lung function
Restrictive defect
Reduced gas diffusion
Hypoxaemia

Clubbing

Blood tests
Rheumatoid factor
Antinuclear factor
Eosinophils
Avian precipitins

High-resolution CT scan

Chest X-ray

DIFFUSE PARENCHYMAL SHADOWING

Bronchoalveolar lavage
Lympocytic: e.g. sarcoidosis
Neutrophilic: e.g. idiopathic pulmonary fibrosis

ALVEOLITIS
(inflammation)

Histology
Transbronchial biopsy
Surgical biopsy

LUNG FIBROSIS
(honeycomb lung)

Organic dusts
Extrinsic allergic alveolitis
e.g. Farmer's lung
Pigeon fancier's lung
Budgie fancier's lung

Inorganic dusts
Asbestosis
Coal miner's pneumoconiosis
(see Chapter 14)

Inhaled toxins
Paraquat

Drugs
Amiodarone
Bleomycin
Nitrofurantoin

Systemic diseases
Rheumatoid disease
Systemic sclerosis
Systemic lupus erythematosus
Dermatomyositis
Amyloidosis
Tuberose sclerosis
Neurofibromatosis
Lymphangitis carcinomatosa

Idiopathic
Idiopathic pulmonary fibrosis
Sarcoidosis
Crytogenic organizing pneumonitis

Figure 13.2 Summary of the clinical investigations and differential diagnosis of interstitial lung disease. CT, computed tomography; VC, vital capacity.

initiation of the disease, and about 30% of patients have autoantibodies (e.g. rheumatoid factor, antinuclear factor) in their serum, suggesting that in some cases it may be a form of connective tissue disease primarily affecting the lungs. Gastro-oesophageal reflux is common in patients with IPF and chronic aspiration into the lungs may aggravate the disease.

Lung biopsy shows a characteristic pattern of '**usual interstitial pneumonia**' with a heterogenous appearance, such that there are alternating areas of normal lung, interstitial inflammation, fibrosis and honeycombing. The changes are more severe subpleurally. **High-resolution CT** scan typically shows evidence of advanced fibrosis, with extensive areas of **reticulation**

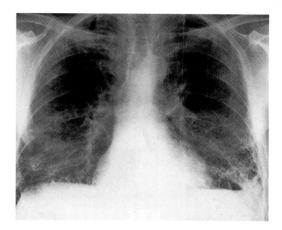

Figure 13.3 This 70-year-old man presented with a 6-month history of progressive breathlessness, crackles and clubbing, with reduced lung volumes and impaired gas diffusion. The chest X-ray shows small lung volumes with reticular shadowing particularly affecting the lung peripheries and bases, suggesting IPF. He failed to respond to prednisolone and died 1 year later of respiratory failure.

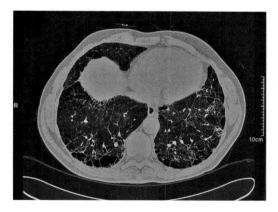

Figure 13.4 High-resolution CT scan of a 70-year-old man with IPF, showing 'honeycombing': a cluster or row of cysts caused by advanced fibrosis in the subpleural area.

and honeycombing in a predominantly lower zone, subpleural distribution and minimal evidence of inflammation as **ground-glass opacities** (Fig. 13.4).

Unfortunately, no drug treatment has been proven to reduce the mortality of IPF. Patients are often given a trial of prednisolone to assess whether any inflammatory component can be suppressed, but there is usually no clinical response and adverse effects are common. Combinations of prednisolone, azathioprine and N-acetyl cysteine have not proven effective. Pirfenidone is an immunosuppressant that is thought to have anti-inflammatory and antifibrotic effects. It is an option in IPF patients at a mild to moderate stage of the disease who have an FVC between 50 and 80% predicted, where it may have a modest effect in slowing the decline in lung function. Lung transplantation is the main option for selected patients who meet the necessary criteria (see Chapter 19).

Idiopathic interstitial pneumonias

The broad term 'idiopathic interstitial pneumonias' is used to describe a spectrum of inflammatory and fibrotic lung diseases of unknown cause, including IPF.

Nonspecific interstitial pneumonia is characterised by more uniform inflammatory changes and less fibrosis on lung biopsy, with correspondingly more ground-glass opacification on CT, a better response to corticosteroids and a more favourable prognosis than IPF. In **cryptogenic organising pneumonia**, histology shows intra-alveolar buds of organising fibrosis. This seems to be a pattern of response in the lungs to a variety of insults. It particularly occurs in association with some drugs (e.g. amiodarone), connective tissue diseases (e.g. rheumatoid disease) and ulcerative colitis, but often no cause is identifiable. Clinically, patients often have cough, malaise, fever, dyspnoea with chest X-ray infiltrates and an elevated erythrocyte sedimentation rate (ESR). Often the patient is thought to have infective pneumonia, but the differential diagnosis is widened when no pathogen is identified and the patient fails to respond to antibiotics. There is typically a dramatic response to corticosteroids, although relapse may occur as the dose is reduced.

Desquamative interstitial pneumonia and **respiratory bronchiolitis–interstitial lung disease** are relatively rare forms of interstitial lung disease that affect smokers. They have particular features of desquamation of alveolar macrophages or bronchiolitis on biopsy. They respond well to smoking cessation and corticosteroids. **Lymphoid interstitial pneumonia** is characterised by the presence of lymphoid cells in the interstitium. It may occur as a complication of human immunodeficiency virus (HIV) infection or connective tissue diseases. **Acute**

interstitial pneumonia is a very aggressive form of interstitial lung disease, characterised by rapidly progressive diffuse alveolar damage.

The idiopathic interstitial pneumonias, therefore, are a complex array of inflammatory and fibrotic lung diseases. The lungs may respond to different insults with a similar pattern of inflammation and fibrosis; conversely, a single agent, such as amiodarone, may produce a range of reactions within the lung. The overall clinical management requires the integration of clinical, radiological and histological features in a multidisciplinary meeting.

Connective tissue diseases

The typical clinical features of IPF with the histopathological pattern of usual interstitial pneumonia can occur in association with a connective tissue disease. When a patient presents with interstitial lung disease, a careful search should be undertaken for features of connective tissue diseases, such as Raynaud's phenomenon, inflammatory arthritis, sicca syndrome (dry eyes, dry mouth), myositis and skin changes. These diseases have a number of other lung complications.

Rheumatoid disease

Involvement of the **crico-arytenoid joint** causes hoarseness and sometimes stridor. **Obliterative bronchiolitis** results in progressive peripheral airway obstruction. **Pleural effusions** are common, and analysis of the pleural fluid characteristically shows a high protein level (exudate), with a low glucose concentration and a high titre of rheumatoid factor. **Rheumatoid nodules** may develop in the lung parenchyma and show the same histological features as the rheumatoid subcutaneous nodules. When rheumatoid disease occurs in association with coalworker's pneumoconiosis, large cavitating pulmonary nodules may develop (**Caplan's syndrome**). Fibrotic lung disease complicating rheumatoid disease is managed in the same way as IPF, but the prognosis is generally better. Drugs (e.g. methotrexate, leflunomide, infliximab) used to treat rheumatoid disease may cause inflammatory reactions within the lung and may also predispose to lung infections. In these circumstances, diffuse infiltrates on chest X-ray could be as a result of infection, a drug reaction, lung involvement by the connective tissue disease or coincidental lung disease (see Table 6.1). Bronchoalveolar lavage is useful in detecting infection. Where a drug reaction is suspected, information is available on the Pneumotox Web site (www.pneumotox.com) and prompt cessation of the drug and treatment with corticosteroids are important. The pulmonary complications of rheumatoid disease are summarised in Fig. 13.5.

Systemic sclerosis (scleroderma)

Diffuse lung fibrosis is the most common complication. **Chest wall restriction** by contraction of the skin is rare. **Aspiration pneumonia** may occur due to oesophageal dysmotility in the CREST variant of the disease: calcinosis, Raynaud's phenomenon, oesophageal dysfunction, sclerodactyly and telangiectasia. **Pulmonary hypertension** may also develop in patients with the CREST syndrome as a primary vascular phenomenon, often in the absence of significant pulmonary fibrosis (see Chapter 15).

Systemic lupus erythematosus

Pleural effusions are common and may cause **pleural thickening**. The phenomenon of '**shrinking lungs**', in which the chest X-ray shows high hemidiaphragms with small lungs, is probably caused by myopathy of the diaphragm. Lung fibrosis may occur. Immunosuppressive treatments predispose to **opportunistic infections** (e.g. *Pneumocystis* pneumonia).

Hypersensitivity pneumonitis

Hypersensitivity pneumonitis (extrinsic allergic alveolitis) is an **immunologically mediated lung disease** in which a hypersensitivity response occurs in an individual **sensitised to an inhaled antigen**. Typical examples of this disease are **farmer's lung** and **bird fancier's lung**. When hay is harvested and stored in damp conditions, it becomes mouldy and generates heat, which encourages the growth of fungi such as *Thermoactinomyces vulgaris* and *Saccharopolyspora rectivirgula*. When the hay is subsequently used as cattle fodder, fungal spores may be inhaled. Likewise, people who participate in the sport of pigeon racing or who keep pet birds, such as budgerigars, can inhale avian antigens. Various water systems in the home or work environment can be contaminated

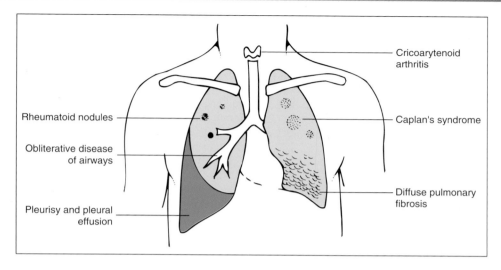

Figure 13.5 Summary of pulmonary complications of rheumatoid disease.

by fungi or mycobacteria, giving rise to hypersensitivity pneumonitis. Metalworking fluid alveolitis, for example, has been described in workers in car manufacturing, caused by contamination of fluid used to cool and lubricate metals. The inhalation of these antigens provokes a complex immune response in susceptible individuals, involving antibody reactions, immune-complex formation, complement activation and cellular responses, resulting in alveolitis. These diseases are less common in smokers, probably because of the immunosuppressive effects of cigarette smoke.

In the **acute form** of the disease, the patient typically experiences recurrent episodes of dyspnoea, dry cough, pyrexia, myalgia and a flu-like sensation, occurring about 4–8 hours after antigen exposure. During such an episode, lung function tests may show a reduction in lung volumes and gas diffusion, and chest X-ray may show diffuse shadowing. Sometimes, however, the chest X-ray may be normal, and CT is more sensitive in detecting the changes of hypersensitivity pneumonitis (Fig. 13.6). The acute illness is often misdiagnosed as pneumonia. The **chronic form** is characterised by the insidious development of dyspnoea and lung fibrosis. Lung biopsies show features of fibrosis, alveolitis and granuloma formation. Bronchoalveolar lavage typically shows evidence of a lymphocytic alveolitis, with a predominance of T-suppressor lymphocytes. Precipitating antibodies to avian or fungal antigens can be detected in serum but are also found in many asymptomatic individuals, so that they are not diagnostic.

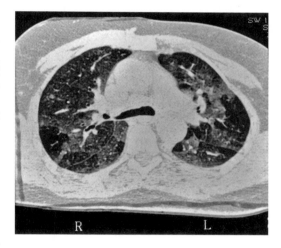

Figure 13.6 This 65-year-old man, who kept 150 racing pigeons, presented with recurrent episodes of dyspnoea, cough, fever and 'flu'. The CT scan shows a characteristic pattern for hypersensitivity pneumonitis of 'ground-glass' shadowing, with areas of decreased attenuation and air trapping on expiratory scans.

Complete **cessation of exposure to the provoking antigen** is the main treatment. However, pigeon fanciers, for example, are very committed to their sport and will often wish to continue keeping pigeons. They can reduce antigen contact by wearing a mask, loft-coat and hat (so as to avoid carrying antigen on their clothing or hair). **Steroids** (e.g. prednisolone 40 mg/day) hasten the resolution of the alveolitis and are often used during severe acute episodes. The immune response in hypersensitivity pneumonitis is complex, and a variety of modulating factors influence the interaction of antigenic stimulus and host response, so that the longitudinal course of the disease is variable, with some patients developing lung fibrosis and others showing spontaneous improvement despite continued antigen exposure.

Sarcoidosis

Sarcoidosis is a mysterious **multisystem disease** characterised by the occurrence in affected organs of **noncaseating granulomatous lesions**, which may progress to cause fibrosis. The aetiology is unknown but the accumulation of CD4 lymphocytes at disease sites is suggestive of an immunological reaction to an unidentified, poorly degradable antigen. The frequent involvement of the lungs raises the possibility that such a putative antigen enters the body via that route. The compartmentalisation of CD4

lymphocytes in affected tissues is associated with a corresponding depletion of CD4 cells in other tissues and depression of some delayed-type hypersensitivity responses, such that patients with sarcoidosis often demonstrate negative reactions to tuberculin (i.e. negative Heaf or Mantoux tests despite previous bacillus Calmette–Guérin (BCG) vaccination). Serum immunoglobulin levels are usually elevated and immune complexes are often present in acute sarcoidosis.

The clinical features of sarcoidosis are very varied, but it is useful to consider two broad categories of disease: an acute form that is usually transient and often resolves spontaneously and a chronic form that is persistent and may cause fibrosis (Fig. 13.7).

Acute sarcoidosis

The acute form typically develops abruptly in young adults with **erythema nodosum** and **bilateral hilar lymphadenopathy (BHL)**, sometimes with **uveitis**, **arthritis** and **parotitis**.

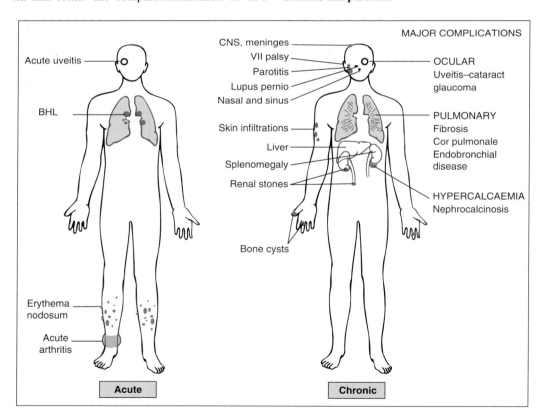

Figure 13.7 Principal clinical features of sarcoidosis. BHL, bilateral hilar lymphadenopathy.

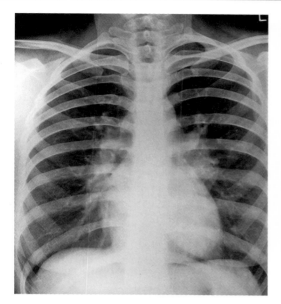

Figure 13.8 This 25-year-old woman presented with uveitis, arthralgia and erythema nodosum of her shins. The chest X-ray shows bilateral hilar lymphadenopathy. She was otherwise well, and lung function tests were normal. A diagnosis of probable acute sarcoidosis was made. The disease resolved spontaneously, without the need for any medical intervention.

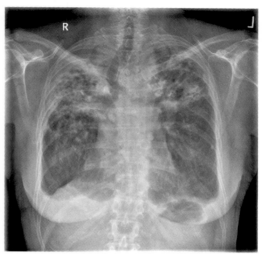

Figure 13.9 This 60-year-old woman presented with cough and progressive breathlessness. There were no crackles on auscultation of her chest, but transfer factor for carbon monoxide and transfer coefficient were reduced to 60% of predicted values. The chest X-ray shows extensive upper lobe fibrosis. Transbronchial lung biopsy showed noncaseating granulomas and lung fibrosis. Tests for tuberculosis were negative. She was treated with prednisolone, with some improvement in lung function.

Erythema nodosum

This appears as **round, red, raised nodules**, typically over the shins. It is a manifestation of hypersensitivity and is also found in other diseases, such as streptococcal infection, tuberculosis, ulcerative colitis and Crohn's disease, and with drugs, such as sulphonamides and the contraceptive pill, but in many cases no cause is identified.

Bilateral hilar lymphadenopathy

BHL is not associated with any signs on examination of the chest or with any loss of lung function and is often found incidentally on a **chest X-ray**, but often the X-ray has been taken in a patient with other features suggestive of sarcoidosis (Fig. 13.8). Although sarcoidosis is the most common cause of BHL, other causes include lymphoma, metastatic carcinoma, tuberculosis, fungal infections such as coccidioidomycosis and histoplasmosis in endemic areas (e.g. North America) and, in the past, berylliosis (e.g. beryllium used in fluorescent lighting).

Chronic sarcoidosis

The chronic form of sarcoidosis pursues a more indolent course, often in an older age group, with involvement of many tissues of the body.

Chronic pulmonary sarcoidosis

This involves the lung parenchyma, with **reticular shadowing** often distributed in a perihilar fashion on chest X-ray (Fig. 13.9). There are often remarkably few signs on examination of the chest, and lung function may be well maintained, but the disease can progress in some patients, causing **progressive fibrosis** and loss of lung function, with impairment of gas diffusion, reduction in lung volumes and sometimes airway obstruction with air trapping and bulla formation.

Chronic extrapulmonary sarcoidosis

Sarcoidosis can affect virtually any organ in the body. **Ocular sarcoidosis** often presents as pain and redness of the eye as a result of anterior uveitis. Chorioretinitis, keratoconjunctivitis sicca and lacrimal gland enlargement may complicate chronic sarcoidosis. **Parotid gland enlargement** may be painful and sometimes causes facial nerve palsy. **Central nervous system** involvement may cause cranial nerve palsies, chronic meningitis, obstructive hydrocephalus and a variety of neurological syndromes. **Posterior pituitary** involvement may rarely cause diabetes insipidus. **Cutaneous sarcoidosis** may cause maculopapular eruptions, plaques, nodules and lupus pernio (a violaceous chronic skin lesion particularly affecting the nose and cheeks). **Bone** cysts are sometimes found and are often asymptomatic. **Cardiac** sarcoid may cause conduction system damage and arrhythmias. **Hypercalcaemia** may result from increased bone resorption, and nephrocalcinosis, hypercalcuria and renal calculi may occur. Sarcoid granulomas and fibrosis may also be found in the liver, spleen, lymph nodes and muscle, for example.

Diagnosis

The diagnosis of sarcoidosis can often be made on **clinical** grounds, particularly when a young adult presents with classic features such as erythema nodosum and BHL. In less typical cases, it is helpful to obtain **biopsy of an affected organ. Bronchial and transbronchial biopsies** are particularly useful and may be combined with **bronchoalveolar lavage**, which typically demonstrates evidence of a CD4 lymphocyte alveolitis. **Mediastinoscopy** and biopsy of hilar lymph nodes is sometimes indicated to exclude other diagnoses, such as lymphoma. Needle aspiration of the mediastinal nodes can also be performed via a bronchoscope with endobronchial ultrasound guidance. The histological appearances must be considered in the clinical context, because they are not in themselves diagnostic, and other granulomatous disease (e.g. tuberculosis) must be excluded. Serum angiotensin-converting enzyme (ACE) levels are elevated in about two-thirds of patients with active sarcoidosis, but this test lacks sensitivity and specificity and is therefore of limited value in diagnosis and in monitoring the course of the disease.

Treatment

In most patients, sarcoidosis is a **self-limiting disease** that **resolves spontaneously** without treatment. However, a minority of patients with chronic sarcoidosis develop progressive fibrosis. Because the cause of sarcoidosis is unknown, no specific treatment is available, but **corticosteroids** suppress inflammation in the affected organs, frequently improving local and systemic symptoms. Their effect on the long-term natural history of sarcoidosis is less clear. They are usually used in patients with progressive disease and studies suggest some benefit from steroid therapy, at the cost of adverse effects (e.g. osteoporosis, Cushing's syndrome). A short course of prednisolone is sometimes used for particularly troublesome acute symptoms, such as parotitis, arthritis or erythema nodosum, if nonsteroidal anti-inflammatory drugs are not sufficient. Uveitis may be treated by topical steroids, and skin manifestations may be amenable to steroid creams or steroid injections. Inhaled steroids have been tried for pulmonary disease, but evidence of efficacy is lacking. In chronic sarcoidosis, deciding who to treat and when to treat requires **careful judgement to balance the benefit and risks of chronic steroid therapy**.

 KEY POINTS

- Interstitial lung disease typically presents with breathlessness, crackles, reduced gas diffusion and VC and diffuse infiltrates on chest X-ray.
- Exclude other diagnoses, such as pulmonary oedema, bronchiectasis, pneumonia and lymphangitis carcinomatosa.
- Seek potential causes, such as drugs (e.g. amiodarone), antigens (e.g. pet birds), occupational dust exposure (e.g. asbestos) and systemic diseases (e.g. rheumatoid disease).
- High-resolution CT shows the pattern and extent of fibrosis and alveolitis, and lung biopsy may be needed to determine the histopathological pattern.
- Treatments such as prednisolone and azathioprine should be used judiciously, carefully assessing the benefits and adverse effects.

 FURTHER READING

American Thoracic Society and European Respiratory Society. Update of the international multidisciplinary classification of the idiopathic interstitial pneumonias. *Am J Respir Crit Care Med* 2013; **188**: 733–48.

Bourke SJ, Dalphin JC, Boyd G, et al. Hypersensitivity pneumonitis: current concepts. *Eur Respir J* 2001; **18**(Suppl. 32): 81–92.

British Lung Foundation. Idiopathic pulmonary fibrosis (IPF) (http://www.blf.org.uk/Page/IPF, last accessed 29 December 2014).

British Thoracic Society Interstitial Lung Disease Guideline Group. Interstitial lung disease guideline. *Thorax* 2008; **63**(Suppl. V): 1–58.

Martin W, Iannuzzi MC, Gail DB, Peavy HH. Future directions in sarcoidosis research. *Am J Respir Crit Care Med* 2004; **170**: 567–72.

National Institute for Health and Care Excellence. Pirfenidone for treating idiopathic pulmonary fibrosis: technology appraisal guidance 282 (http://www.nice.org.uk/guidance/ta282, last accessed 29 December 2014).

Pneumotox Web site (www.pneumotox.com, last accessed 29 December 2014).

Raghu G, Collard HR, Egan JJ, et al. An official ATS/ERS/JRS/ALAT statement: idiopathic pulmonary fibrosis: evidence-based guidelines for diagnosis and management. *Am J Resp Crit Care Med* 2011; **183**: 788–824.

Strieter RM, Mehrad B. New mechanisms of pulmonary fibrosis. *Chest* 2009; **136**: 1364–70.

Vij R, Strek ME. Diagnosis and treatment of connective tissue disease-associated interstitial lung disease. *Chest* 2013; **143**: 814–24.

Multiple choice questions

13.1 Bilateral hilar lymphadenopathy and erythema nodosum suggest a diagnosis of:
- A hypersensitivity pneuminitis
- B sarcoidosis
- C lymphoid interstitial pneumonia
- D systemic sclerosis
- E systemic lupus erythematosis

13.2 A 70-year-old man, who has smoked heavily, presents with progressive breathlessness, clubbing, bibasal crackles and reticular shadowing on chest X-ray. The most likely diagnosis is:
- A cryptogenic organising pneumonia
- B lympoid interstitial pneumonia
- C desquamative interstitial pneumonia
- D idiopathic pulmonary fibrosis
- E respiratory bronchiolitis/interstitial lung disease

13.3 In sarcoidosis, bronchoalveolar lavage typically shows a high count of:
- A lymphocytes
- B eosinophils
- C neutrophils
- D macrophages
- E histiocytes

13.4 Ground-glass shadowing with areas of decreased attenuation and air trapping on high-resolution CT scanning are characteristic features of:
- A sarcoidosis
- B lymphocytic interstitial pneumonia
- C nonspecific interstitial pneumonia
- D hypersensitivity pneumonitis
- E idiopathic pulmonary fibrosis

13.5 The worst prognosis is associated with a diagnosis of:
- A nonspecific interstitial pneumonia
- B cryptogenic organising pneumonia
- C idiopathic pulmonary fibrosis
- D sarcoidosis
- E hypersensitivity pneumonitis

13.6 In the UK, the number of new cases of idiopathic pulmonary fibrosis diagnosed each year is about:
- A 500
- B 1000
- C 2000
- D 4000
- E 5000

13.7 Erythema nodosum is a characteristic feature of:
- A hypersensitivity pneumonitis
- B Caplan's syndrome
- C rheumatoid disease
- D sarcoidosis
- E systemic sclerosis

13.8 Interstitial lung disease is typically associated with:
- A impaired gas diffusion
- B hypercapnic respiratory failure
- C reduced FEV_1/VC ratio
- D hyperinflated lungs
- E wheeze

13.9 A classic example of hypersensitivity pneumonitis is:
- A cryptogenic organizing pneumonia
- B farmer's lung
- C sarcoidosis
- D systemic lupus erythematosis
- E Caplan's syndrome

13.10 Pirfenidone is a treatment option for patients with:
- A sarcoidosis
- B idiopathic pulmonary fibrosis
- C hypersensitivity pneumonitis
- D cryptogenic organizing pneumonia
- E nonspecific interstitial pneumonia

Multiple choice answers

13.1 B

Bilateral hilar lymphadenopathy (BHL) on chest X-ray is a characteristic feature of sarcoidosis. It may also be caused by lymphoma, metastatic carcinoma, tuberculosis and fungal infections such as histoplasmosis. Erythema nodosum consists of round, red, raised nodules, often on the shins. It is a feature of hypersensitivity and is also found in streptococcal infections, tuberculosis, ulcerative colitis and Crohn's disease and with drugs (e.g. contraceptive pill). The combination of BHL and erythema nodosum is highly suggestive of sarcoidosis, and this form of the disease has an excellent prognosis, often resolving spontaneously.

13.2 D

Idiopathic pulmonary fibrosis is a severe form of interstitial lung disease. The fibrosis is predominantly basal and subpleural, giving rise to crackles on auscultation and reticular shadowing on X-ray. Approximately 60–70% has clubbing.

13.3 A

Both sarcoidosis and hypersensitivity pneumonitis are characterised by high lymphocyte counts in bronchoalveolar lavage fluid. Bronchoalveolar lavage is also useful in excluding infection in patients presenting with diffuse shadowing on chest X-ray.

13.4 D

High-resolution CT is a key investigation in interstitial lung disease. Diagnosis is based on the integration of clinical, radiological and histopathology features in a multidisciplinary meeting. Hypersensitivity pneumonitis has a characteristic CT pattern of ground-glass shadowing, with areas of decreased attenuation and air trapping, best seen on expiratory views.

13.5 C

Idiopathic pulmonary fibrosis is a serious disease that usually progresses relentlessly and responds poorly to treatment. In contrast, diseases such as cryptogenic organising pneumonia and nonspecific interstitial pneumonia have a greater inflammatory component, which usually responds to prednisolone.

13.6 E

About 5000 new cases of idiopathic pulmonary fibrosis are diagnosed each year in the UK.

13.7 D

Erythema nodosum is a characteristic feature of sarcoidosis.

13.8 A

Impaired gas diffusion with reduced transfer factor for carbon monoxide and transfer coefficient is a characteristic feature of diseases of the lung parenchyma, such as interstitial lung disease.

13.9 B

Farmer's lung is a hypersensitivity pneumonitis in which repeated inhalation of antigens in mouldy hay provokes an immune response in the alveoli and distal airways.

13.10 B

Pirfenidone is an immunosuppressant that is thought to have anti-inflammatory and antifibrotic effects. It is an option in idiopathic pulmonary fibrosis patients at a mild to moderate stage of the disease, who have an FVC between 50 and 80% predicted, where it may have a modest effect in slowing the decline of lung function.

14

Occupational lung disease

Introduction

The importance of the work environment as a cause of lung disease has been recognised since ancient times. Hippocrates (460–377 BCE) taught his pupils to observe the environment of their patients. In the 18th century, Ramazzini urged physicians to ask patients what work they did and to visit their workplace; in 1713, he published a treatise on work-related diseases (*De Morbis Artificium*), which included descriptions of baker's asthma and what is now known as extrinsic allergic alveolitis.

Occupational lung diseases result from the inhalation of vapours, gases, dusts or fumes encountered in the workplace. The hazards of the work environment are constantly changing as old industries are replaced by new ones. The effects of inhaled substances depend on many factors, including particle size, physical characteristics (e.g. solubility), toxicity, the intensity and duration of exposures and the individual's susceptibility. Particles >10 µm in diameter are usually filtered out of the inhaled airstream in the nose, particles of 1–10 µm are mainly deposited in the bronchi and particles <1 µm penetrate to the alveoli. Inhaled substances may exert their effects in various ways, and in many circumstances the precise mechanisms involved are incompletely understood. We know, for example, that at an epidemiological level, occupational exposure to vapours, gases, dusts and fumes increases the risk of developing chronic obstructive pulmonary disease (COPD), but we don't know exactly why. Some substances are **toxic** to the airways (e.g. chlorine, ammonia), with all workers exposed being similarly affected. Others induce **hypersensitivity** or allergic reactions in susceptible individuals, giving rise to asthma or extrinsic allergic alveolitis (see Chapter 10). Some inhaled dusts **promote fibrosis** in the lung parenchyma (e.g. silica, asbestos, coal dust) and some are **carcinogenic** (e.g. cigarette smoke, asbestos). Occasionally, **infective organisms** are inhaled (e.g. *Mycobacterium tuberculosis* in healthcare workers, *Legionella pneumophila* and *Chlamydophila psittaci* in bird handlers). Smoking bans have now reduced the risk of occupational exposure to **tobacco smoke** for those working in places such as bars, restaurants and nightclubs.

Work-related asthma

Work-related asthma encompasses **occupational asthma**, where an exposure at work has *caused* the asthma, and **work-exacerbated asthma**, where the asthma existed prior to the occupational exposure but was *exacerbated* by the work environment. The latter is more common and has just as great an impact on an individual's ability to continue to work in their work environment. Work-related asthma may be defined as **variable airway obstruction caused by workplace exposures**.

Occupational asthma is now the most common type of occupational lung disease. In the UK, approximately 1000 new cases are diagnosed each year. In most cases, it is the result of a **hypersensitivity reaction** to a substance at work, but it may result from an **irritant effect** following acute exposure to a gas, fume or vapour at work. Occupational asthma accounts for about 10–15% of cases of asthma in adults. The list of causes is long, and new agents are being continuously added. Broadly, the agents can be divided into two categories: **high-molecular-weight allergens**

Respiratory Medicine Lecture Notes, Ninth Edition. Stephen J. Bourke and Graham P. Burns.
© 2015 John Wiley & Sons, Ltd. Published 2015 by John Wiley & Sons, Ltd.
Companion Website: www.lecturenoteseries.com/Respiratory

Table 14.1 Common causes of occupational asthma

Agent	Occupational exposure
Isocyanates	Spray paints, varnishes, adhesives, polyurethane foam manufacture
Flour	Bakery
Colophony	Electronic soldering flux
Epoxy resins	Hardening agents, adhesives
Animals (rats, mice)	Laboratory
Wood dust	Sawmills, carpentry
Azodicarbonamide	Polyvinyl plastics manufacture
Persulphate salts	Hair salons
Latex	Healthcare industry
Drugs (penicillin, cephalosporins)	Pharmaceutical industry
Grain dust (mites, moulds)	Farms, mills, bakeries

(e.g. flour (bakers), animal dander, shell fish) and **low-molecular-weight chemicals (**e.g. isocyanates (spray painters), persulphates (hairdressers), epoxy resins, azodicarbonamide (cleaners and workers in the plastics and chemical industries)) (Table 14.1).

Diagnosis

To establish a diagnosis of occupational asthma, it is first necessary to **confirm the presence of asthma** and, then, to show a **causal relationship between the asthma and the work environment**. Although the suspicion of occupational asthma is often based upon a **patient's history**, the diagnosis should be confirmed by **objective tests** wherever possible. Not only is security of diagnosis important in terms of managing the patient but identification of the causative agent facilitates reduction of the risk to other workers and may be relevant in the medico-legal and compensation aspects of the case. Characteristically, there is an initial latent interval of asymptomatic exposure to the agent before symptoms develop. This **latent interval** varies from a few weeks to several years. Once the worker has developed sensitisation to the agent, further exposure may provoke an **early asthmatic response** (reaching a peak within 30 minutes), a **late asthmatic response**

(occurring 4–12 hours later) or a **dual response**. If an early response occurs, the relationship of symptoms to the work environment is usually apparent. Late responses typically develop the evening after exposure, disturbing sleep and causing cough and wheeze the following morning. Initially, symptoms **improve away from work** on holidays or at weekends and **deteriorate on return to work**. Once asthma becomes established, symptoms may persist even when away from the work environment and can be triggered by other factors, such as exercise or cold air. Sometimes, the sensitising agent also causes rhinitis and dermatitis. In work-exacerbated asthma, where the asthma existed prior to the exposure, the link to the working environment may be missed. Some agents are well recognised by doctors (e.g. isocyanates used by paint sprayers), but they must still be constantly alert to new causes of occupational asthma. Atopy increases the risk of developing occupational asthma, but principally only in response to the high-molecular-weight allergens (i.e. where a specific IgE response will be mounted). Smoking increases the risk of occupational asthma in workers exposed to isocyanates.

In some cases, a typical history combined with evidence of a positive immunological response (in the form of specific IgE or skin-prick tests) can be sufficient to secure the diagnosis. Care is required, however, as a positive immunological response can be seen in individuals who are sensitised but remain asymptomatic.

Serial measurement of **peak expiratory flow** (PEF) or **spirometry** over several days at work and away from work will usually show evidence of variable airway obstruction (the hallmark of asthma) and may demonstrate a relationship between symptoms, airway obstruction and the work environment. Lung function tests may be normal when the patient is seen away from the work environment. Assessment and management of work-related asthma is notoriously difficult as some workers may be reluctant to admit to symptoms in case it jeopardises their employment, while others may exaggerate symptoms in an attempt to gain compensation. Patients with suspected work-related asthma should therefore be referred for specialist assessment.

One of the best ways of showing a relationship between asthma and the work environment is to perform a carefully supervised **workplace challenge study**. This involves removing the patient from the work environment for about 2 weeks and then returning them to work under supervision. Serial measurements of spirometry or PEF are performed on control days away from work and then

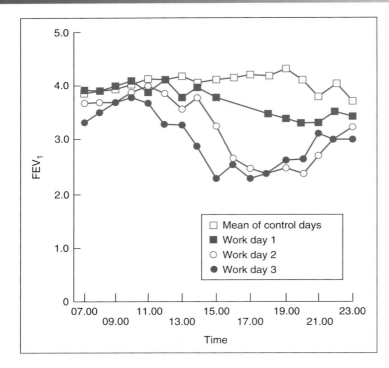

Figure 14.1 Workplace challenge study showing the mean forced expiratory volume in 1 second (FEV$_1$) on control days away from the workplace and progressive falls in FEV$_1$ over 3 days at work, indicating late asthmatic reactions of increasing severity occurring in relation to exposure to a biocide in the workplace.

over about 3 days on return to the patient's normal work environment. Serial measurements of **airway responsiveness** to methacholine or histamine (see Chapter 10) typically show sequential improvement away from work and rapid deterioration on return to work. Fig. 14.1 shows a typical late asthmatic reaction occurring during a workplace challenge study in a worker in a biocide manufacturing plant. The agent inducing the patient's asthma can often be identified with reasonable confidence by a **visit to the workplace** and an assessment of the materials used. However, workers may be exposed to many agents and it can be difficult to know which is causing asthma.

Laboratory challenge studies involve the patient inhaling the specific suspect agent under double-blind, carefully controlled circumstances, with serial measurements of spirometry and airway responsiveness. These studies are particularly useful in identifying previously unrecognised causes of occupational asthma but they should only be undertaken in specialist units, as they are potentially hazardous.

Management

Treatment of occupational asthma involves management of both the **affected individual** and the **affected industry**. Early cessation of exposure to

the inducing agent may result in complete resolution of the patient's asthma. The key factor in the patient's treatment is therefore not the institution of bronchodilator and steroid treatments, as in conventional asthma, but the **avoidance of exposure** to the inducing agent. This can be achieved in a number of ways, but often involves moving the patient to a different job within the workplace. Where there has been a delay in recognising the nature of the patient's asthma and in ceasing exposure, chronic asthma that persists even after cessation of contact with the inducing agent may develop, and long-term inhaled steroid and bronchodilator drugs are then required.

Substitution of an alternative nonasthmagenic substance in the industrial process is the ideal solution, as this also removes the risk to other workers. Where this is not possible, **enclosure** of the process in a confined booth with **exhaust ventilation** may be possible. **Segregation** of the hazardous process may be useful in limiting exposure to a small group of workers, who can then be provided with appropriate personal **protective devices**, such as respirator masks. **Surveillance** of other workers should be undertaken where a work environment has been shown to cause asthma. This typically involves a pre-employment medical examination, combined with periodic assessment of asthma symptoms, spirometry and, ideally, serial measurements of airway responsiveness. Institution of these measures in the workplace requires the cooperation of the factory safety officer, management, occupational health department and industrial hygienist. Hazards within the workplace fall within the remit of governmental agencies, such as the Health and Safety Executive (HSE) in the UK. Workers suffering disability as a result of their employment are entitled to **compensation** from the Department for Work and Pensions (DWP) in the UK, and may also wish to pursue legal action against their employer where there has been negligence in causing the disease. Under the Reporting of Injuries, Diseases and Dangerous Occurrences Regulations 2013 (RIDDOR), employers have a duty to report diagnoses of industrial diseases to the HSE, as well as work-related accidents and 'dangerous occurrences' that cause death or serious injury.

Berylliosis

Beryllium is a rare metal that is unusually light for its strength. It has special application in the aerospace industry, nuclear weapons manufacturing, electronic parts and dental alloys.

Inhaled beryllium, in some exposed individuals, causes berylliosis, a **systemic** disease with a predominant respiratory component. With exposure, the lungs can become hypersensitive, causing the development of small inflammatory non-necrotising (noncaseating) granulomas, similar to those seen in sarcoidosis. These occur in the lungs and hilar nodes but can also be seen in the liver and skin. Clinically, patients experience cough and shortness of breath. Other symptoms include chest pain, joint aches, weight loss and fever. The onset of symptoms can range from weeks up to decades following initial exposure, which may have been relatively brief. Ultimately, this process leads to a **restrictive deficit** (reduced lung volumes) and **impaired gas diffusion** (reduced transfer factor for carbon monoxide) (see Chapter 3). The disease can be fatal.

Apart from the aerospace industry, the occupations most commonly associated with berylliosis are beryllium mining and the manufacture of fluorescent light bulbs (which used to contain beryllium compounds in their internal phosphor coating).

Diagnosis relies on a history of beryllium exposure, exclusion of other causes of granulomatous disease and immunological evidence of beryllium sensitisation. The chest X-ray typically demonstrates small, round opacities, which may become irregular as the disease progresses. The features on high-resolution computed tomography (CT) scanning are indistinguishable from sarcoidosis.

Popcorn worker's lung

Recently, cases of severe **obliterative bronchiolitis** have been reported in workers in popcorn production plants, due to inhalation of diacetyl, a ketone with butter flavour characteristics. Patients develop progressive cough, breathlessness and wheeze, with fixed airway obstruction. CT scans show bronchial wall thickening and air trapping, and lung biopsies show inflammation and occlusion of the small airways in the form of obliterative bronchiolitis. Further cases of '**food flavourer's lung**' have been identified in other areas of the food industry. Doctors need to be vigilant to detect new causes of occupational lung disease.

Pneumoconiosis

Pneumoconiosis is a general term used to describe lung fibrosis resulting from inhalation of dusts such as coal, silica and asbestos.

Coal worker's pneumoconiosis

Although there has been a marked decline in coal production in the UK in recent decades, worldwide coal production has almost doubled in the past 25 years, with the fastest growth in Asia, especially China. The industry employs over 7 million people worldwide, 90% of whom are in developing countries. More than 5 billion tons of coal are currently produced annually, with 60% extracted from underground mines. The development of pneumoconiosis is directly related to a worker's total exposure to coal dust. Dust exposure varies in different parts of a coal mine and is heaviest at the coalface. Improvements in ventilation and working conditions have considerably reduced the level of dust in modern coal mines.

Coal dust inhaled into the alveoli is taken up by macrophages, which are then cleared via the lymphatic drainage system or the mucociliary escalator of the bronchial tree. If there is heavy prolonged exposure to dust, the clearance mechanisms are overwhelmed and dust macules arise, particularly in the region of the respiratory bronchioles. Release of dust from dying macrophages induces fibroblast proliferation and fibrosis. There is an important distinction to be made between the two major categories of coal worker's pneumoconiosis:

- **Simple coal worker's pneumoconiosis** consists of the accumulationwithin the lung tissueof small (<5 mm) aggregations of coal particles, which are uniformly dispersed and are evident on chest X-ray as a delicate micronodular mottling. **Simple pneumoconiosis is not associated with any significant symptoms, signs, impairment of lung function or alteration to prognosis, such as of life expectancy.** The benign nature of simple pneumoconiosis is sometimes not appreciated and there is often a tendency to attribute any respiratory symptoms to it, whereas alternative explanations such as COPD, asthma or heart disease are more likely to account for the patient's symptoms.
- **Complicated coal worker's pneumoconiosis (progressive massive fibrosis)** is characterised by the occurrence of large black fibrotic masses in the lung parenchyma, consisting of coal dust and bundles of collagen. These are typically situated in the upper zones and appear as rather **bizarre opacities on chest X-ray** against the background of simple pneumoconiosis (Fig. 14.2). **Cavitation** of these lesions may occur and can result in the expectoration of black sputum (melanoptysis). Complicated pneumoconiosis often results in **dyspnoea**, a **restrictive ventilatory defect** and **impaired gas diffusion**, and in **reduced life expectancy**.

Distinguishing the radiological features of pneumoconiosis from other possible diagnoses is key in management of the patient. Appearances can be similar to those seen in sarcoidosis, tuberculosis or lung cancer.

Caplan's syndrome (rheumatoid pneumoconiosis)

Coal workers with **rheumatoid arthritis** may develop **multiple nodules** of about 0.5–2.0 cm diameter in the lungs. These lung nodules are often accompanied by subcutaneous rheumatoid nodules. They are rarely seen in the UK today.

Chronic obstructive pulmonary disease

A number of occupational exposures are linked to the development of COPD, with coal mining being the most well established and thoroughly investigated.

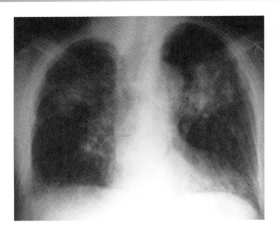

Figure 14.2 This 78-year-old man, who had been a faceworker in a coalmine for 40 years, presented with progressive breathlessness. Chest X-ray shows irregular opacities of progressive massive fibrosis in both upper lobes, with extensive background nodular shadowing of coal worker's pneumoconiosis.

Coal miners have a high prevalence of **chronic bronchitis**, with 45% of nonsmoking workers reporting relevant symptoms. In miners, coal macules can develop around the terminal bronchioles, which can be associated **centrilobular emphysema**. A number of studies have shown that emphysema is more common in miners than in control populations. Most epidemiological studies have also demonstrated an association with **airway obstruction**, independent of the effects of smoking. The establishment of a link between COPD and exposure to mixed mine dust and nitrous fumes in the coal mining industry led to the British Coal Respiratory Disease Litigation, the largest ever personal injury action in the UK. Over 315 000 claims were received before the scheme's cut-off of 31 March 2004.

Other occupational exposures linked to the development of COPD include **other mineral dusts** (e.g. silica in hard rock and gold mines), **fumes** (e.g. welding and cadmium in the production of alloys) and **organic dusts** (e.g. cotton, grain and wood dusts).

Silicosis

Silicosis is a form of pneumoconiosis resulting from the inhalation of crystalline silica (silicon dioxide). It is now less common in developed countries, due to widespread recognition and control of the hazards of respirable silica dust in the mining and quarrying

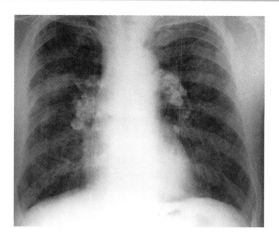

Figure 14.3 This 65-year-old man had extensive exposure to silica when working in a stone quarry. Chest X-ray shows eggshell calcification (a rim of calcification around the outer margin) of the hilar lymph nodes with upper lobe fibrosis. Tests for tuberculosis were negative.

industries. There is a risk of silicosis in workers involved in: **quarrying**, **grinding** and dressing of **sandstone**, granite and slate; development of **tunnels** and sinking of shafts (e.g. coal mines); **boiler scaling**; **sandblasting** of castings in iron and steel foundries; and the **pottery** industry, where silica may be used in the lining of kilns and the dry-grinding of ceramic products.

Simple nodular silicosis, like simple coal worker's pneumoconiosis, causes no symptoms and is an X-ray phenomenon. Complicated silicosis, however, results in **progressive fibrosis**, loss of lung function and breathlessness. The silicotic nodule consists of concentric layers of collagen surrounding a central area of dust, including quartz crystals and dying macrophages. There is a significantly increased risk of **tuberculosis** in patients with silicosis, as silica interferes with the ability of macrophages to kill tubercle bacilli. Patients with silicosis are also at increased risk of developing **lung cancer and COPD**.

A chest X-ray typically shows **nodular opacities**, particularly affecting the **upper lobes**. Eggshell **calcification** of **hilar lymph nodes** is a particularly characteristic feature (Fig. 14.3). **Pleural thickening** may also occur.

Siderosis

Dust containing **iron** and its oxides is encountered at various stages in the iron and steel industry and in welding. It gives rise to a simple pneumoconiosis (siderosis), which produces a striking mottled appearance on the chest X-ray because of the high radiodensity of iron, but is not accompanied by symptoms, signs or any physiological defect. Other metals, such as antimony and tin, may produce a similar picture.

Asbestos-related lung disease

'Asbestos' is a collective term for a number of naturally occurring fibrous mineral silicates that were once widely used in construction for their fire-resistant and insulation properties. Asbestos fibres come in two main types, which have different physical and chemical properties: **serpentine asbestos fibres** (**chrysotile** (**white asbestos**)) are wispy, flexible and relatively long, such that they are less easily inhaled to the periphery of the lung; while **amphibole asbestos fibres** (e.g. **crocidolite** (**blue asbestos**), **amosite** (**brown asbestos**), **tremolite**) are straighter, stiffer and more brittle, and penetrate more deeply into the lung. They are also more resistant to breakdown within the lung.

Workers may have been exposed to asbestos in many different settings, so it is important to take a detailed history of all of a patient's occupations over the years and of the tasks they undertook. **Pipe laggers** and industrial **plumbers** often had heavy exposure to asbestos, because it used to be widely used for **thermal insulation** in **ships**, **power stations** and factories. Many workers in the **shipbuilding** industry were heavily exposed to asbestos when they worked alongside pipe laggers in confined spaces, such as engine rooms. Women washing their husbands' work overalls could inhale significant amounts of asbestos. Workers in the **insulation industry** and those producing **asbestos products** may have been heavily exposed. Chrysotile asbestos was used in **brake-pad linings**, in **cement products** and in **pipes**, **tiles** and **roofing** materials. In many circumstances, the asbestos was safely bound within composite materials, but respirable dust could be produced by the **cutting of asbestos sheets** or in demolition work involving the removal, or **stripping off**, of asbestos insulation from pipes or boilers.

Strict precautions were eventually widely introduced in the 1970s to restrict exposure to asbestos through the use of protective respirators and exhaust ventilation, and through the substitution of other materials where possible. However, the long lag interval between the inhalation of asbestos and the development of disease means that asbestos-related lung disease is still all too common. Several different diseases are related to asbestos exposure (Fig. 14.4), and each has very different manifestations and prognoses.

- **Asbestosis.** Asbestosis is a pneumoconiosis in which **diffuse parenchymal lung fibrosis** develops as a result of *heavy* prolonged exposure to asbestos. The lag interval between exposure and the onset of disease is now typically 30–40 years, although the previous generation of workers, who experienced more intense exposure, presented earlier and often with rapidly progressive disease. The clinical features are similar to those of idiopathic pulmonary fibrosis, with **cough**, progressive **dyspnoea**, bibasal **crackles**, **clubbing** (in advanced disease) and a **restrictive ventilatory defect** (reduced lung

volumes) with **impaired gas diffusion** (reduced transfer factor for carbon monoxide). Chest X-ray shows bilateral, predominantly basal **reticulonodular shadowing**. CT is more sensitive in detecting early changes. Fibrosis is usually first evident around the respiratory bronchioles at the lung bases, becoming more diffuse as the disease progresses. **Asbestos bodies**, consisting of an asbestos fibre coated with an iron-containing protein, are usually seen within areas of fibrosis on light or electron microscopy. The disease is usually slowly progressive even after exposure has ceased, and it is not usually responsive to corticosteroids. Patients with asbestosis are at substantial risk of developing lung cancer. It seems likely that some individuals have an increased susceptibility to developing asbestosis, although the nature of this susceptibility is unknown.

- **Pleural plaques.** Pleural plaques are often visible as an incidental finding on chest X-rays of

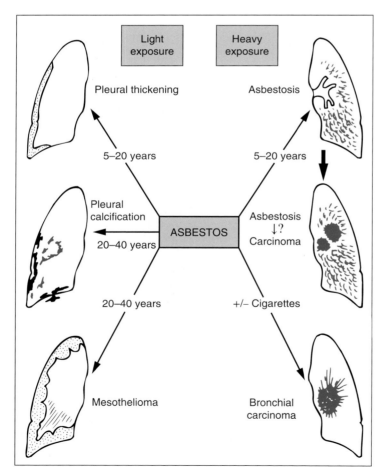

Figure 14.4 Pulmonary diseases relating to exposure to asbestos.

workers who have been exposed to asbestos. They are often calcified and appear as **dense, white, irregularly shaped lines** on the pleura of the chest wall, diaphragm, pericardium and mediastinum. When seen face-on, they form a well-defined but irregularly shaped **'holly leaf' pattern** (Fig. 14.5). They consist of white fibrous tissue, usually situated on the parietal pleura. They **do not give rise to any impairment** of lung function or disability.

- **Asbestos pleuritis and pleural effusions.** Many years after first exposure to asbestos, patients may develop a **pleural effusion**, which can occasionally be associated with pleuritic pain. The pleural fluid is an **exudate** and can be **bloodstained** even in the absence of malignancy. There is sometimes associated elevation of erythrocyte sedimentation rate (ESR). Other causes of pleural effusion need to be excluded. Pleural biopsy shows evidence of inflammation and fibrosis without any specific diagnostic features. There is usually spontaneous resolution, but recurrent episodes affecting both sides may occur and can lead to pleural thickening.
- **Pleural thickening.** Localised or diffuse thickening and fibrosis of the pleura may develop as a result of asbestos exposure. There may be a history of recurrent episodes of acute pleurisy, although these are often subclinical. The pleural thickening is usually most marked at the lung bases, with **obliteration of the costophrenic angles**. It may initially be unilateral but often becomes bilateral. Areas of fibrous strands extending from the thickened pleura may give the appearance of '**crow's feet**' on X-ray and **rolled atelectasis** may appear as a rounded opacity, caused by puckering of the lung by the thickened pleura. When the pleural thickening is extensive, it causes **restrictive ventilatory defect**, which can give rise to **dyspnoea**.
- **Asbestos-related lung cancer.** Epidemiology studies show an increased risk of lung cancer in workers in the asbestos industry, with an approximately linear relationship between the dose of asbestos and the occurrence of lung cancer. The interaction between **asbestos** and **smoking** is **multiplicative**. The clinical features, distribution of cell types, investigation and treatment of asbestos-related lung cancers are the same as for those not associated with asbestos exposure (see Chapter 12), but impairment of lung function as a result of asbestosis may preclude surgery. In the UK, workers are entitled to compensation from the

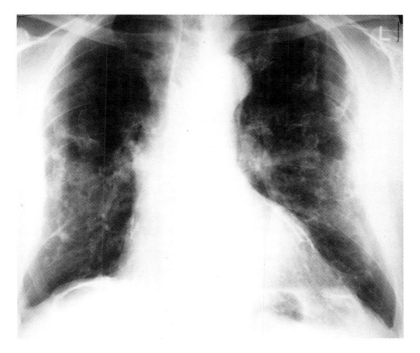

Figure 14.5 This 70-year-old man had extensive exposure to asbestos when he worked as a pipe lagger in shipyards. His chest X-ray shows extensive calcified pleural plaques, seen as dense white lines over the diaphragm and pericardium and demonstrating a 'holly leaf' pattern when seen face-on over the mid zones of the lungs. There is pleural thickening in both mid zones, with some blunting of the costophrenic angles.

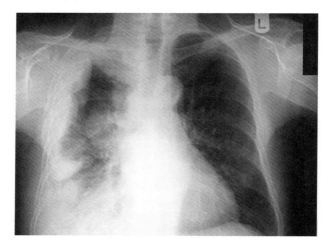

Figure 14.6 This 74-year-old man presented with right-sided chest pain and progressive breathlessness. He had been exposed to asbestos 40 years previously in his job as a plumber. His chest X-ray shows extensive lobulated pleural masses encasing the right lung. Percutaneous pleural biopsy showed malignant mesothelioma.

DWP for asbestos-related lung cancer if it occurs in association with asbestosis. In the absence of asbestosis, if there is a work history of exposure in certain occupations, they may still be entitled to compensation, depending on the type of work they did (e.g. applying or removing asbestos in shipbuilding, asbestos insulation work) and the duration of their exposure (5 years if it began before 1 January 1975, 10 years if later).

- **Mesothelioma.** Mesothelioma is a **malignant tumour of the pleura**, in which there is an identifiable history of asbestos exposure in at least 90% of cases. It may be that in the other 10%, exposure occurred but could not be recalled. The risk is greatest in those exposed to **crocidolite (blue asbestos)**. In some cases, the period of exposure to asbestos may have been very brief. At present there are over 2000 deaths each year in the UK from mesothelioma and the incidence is expected to continue to rise until about the year 2020, because effective controls on asbestos exposure were only widely introduced in the 1970s and there is an average **lag interval of 20–40 years** between exposure to asbestos and the development of mesothelioma. It usually presents with **pain, dyspnoea, weight loss** and **lethargy**, and features of a **pleural effusion** are sometimes associated with a lobulated pleural mass on X-ray (Fig. 14.6). **CT scan** typically shows nodular pleural thickening encasing the lung and involving the mediastinal pleura. Video-assisted thoracoscopic **pleural biopsy** may be needed for definitive histopathological diagnosis, and

pleurodesis can be performed at the same time for control of a pleural effusion. As the tumour progresses, it encases the lung and may involve the pericardium and peritoneum, and can give rise to bloodborne metastases. Radical surgery in the form of **extrapleural pneumonectomy** has been attempted but has generally not proved successful. **Radiotherapy** is sometimes employed in an attempt to reduce the risk of spread of the tumour through biopsy tracks and may relieve pain. **Chemotherapy**, using drugs such as pemetrexed and cisplatin, results in tumour shrinkage in about 40% of patients, although its impact on survival is unclear. Unfortunately, prognosis is poor, with most patients **dying within 2 years** of diagnosis.

Patients who have suffered disability as a result of occupational lung disease have a statutory right to receive **compensation** from governmental agencies such as the DWP in the UK. In some cases, they may wish to pursue **litigation** against their employer. The death of a patient with a suspected occupational lung disease should be reported to the relevant authority, such as the **coroner**, who may wish to undertake a **post mortem examination**.

 KEY POINTS

- Asthma is the most common type of occupational lung disease.

- Occupational asthma accounts for 10–15% of all cases of asthma in adults.
- Avoidance of exposure to the inducing agent is the main treatment for occupational asthma.
- Pneumoconiosis is a form of lung fibrosis caused by inhalation of dusts such as asbestos, coal and silica.
- Mesothelioma is a malignant tumour of the pleura caused by inhalation of asbestos 20–40 years previously.

 FURTHER READING

British Lung Foundation Web site (www.lunguk.org, last accessed 29 December 2014).

British Thoracic Society. Statement on malignant mesothelioma in the United Kingdom. *Thorax* 2007; **62**(Suppl. II): 1–19.

Edwards PR, Tongeren M, Watson A, et al. Environmental tobacco smoke. *Occup Environ Med* 2004; **61**: 385–6.

Fishwick D, Barber CM, Bradshaw LM, et al. Standards of care for occupational asthma. *Thorax* 2008; **63**: 240–50.

Hendrick DJ. Popcorn worker's lung in Britain in a man making potato crisp flavouring. *Thorax* 2008; **63**: 267–8.

McDonald JC, Chen Y, Zekveld C, Cherry NM. Incidence by occupation and industry of acute work related respiratory diseases in the UK, 1992–2001. *Occup Environ Med* 2005; **62**: 836–42.

Nicholson PJ, Cullinan P, Newman Taylor AJ, et al. Evidence based guidelines for the prevention, identification, and management of occupational asthma. *Occup Environ Med* 2005; **62**: 290–9.

Oasys Web site (http://www.occupationalasthma.com/, last accessed 29 December 2014).

Sigsgaard T, Nowak D, Annesi-Maesano I, et al. European Respiratory Society position paper: work-related respiratory diseases in the EU. *Eur Resp J* 2010; **35**: 234–8.

Multiple choice questions

14.1 The most common work-related lung disease in the UK is:
A coalminer's pneumoconiosis
B asbestosis
C extrinsic allergic alveolitis
D asthma
E silicosis

14.2 Isocyanate-induced occupational asthma is a substantial hazard for:
A healthcare workers
B cleaners
C paint sprayers
D hairdressers
E coalminers

14.3 A 70-year-old man who has smoked 20 cigarettes/day for 50 years and who has worked for 10 years as a pipe lagger in shipyards presents with right chest pain and breathlessness. Chest X-ray shows a right pleural effusion. CT shows nodular pleural thickening extending onto the mediastinal pleura. The most likely diagnosis is:
A mesothelioma
B benign asbestos pleurisy
C lung carcinoma
D diffuse pleural thickening
E pleural plaques

14.4 Eggshell calcification of mediastinal nodes on chest X-ray is a characteristic feature of:
A simple coalminer's pneumoconiosis
B coalminer's progressive massive fibrosis
C silicosis
D asbestos pleural plaques
E Caplan's syndrome

14.5 There is an increased risk of tuberculosis in patients with:
A asbestosis
B coalminer's pneumoconiosis
C siderosis
D byssinosis
E silicosis

14.6 Particles of approximately 5 μm in inspired air will:
A be filtered out of the inhaled airstream in the nose
B mainly be deposited in the bronchi
C penetrate to the alveoli

D be too small to deposit and will immediately be expired with the next breath

14.7 By which of the following mechanisms can inhaled substances lead to occupational lung disease?
A direct toxicity
B hypersensitivity
C promotion of fibrosis
D infection
E carcinogenesis

14.8 In relation to occupational asthma:
A the initial latent interval of asymptomatic exposure is often decades
B an early asthmatic response (<30 minutes after exposure) is never seen
C a late asthmatic response (4–12 hours after exposure) is always present
D permanent removal of the patient from the working environment leads to resolution of the asthma
E atopy is not a factor

14.9 A 42-year-old man presents with a 3-month history of cough, shortness of breath, chest pains, joint aches and weight loss. He has smoked 5 cigarettes/day for 20 years, has a pet cat and works in the aerospace indus-try. His chest X-ray reveals small round opacities. The most likely diagnosis is:
A berylliosis
B tuberculosis
C sarcoidosis
D lung cancer
E occupational asthma

14.10 A 68-year-old man presents with a 2-month history of increasing breathlessness and left-sided chest pain. He has just retired from his own successful electrical business – a business he set up at the age of 22 after qualifying as an electrician in the shipyards. He stopped smoking 30 years ago, with a 22 pack year history. His chest X-ray reveals a large left-sided effusion. The most likely diagnosis is:
A pneumonia
B benign pleural thickening
C asbestosis
D mesothelioma
E lung cancer

Multiple choice answers

14.1 D

Occupational asthma is now the most common type of occupational lung disease. In the UK, about 1000 new cases are diagnosed each year.

14.2 C

Isocyanates are a potent cause of occupational asthma. They are used in spray paints, varnishes, adhesives and polyurethane foams.

14.3 A

The CT scan features of nodular pleural thickening extending on to the mediastinal pleura are a characteristic feature of mesothelioma. The patient has had heavy exposure to asbestos, which was used for pipe lagging in shipyards.

14.4 C

Eggshell calcification of mediastinal nodes is a characteristic feature of silicosis. It may also occur in longstanding sarcoidosis. Asbestos causes calcified pleural plaques (but not calcification of mediastinal nodes).

14.5 E

Silica interferes with the ability of macrophages to kill tubercle bacilli. There is a significantly increased risk of tuberculosis in patients with silicosis.

14.6 B

Therefore, if they do cause a problem, it is likely to be a disease of the airways rather than the alveoli.

14.7 All

14.8 None

The latent interval varies from a few weeks to several years. Once the worker has developed sensitisation to an agent, further exposure may provoke an early asthmatic response (reaching a peak within 30 minutes), a late asthmatic response (occurring 4–12 hours later) or a dual response. Once asthma becomes established, symptoms may persist even when away from the work environment.

14.9 A

14.10 D

Mesothelioma typically presents many years after asbestos exposure. The X-ray suggests either benign asbestos pleural disease (thickening/effusion) or mesothelioma. The chest pain makes a malignant cause much more likely.

15

Pulmonary vascular disease

Pulmonary embolism

It is estimated that pulmonary emboli occur in about 1% of patients admitted to hospital and are directly responsible for about 5% of all deaths in hospital. The thrombus typically develops in the deep veins of the legs and then travels to the lungs, causing obstruction of the pulmonary vasculature. Patients who are immobilised in the community or in hospital are particularly vulnerable to developing deep vein thrombosis (DVT) and then pulmonary embolism. It is a major cause of death following elective surgery and is one of the leading causes of maternal death in the UK. Strategies to defend against this killer rely on widespread use of subcutaneous heparin prophylaxis against DVT and rapid resort to full anticoagulation pending definitive investigations in patients showing features suggesting DVT or pulmonary embolism.

Deep vein thrombosis

Factors predisposing to venous thrombosis were described by Virchow as a triad of venous stasis, damage to the wall of the vein and hypercoagulable states:

- **Venous stasis** occurs as a result of **immobility** (e.g. bed-bound patients on medical, surgical or obstetric wards, airplane flights), **local pressure** (e.g. tight plaster of Paris), **venous obstruction** (e.g. pressure of a pelvic tumour, pregnancy, obesity, varicose veins), congestive **cardiac failure** and **dehydration**.
- **Damage to a vein** occurs from local **trauma** to the vein, **previous thrombosis** and **inflammation** (phlebitis).

- **Hypercoagulable states** arise as part of the body's response to **surgery**, **trauma** and **childbirth** and are found in association with **malignancy** and use of **oral oestrogen contraceptives**. Recurrent thrombosis is particularly likely to occur where there are specific inherited abnormalities of the clotting system, such as **factor V Leiden gene mutation, antithrombin III, protein S** or **protein C deficiencies**, and in **anticardiolipin antibody** disease.

Pulmonary embolism is particularly common when thrombosis occurs in the proximal femoral or iliac veins and is less likely to occur when thrombosis is confined to the calf veins. Most pulmonary emboli arise in the deep veins of the legs, but they may occasionally arise from thrombus in the inferior vena cava or the right side of the heart, or from indwelling catheters in the subclavian or jugular veins. DVT may cause permanent damage to the vein, with impairment of venous drainage, oedema, pigmentation, ulceration and an increased risk of further thrombosis.

The classic signs of DVT are oedema of the leg, with tenderness, erythema and pain on flexing the ankle (Homan's sign). However, thrombosis in the deep veins of the leg, pelvis or abdomen may be completely silent. DVT must be distinguished from other conditions such as cellulitis, muscle injury and ruptured cysts of the knee, and **compression ultrasound** of the leg veins is the usual investigation used to confirm or exclude the diagnosis.

Clinical features

The clinical features of pulmonary embolism depend upon the size and severity of the embolism, as

Respiratory Medicine Lecture Notes, Ninth Edition. Stephen J. Bourke and Graham P. Burns.
© 2015 John Wiley & Sons, Ltd. Published 2015 by John Wiley & Sons, Ltd.
Companion Website: www.lecturenoteseries.com/Respiratory

summarised in Fig. 15.1, although there is overlap between the different presentations. In **acute massive pulmonary embolism**, the picture is often of a patient recovering from recent surgery who suddenly collapses. Attempts at resuscitation are often unsuccessful and there is a rapid high mortality, with very limited opportunity for intervention. Occlusion of a large part of the pulmonary circulation produces a catastrophic drop in cardiac output and the patient collapses with hypotension, cyanosis, tachypnoea and engorged neck veins. Sometimes, the presentation is more **subacute**, as a series of

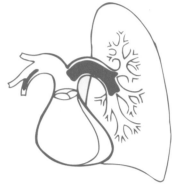
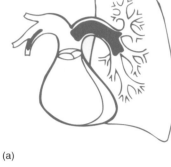

(a)

Massive pulmonary embolism

Acute
>50% occlusion of circulation
Sudden circulatory collapse. Cyanosis
Central chest pain
Hyperventilation. Engorged neck veins
ECG: sometimes S1, Q3, T3 pattern
CXR: usually unhelpful
CTPA shows occlusion of central pulmonary arteries

Subacute
>50% occlusion of circulation
Progressive severe dyspnoea over few weeks without
    obvious cause. Dyspnoea even at rest
Raised jugular vein pulse, sometimes loud P2
ECG: may show right ventricular hypertrophy (RVH)
CXR: may show infarcts
CTPA shows a high burden of clot

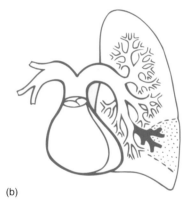

(b)

Acute minor pulmonary embolism
With infarction
Pleural pain haemoptysis, effusion, fever, hyperventilation
CXR: segmental collapse/consolidation

Without infarction
May be 'silent'
? Dyspnoea, hyperventilation
? Fever
CXR: may be normal
ECG: unhelpful
CTPA shows thrombus peripherally with a lower burden
    of clot

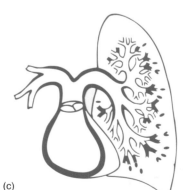

(c)

Chronic thromboembolic pulmonary hypertension
(repeated small emboli)
Progressive breathlessness, hyperventilation
? Effort syncope
Clinical features of pulmonary hypertension
ECG: right ventricular hypertrophy and axis deviation
CXR: prominent pulmonary artery
CTPA shows large pulmonary arteries and right
    ventricular hypertrophy with organised clot
and mosaic perfusion of the lungs

Figure 15.1 Synopsis of pulmonary embolism. CTPA, computed tomography pulmonary angiography; CXR, chest X-ray; ECG, electrocardiogram.

emboli progressively occlude the pulmonary circulation over a longer period of time, with the patient developing progressive dyspnoea, tachypnoea and hypoxaemia. **Acute minor pulmonary embolism** presents as dyspnoea, typically accompanied by pleuritic pain, haemoptysis and fever if there is associated **pulmonary infarction**. Prompt recognition and treatment of an acute minor embolism may prevent the occurrence of a massive embolism. **Chronic thromboembolic pulmonary hypertension** is a condition in which recurrent emboli progressively occlude the pulmonary circulation, giving rise to progressive dyspnoea, pulmonary hypertension and right heart failure.

Pulmonary embolism is both under- and over-diagnosed in clinical practice, leading to some patients failing to receive treatment for a potentially life-threatening condition and others being unnecessarily subjected to the risks of anticoagulant therapy. Although it is crucial to confirm a clinical suspicion of pulmonary embolism by a definitive test, it is also important to avoid subjecting large numbers of patients to unnecessary and expensive investigations. Dyspnoea, tachypnoea (respiratory rate >20/min) and pleuritic pain are the three cardinal features of pulmonary embolism. If none of these features is present, a diagnosis of pulmonary embolism is very unlikely.

Investigations

General investigations

General investigations may yield clues that point towards a diagnosis of pulmonary embolism. They are particularly useful in excluding alternative diagnoses:

- **Chest X-ray** is often normal, but **elevation of a hemidiaphragm** and areas of **linear atelectasis** may be seen as a result of pulmonary emboli. A small **pleural effusion** with **wedge-shaped peripheral opacities** may occur in association with pulmonary infarction, and an area of lung infarction may rarely undergo cavitation. In massive embolism, an **area of underperfusion** with few vascular markings may be apparent. **Enlarged pulmonary** arteries are a feature of pulmonary hypertension in chronic thromboembolic disease. The chest X-ray helps exclude alternative diagnoses, such as pneumothorax, pneumonia and pulmonary oedema.
- **Electrocardiogram (ECG)** is often normal, apart from showing a **sinus tachycardia**. In major pulmonary embolism, there may be features of **right heart strain**, with depression of the ST segment and T wave in leads V_1–V_3 and evidence of right axis deviation with an **S1 Q3 T3** pattern. The ECG helps exclude myocardial infarction and cardiac arrhythmias.
- Characteristically pulmonary embolism is associated with ventilation of underperfused areas of lung, resulting in hypoxaemia and hyperventilation, so that **arterial blood gases** show a reduced Po_2 and Pco_2.
- **Lung function tests** are not usually helpful in the acute situation, but in patients with dyspnoea caused by chronic or subacute pulmonary emboli there is reduced gas diffusion and a reduction in the transfer factor for carbon monoxide. Lung function tests may also help identify other lung diseases (e.g. chronic obstructive pulmonary disease (COPD) and emphysema).
- **Blood tests** may show evidence of intravascular thrombosis (thrombin–antithrombin III complex assay) and fibrinolysis (fibrin degradation products). **D-dimer** is a breakdown product of crosslinked fibrin and levels are elevated in patients with thromboembolism. However, levels are also often elevated in other hospitalised patients, so that **D-dimer assays can be used to exclude, but not to confirm, venous thromboembolism**. A normal D-dimer level can be particularly useful in certain clinical settings. For example, a young woman on oral contraception who presents with isolated pleuritic pain is very unlikely to have pulmonary embolism if her respiratory rate is below 20/min and chest X-ray, arterial blood gases and D-dimer are normal. She can be reassured without the need for admission to hospital or further investigation.

Specific investigations

- **Pulmonary angiography** is the definitive test for diagnosing pulmonary embolism but is an invasive test requiring specialist expertise and equipment that is not widely available, and it is associated with a small risk, particularly in critically ill patients. A catheter is passed from a peripheral vein (e.g. femoral vein) through the right side of the heart and into the pulmonary arteries. Radiocontrast material is then injected and a rapid sequence of X-rays is taken. The angiographic features of embolism are intraluminal filling defects, abrupt cut-off of vessels, peripheral pruning of vessels and areas of reduced perfusion.
- **Computed tomography pulmonary angiography (CTPA)** (Fig. 15.2) is increasingly being used as the definitive initial noninvasive imaging modality

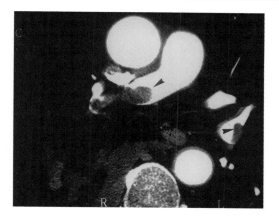

Figure 15.2 Computed tomography pulmonary angiogram (CTPA) showing clot in the main pulmonary artery of the right lung (upper arrow) and the lower lobe pulmonary artery of the left lung (lower arrow).

for pulmonary embolism. Very rapid spiral images are obtained during the injection of iodinated contrast medium into a peripheral vein. It has better specificity than ventilation–perfusion isotope scanning in the diagnosis of pulmonary embolism, although it does involve a higher radiation dose. It also provides information on a potential alternative diagnosis when pulmonary embolism is excluded. The increased use of CTPA has been associated with a rise in the incidence of the diagnosis of pulmonary emboli, as it is more sensitive than V/Q scanning in detecting small subsegmental emboli.

- In a **ventilation/perfusion (V/Q) lung scan**, macroaggregated particles or microspheres of human albumin, labelled with a gamma-emitting radioisotope (technetium-99m) are injected intravenously. These particles impact in the pulmonary capillaries and the radioactivity emitted from the lung fields is detected by a gamma camera, outlining the distribution of pulmonary perfusion. The distribution of ventilation in the lungs is similarly outlined after the patient has inhaled radiolabelled xenon. A completely normal pattern of pulmonary perfusion is strong evidence against pulmonary embolism. 'Cold areas' are evident on the scan where there is defective blood flow. These may occur in association with localised abnormalities apparent on a chest X-ray (e.g. pleural effusion, carcinoma, bulla), in which case ventilation is usually decreased in the same areas, resulting in 'matched defects' in ventilation and perfusion scans. The classic pattern seen in pulmonary embolism consists of multiple areas of perfusion defects that are not matched with defects in ventilation. A V/Q scan may therefore show: normal perfusion, in which case pulmonary embolism is unlikely ('low probability'); areas of perfusion defects not matched with ventilation defects in the presence of a normal chest X-ray, in which case there is a 'high probability' of pulmonary embolism; or matched ventilation and perfusion defects, in which case interpretation is difficult and the scan is regarded as 'indeterminate'. Patients with a suspected pulmonary embolism but an indeterminate scan require further imaging, such as CTPA.

- Demonstration of thrombus in the peripheral veins by **Doppler ultrasound** provides support for the decision to anticoagulate a patient who has clinical features of pulmonary embolism but an 'indeterminate' V/Q scan.

Diagnosing pulmonary embolism

The British Thoracic Society recommends a stepwise approach and use of a probability scoring system in diagnosing pulmonary embolism:

- **Assess the probability of pulmonary embolism.** The main clinical features are breathlessness, increased respiratory rate (>20/min), pleuritic pain, haemoptysis and sudden collapse.
- **Are other diagnoses unlikely?** (e.g. pneumothorax, COPD, pneumonia etc.). If yes, score +1.
- **Is a major risk factor for venous thrombosis present?** (e.g. surgery, pregnancy, previous venous thrombosis, immobility, major medical illness). If yes, score +1.

Patients scoring 2 have a high probability of pulmonary embolism. Heparin should be started immediately and CTPA should be organised to confirm the diagnosis. Patients scoring 1 have an intermediate probability of pulmonary embolism. Measurement of D-dimer is then useful, as a negative D-dimer in this situation makes pulmonary embolism unlikely. If D-dimer is positive then heparin should be started and CTPA should be arranged. Patients scoring 0 may have an alternative diagnosis accounting for their symptoms. A negative D-dimer in these circumstances would make pulmonary embolism unlikely. However, if D-dimer is positive then further investigations by CTPA may be needed. **D-dimer assays can be used to exclude but not to confirm venous thromboembolism** and can reduce the need for CTPA in some circumstances.

Pregnancy

The diagnosis of pulmonary embolism in a woman who is pregnant requires particular consideration. Pulmonary embolism is a leading cause of maternal death and accurate diagnosis is essential. CTPA exposes the foetus to less radiation than an isotope perfusion scan but exposes the mother's breasts to a significant dose of radiation at a time when they are particularly vulnerable, increasing the risk of future breast cancer. **Ultrasound of the legs for DVT** is a useful initial investigation. If this is negative and chest X-ray is normal then a **half-dose perfusion scan** is recommended. **CTPA** is reserved for patients with indeterminate initial investigations.

Treatment

Anticoagulant therapy

When a clinical diagnosis of suspected pulmonary embolism or DVT has been made, anticoagulants should be started at once unless there is a strong contraindication (e.g. active haemorrhage). The decision as to whether anticoagulants should be continued in the long term is made later, based upon the results of subsequent investigations. **Low-molecular-weight heparin** (e.g. **tinzaparin 175 units/kg subcutaneously once daily**) is now the standard initial treatment for patients with pulmonary embolism. The dose is determined by the patient's weight and anticoagulant monitoring is not needed. An alternative is unfractionated heparin (e.g. heparin given as an initial intravenous bolus followed by an infusion); this requires monitoring of the activated partial thromboplastin time (APTT), with adjustment of the dose to maintain the APTT at 1.5–2.5 times the control value. Intravenous heparin may be preferred to subcutaneous heparin in patients with a massive pulmonary embolism or where rapid reversal of anticoagulation may be needed (e.g. in patients at risk of haemorrhage). Adverse effects of heparin include haemorrhage, bruising and thrombocytopenia. Once the clinical suspicion of pulmonary embolism or DVT has been supported by subsequent investigations, **oral anticoagulation** is commenced using **warfarin**. Usually, 5 mg is given on day 1 and day 2 as a loading dose, and then the international normalised ratio (INR) is measured and the dosage adjusted to maintain a ratio of about 2–3. Since warfarin takes at least 48 hours to establish its anticoagulant effect, heparin needs to be continued for this period. The optimal duration of warfarin treatment is uncertain, but it is usually continued for 3–6 months after a first episode of idiopathic venous thromboembolism.

Newer oral anticoagulants are also an option in treating thromboembolic disease. **Rivaroxaban** is a direct inhibitor of activated factor X that interrupts the intrinsic and extrinsic coagulation pathways, inhibiting both thrombin formation and development of thrombi. It has a rapid onset of action. No routine coagulation monitoring is required. Patients with recurrent or unexplained thromboembolic disease should have investigations for hypercoagulable states (e.g. antithrombin III, protein S or C deficiencies, anticardiolipin antibody disease) or predisposing diseases (e.g. malignancy) and may require long-term anticoagulation.

The patient should be given an **anticoagulant information booklet** that explains the nature and side effects of treatment, states the indication for and proposed duration of treatment and provides contact numbers for obtaining advice and instructions on avoiding medications that interfere with therapy. This provides a useful means of communication with the patient and with all involved in their care (e.g. general practitioner, dentist, nurses etc.). Many drugs enhance the effect of warfarin (e.g. nonsteroidal anti-inflammatory drugs, aspirin, ciprofloxacin, erythromycin etc.), while others reduce it (e.g. carbamazepine, barbiturates, rifampicin etc.). Warfarin is teratogenic and women of child-bearing age should be warned of this danger, and may require specialist contraceptive advice. Precise details of INR, warfarin dosage and clinic appointments should thus be included in the booklet.

Thrombolytic therapy

The aim of thrombolytic therapy is to actively dissolve clots, but its use is reserved for those patients with acute massive pulmonary embolism who remain in severe haemodynamic collapse (e.g. hypotensive, poorly perfused, hypoxaemic). These patients have survived the immediate impact of the pulmonary embolism but remain critically ill. If all the clinical features and bedside tests (e.g. ECG, chest X-ray) suggest a massive pulmonary embolism and exclude alternative diagnoses (pneumothorax, postoperative haemorrhage, myocardial infarction, aortic dissection etc.), a decision may have to be taken that the circumstances justify the use of thrombolytic therapy. Contraindications to thrombolytic therapy include active haemorrhage, recent major surgery and trauma. Typically, **alteplase 50 mg** is given as a bolus via a peripheral vein. Thereafter, heparin anticoagulation is commenced. In some specialist centres, **transcatheter clot removal** or surgical **embolectomy** can be performed.

Patients with acute pulmonary embolism require **high-flow oxygen** to correct hypoxaemia and **analgesia** (e.g. diamorphine) to relieve pain and distress. In patients with active haemorrhage contraindicating the use of anticoagulant, or with recurrent pulmonary emboli despite adequate anticoagulation, **a venous filter** procedure may be useful. This involves the passing of a specially designed filter into the inferior vena cava to prevent further emboli from reaching the lungs due to DVT in the pelvis or lower limbs (Fig. 15.3).

DVT prophylaxis

A variety of measures are directed against Virchow's triad of factors predisposing to DVT. Early **ambulation**, use of graded elastic **compression stockings** and leg **exercises** reduce venous stasis. Prophylactic **low-dose heparin** is now widely used to reduce the risk for patients on surgical, obstetric and medical wards. Typically, **tinzaparin 3500 units/day** is given subcutaneously. For patients undergoing surgery with a higher risk of DVT (e.g. hip replacement), the dosage may be increased to 4500 units given 12 hours before surgery and then daily until the patient is mobile again.

Other materials that may occasionally embolise to the lungs include **fat** (after fracture of long bones), **amniotic fluid** (post-partum), **air** (e.g. from disconnected central venous lines), **tumour** (from tumour invasion of venous system), **infected vegetations** (from tricuspid endocarditis) and **foreign materials** (from contamination of drugs injected by drug misusers).

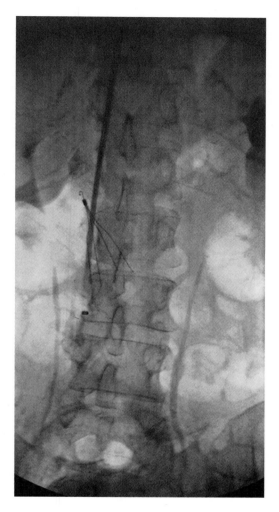

Figure 15.3 Inferior vena caval filter. Most pulmonary emboli arise from thrombi in the deep veins of the leg. An inferior vena caval filter can be used to prevent emboli from reaching the lungs. They are used in patients who have suffered recurrent pulmonary emboli despite adequate anticoagulation and in those in whom anticoagulant therapy is contraindicated. This 64-year-old woman had had major pulmonary emboli from a DVT in her right femoral vein. She then suffered major haemorrhage from a gastric ulcer while on heparin therapy, which was discontinued. A filter device was passed through the venous system from the internal jugular vein to be placed in the inferior vena cava.

Pulmonary hypertension

In normal lungs, the pulmonary arterial pressure is about 20/8 mmHg (compared with typical systemic artery systolic/diastolic pressures of 120/80 mmHg) and the mean pulmonary artery pressure is 12–15 mmHg. Pulmonary hypertension is defined as a mean pulmonary artery pressure >25 mmHg at rest. It may occur as a result of hypoxaemia and chronic lung disease, when it is often referred to as **cor pulmonale**, but in some cases there is no demonstrable cause, which is termed **idiopathic pulmonary hypertension**.

Cor pulmonale

Some confusion arises from the differing ways in which the term 'cor pulmonale' is used, but it essentially refers to the development of pulmonary hypertension and right ventricular hypertrophy secondary to disease of the lungs. **Hypoxaemia** is a powerful stimulus for pulmonary vasoconstriction, and this is the most common mechanism giving rise to cor pulmonale (e.g. chronic hypercapnic respiratory failure in COPD). Other mechanisms giving rise to pulmonary hypertension include **vascular obstruction** (e.g. chronic pulmonary emboli, pulmonary artery stenosis), **increased blood flow** (e.g. left-to-right intracardiac shunts – atrial and ventricular septal defects) and **loss of pulmonary vascular bed** (e.g. fibrotic lung disease, emphysema).

The clinical features of cor pulmonale are **elevation of jugular venous pressure**, **hepatomegaly** (as a result of congestion), peripheral **oedema**, a prominent left **parasternal heave**, a **loud pulmonary secondary sound** and a systolic murmur of **tricuspid regurgitation**. A chest X-ray may show large pulmonary arteries with pruning of the vessels in the lung fields. ECG typically shows p pulmonale (tall p-wave in leads II III AVF), with a tall R-wave in V_1 and ST segment depression with T-wave inversion in V_1–V_3. Echocardiography can assess the structure and dimension of the right heart chambers and the pulmonary artery pressure can be estimated from the velocity of the tricuspid regurgitation jet.

Idiopathic pulmonary hypertension

This is a rare disease, affecting about 2 per million of the population per annum, in which pulmonary hypertension occurs **without a demonstrable cause**. It particularly affects young women. Some cases of familial pulmonary hypertension are inherited as an autosomal dominant trait due to mutations in the bone morphogenetic protein receptor 2 gene. Some cases are associated with **human immunodeficiency virus (HIV)** infection or with use of **appetite-suppressant drugs** (e.g. aminorex, fenfluramine), but in most cases no cause is apparent. Pulmonary hypertension also occurs as a complication of **collagen vascular diseases**, such as systemic sclerosis (scleroderma), mixed connective tissue disease and systemic lupus erythematosus (SLE). Some patients with generalised systemic sclerosis develop severe pulmonary fibrosis (see Chapter 13), but

there is also a limited cutaneous variant of systemic sclerosis characterised by subcutaneous calcinosis, Raynaud's phenomenon, oesophageal involvement, sclerodactyly and telangiectasia (CREST syndrome). Patients with the CREST syndrome usually have anti-centromere antibodies and may develop pulmonary hypertension as a primary vascular phenomenon, often in the absence of significant pulmonary fibrosis. Patients present with dyspnoea, fatigue, angina and syncope on exertion. Investigations (e.g. echocardiography, V/Q scans, pulmonary artery catheterisation) are particularly directed towards excluding other causes of pulmonary hypertension, such as left-to-right cardiac shunts and chronic thromboembolic disease. The pathophysiology of the disease involves pulmonary artery vasoconstriction, vascular wall remodelling and thrombosis in situ. Treatment of patients with pulmonary hypertension is complex and is delivered from specialist centres. Supportive treatments include warfarin, diuretics and oxygen therapy. Pulmonary endarterectomy is a surgical procedure in which organised thrombi are removed from the proximal pulmonary arteries in appropriate patients with chronic thromboembolic disease. Calcium channel-blocker drugs (e.g. nifedipine) produce useful vasodilatation in a small number of these patients. Prostacycline drugs produce vascular smooth-muscle relaxation and inhibit vascular smooth-muscle growth. These include epoprostenol given as a continuous intravenous infusion via an indwelling central venous catheter, iloprost given by inhalation and treprostinil given as a subcutaneous infusion. Endothelial receptor antagonists (e.g. bosentan) reduce vascular tone and proliferation in pulmonary hypertension. Selective phosphodiesterase-5-inhibitors (e.g. sildenafil) also reduce pulmonary artery pressure. Atrial septostomy involves the creation of a right-to-left interatrial shunt and can be used to decompress the failing right heart. Heart–lung or lung transplantation also needs to be considered, as the disease is usually progressive (see Chapter 19).

Pulmonary vasculitis

When pulmonary vasculitis occurs, it is usually as part of a more widespread systemic vasculitis such as Wegener's granulomatosis, Churg–Strauss syndrome, polyarteritis nodosa, Goodpasture's disease or collagen vascular diseases (e.g. scleroderma, SLE; see also Chapter 13).

Wegener's disease (granulomatosis with polyangiitis)

This is characterised by necrotising granulomatous inflammation and vasculitis, affecting in particular the **upper airways** (rhinitis, sinusitis, bloodstained nasal discharge), **lungs** (cavitating nodules, endobronchial disease) and **kidneys** (glomerulonephritis). **Antineutrophil cytoplasmic antibodies** (ANCAs) are usually present in the serum. It is treated with a combination of corticosteroids and cyclophosphamide.

Churg–Strauss syndrome

This is an unusual disease consisting of allergic granulomatosis and angiitis. It consists of an initial phase of **asthma** followed by marked peripheral blood **eosinophilia** and **eosinophilic vasculitis**, giving rise to pulmonary infiltrates, myocarditis, myositis, neuritis, rashes and glomerulonephritis. It usually responds rapidly to corticosteroids.

Polyarteritis nodosa

This consists of a vasculitis of medium and small arteries resulting in **aneurysm** formation, **glomerulonephritis** and **vasculitic lesions** in various organs. Pulmonary involvement is unusual but may result in haemoptysis, pulmonary haemorrhage, fibrosis and pleurisy. There is often considerable overlap in the clinical features of the various vasculitic syndromes.

Goodpasture's syndrome

This consists of a combination of **glomerulonephritis** and **alveolar haemorrhage** in association with circulating **anti-basement-membrane antibody**, which binds to lung and renal tissue. Pulmonary involvement is more common in smokers and may cause severe pulmonary haemorrhage, resulting in haemoptysis, infiltrates on chest X-ray, hypoxaemia and anaemia. Transfer factor may be elevated by binding of the inhaled carbon monoxide to haemoglobin in the alveoli. Treatment consists of corticosteroids and cyclophosphamide, with plasmapheresis to remove circulating antibodies.

Respiratory emergencies Pulmonary embolism

- Consider the **diagnosis** of pulmonary embolism in all patients with unexplained breathlessness, pleuritic pain, haemoptysis or sudden collapse.
- Chest X-ray, electrocardiogram and arterial gases are the key initial tests.
- Assess the probability of pulmonary embolism:
  - Are other diagnoses unlikely?
  - Is a major risk factor present?
- **D-dimer** is useful in excluding the diagnosis but not in confirming it, as it is often elevated in patients with infection or systemic illness and following surgery.
- **Computed tomography pulmonary angiography** (CTPA) is the definitive test by which to confirm or exclude pulmonary embolism.
- **Tinzaparin 175 units/kg subcutaneously once daily** should be started immediately when pulmonary embolism is suspected.
- **Warfarin** should be started when the diagnosis is confirmed, and continued for 3–6 months after the first episode.
- **High-flow oxygen** and **analgesia** (e.g. diamorphine) should be given as needed.
- **Thrombolysis (e.g. alteplase 50 mg)** intravenous bolus should be considered for patients with acute massive pulmonary embolism who have severe haemodynamic compromise.

 KEY POINTS

- Most pulmonary emboli arise from thrombosis in the deep veins of the legs, which is common in immobilised patients in the community and in hospital on medical, surgical and obstetric wards.
- Assessing patients with suspected pulmonary emboli involves an appraisal of compatible clinical features and risk factors, exclusion of alternative diagnoses and measurement of D-dimer levels.
- CTPA is the main imaging modality used to confirm or exclude the diagnosis of pulmonary embolism.

- Heparin is used to achieve rapid anticoagulation, followed by warfarin. Thrombolytic therapy is only given to patients with circulatory compromise from a massive pulmonary embolism.
- Pulmonary hypertension (mean pressure >25 mmHg) may arise from chronic thromboembolic disease, as a result of chronic hypoxic lung disease or in the form of idiopathic pulmonary hypertension.

 FURTHER READING

Blann AD, Lip GYH. Venous thromboembolism. *BMJ* 2006; **332**: 215–19.

British Thoracic Society Standards of Care Committee Pulmonary Embolism Guideline Development Group. British Thoracic Society guidelines for the management of suspected acute pulmonary embolism. *Thorax* 2003; **58**: 470–84.

Condliffe R, Elliot CA, Hughes RJ, et al. Management dilemmas in acute pulmonary embolism. *Thorax* 2014; **68**: 174–80.

Ghuysen A, Ghaye B, Willems V. Computed tomographic pulmonary angiography and prognostic significance in patients with acute pulmonary embolism. *Thorax* 2005; **60**: 956–61.

Leung AN, Bull TM, Jaeschke R, et al. An official American Thoracic Society/Society of Thoracic Radiology clinical practice guideline: evaluation of suspected pulmonary embolism in pregnancy. *Am J Resp Crit Care Med* 2011; **184**: 1200–8.

National Institute for Health and Care Excellence. Rivaroxiban for treating pulmonary embolism and preventing recurrent venous thromboembolism (http://www.nice.org.uk/guidance/TA287, last accessed 29 December 2014).

National Pulmonary Hypertension Centres of the UK and Ireland. Consensus statement on the management of pulmonary hypertension in clinical practice. *Thorax* 2008; **63**(Suppl. II): 1–41.

Pulmonary Hypertension Association Web site (www.phassociation.uk.com, last accessed 29 December 2014).

Multiple choice questions

15.1 A 24-year-old woman using a combined oestrogen–progesterone contraceptive pill complains of pleuritic pain. Her pulse is 90/min, blood pressure 120/70 mmHg, respiratory rate 16/min. Chest X-ray is normal. D-dimer level is normal. The best next course of action is:

   A proceed to CT pulmonary angiography
   B reassure her that no further tests are needed
   C proceed to ultrasound of legs
   D commence heparin
   E commence warfarin

15.2 A 26-year-old woman who is 32-weeks pregnant presents with pleuritic pain and breathlessness. Pulmonary embolism is suspected. Chest X-ray is normal. The best next investigation is:

   A ultrasound of the legs
   B D-dimer
   C isotope perfusion scan
   D CT pulmonary angiography
   E pulmonary angiography

15.3 A 60-year-old man presents with a 6-month history of bloodstained nasal discharge, arthralgia and general malaise. He is admitted to hospital with renal failure. Chest X-ray shows cavitating nodules. Antineutrophil cytoplasmic antibodies are present in the serum. The most likely diagnosis is:

   A pulmonary embolism with infarction
   B Wegener's disease
   C Churg–Strauss syndrome
   D metastataic lung cancer
   E systemic lupus erythematosis

15.4 A 70-year-old man has confirmed deep vein thrombosis with pulmonary emboli and has been started on warfarin. Seven days later, he develops haemetemesis, with haemoglobin falling to 5 g/dl. Endoscopy confirms a bleeding duodenal ulcer. His thromboembolic disease is best managed by:

   A subcutaneous tinzaparin
   B intravenous heparin
   C aspirin
   D insertion of an inferior vena caval filter
   E warfarin

15.5 A 50-year-old woman presents with breathlessness. Investigations confirm pulmonary arterial hypertension. She has Raynaud's phenomenon, facial telangiectasia and scerodactyly, with positive anticentromere antibodies. The most likely cause of her pulmonary hypertension is:

   A mitral stenosis
   B chronic thromboembolic disease
   C CREST syndrome
   D Wegener's granulomatosis
   E HIV infection

15.6 A 48-year-old man, presents with a massive pulmonary embolism, confirmed on CT pulmonary angiography, 3 weeks after surgery for a fractured tibia. He is severely hypoxic and has an elevated jugular venous pressure and a systolic blood pressure of 80 mmHg. The most appropriate treatment is:

   A intravenous heparin
   B insertion of an inferior vena caval filter
   C subcutaneous tinzaparin
   D rivaroxaban
   E thrombolysis

15.7 Patients with a first pulmonary embolism caused by a deep vein thrombosis following a precipitating factor such as surgery are usually given warfarin for:

   A 1–2 weeks until mobile
   B 1 month
   C 3–6 months
   D 1 year
   E their lifetime

15.8 Pulmonary emboli account for death in a percentage of hospital patients of:

   A 1%
   B 5%
   C 15%
   D 25%
   E 30%

15.9 At midnight, a patient has developed a painful swollen leg 1 week after abdominal surgery. The most appropriate course of action would be to start treatment with:

A subcutaneous therapeutic tinzaparin 175 units/kg

B subcutaneous prophylactic tinaparin 2500 units

C warfarin in accordance with the INR

D no treatment, pending ultrasound of the leg the next day

E thromobolysis with alteplase

15.10 An appropriate analgesic that does not interefere with warfarin therapy is:

A asprin

B clopidogrel

C ibuprofen

D paracetamol

E diclofenac

Multiple choice answers

15.1 B

The combined low-dose oestrogen contraceptive pill is associated with only a mildly increased risk of venous thrombosis. This patient does not have breathlessness and has a normal respiratory rate. The negative D-dimer provides strong evidence of a lack of pulmonary embolism in these circumstances. She should be reassured and does not need further imaging or anticoagulation.

15.2 A

There is a high probability of pulmonary embolism here, as the patient has a major risk factor (pregnancy) and typical symptoms. CTPA exposes the mother's breasts to radiation, providing an increased risk of future breast cancer. Isotope perfusion scan exposes the foetus and mother to a small radiation dose. Ultrasound of the legs may be useful if it confirms DVT, thereby avoiding the need for CTPA or perfusion scanning.

15.3 B

Wegener's granulomatosis characteristically involves the nose, lungs and kidneys and is an ANCA-associated vasculitis.

15.4 D

This patient has conflicting problems of haemorrhage and thrombosis. Anticoagulation poses a major risk of provoking further bleeding from his duodenal ulcer. Insertion of an inferior vena caval filter prevents major emboli from reaching the lungs, and is indicated in these circumstances.

15.5 C

This patient has some clinical features of CREST syndrome (calcinosis, Raynaud's phenomenon, oesophageal dysmotility and telangiectasia), which is a particular, limited form of systemic sclerosis. It is a recognised cause of pulmonary hypertension and is often associated with anticentromere antibodies.

15.6 E

Thrombolysis is recommended for patients with acute massive pulmonary embolism who remain severely ill with hypoxia, hypotension and right heart strain.

15.7 C

Warfarin is usually continued for 3–6 months after a first episode of DVT.

15.8 B

It is estimated that pulmonary emboli are directly responsible for about 5% of all deaths in hospital.

15.9 A

It is important to start anticoagulation with subcutaneous tinzaparin immediately in order to reduce the risk of the patient developing a pulmonary embolism.

15.10 D

Patients taking warfarin should be advised not to take medications that can interfere with therapy. Nonsteroidal anti-inflammatory drugs enhance the effect of warfarin and are associated with a risk of bleeding. Paracetamol does not affect warfarin therapy.

16

Pneumothorax and pleural effusion

Pneumothorax

Pneumothorax is the presence of air in the pleural space. Usually the air enters the pleural space as the result of a leak from a hole in the underlying lung, but rarely it enters from outside as a result of a penetrating chest injury. Pneumothoraces may be classified as **spontaneous** or **traumatic**, and spontaneous pneumothoraces may be **primary**, without evidence of other lung disease, or occur **secondary** to underlying lung disease (e.g. chronic obstructive pulmonary disease (COPD), cystic fibrosis).

Pathogenesis

Spontaneous primary pneumothorax typically occurs in a previously healthy young adult and is most common in tall, thin men. It normally arises from the rupture of **subpleural blebs or bullae** at the apex of an otherwise normal lung. The aetiology of these blebs is uncertain, but they may represent congenital lesions aggravated by the more negative pleural-space pressure at the apex of the lung. Smoking is associated with a greatly increased risk of pneumothorax. The intrapleural pressure is normally negative because of the retractive force of lung elastic recoil, so that when a communication is established between the atmosphere and the pleural space, air is sucked in and the lung deflates. A small hole in the lung often closes off as the lung deflates. Sometimes the hole remains open, and the air leak will then continue until the pressure equalises. Occasionally, the opening from the lung to the pleural space functions as a valve, allowing air to leak into the pleural space during inspiration but not to re-enter the lung on expiration. This is a potentially lethal situation, as the air accumulates in the pleural space under increasing pressure, giving a **tension pneumothorax** in which the lung is pushed down, the mediastinum is shifted to the opposite side and the venous return to the heart and cardiac output is impaired.

There is an increased risk of pneumothorax in association with almost all lung diseases. These spontaneous secondary pneumothoraces are particularly common in patients with COPD and bullous emphysema. A pneumothorax resulting from rupture of a bulla may render an already disabled patient critically ill. Pneumothorax is a well-recognised complication of positive-pressure endotracheal ventilation in patients on intensive therapy units (ITUs) with underlying lung disease. Traumatic pneumothorax usually arises from puncture of the lung by a fractured rib, but air may enter the pleural space from outside via a penetrating injury or from rupture of alveoli, oesophagus, trachea or bronchi. **Iatrogenic** ('doctor-induced') pneumothorax may arise as a complication of invasive chest procedures such as the insertion of a catheter into the subclavian vein, percutaneous needle aspiration of a lung lesion or transbronchial lung biopsy.

Clinical features

Pneumothorax typically presents with acute **pleuritic pain** and **breathlessness**. An otherwise healthy young adult may tolerate a pneumothorax quite well, but older patients with underlying lung disease often develop severe respiratory distress with cyanosis. The clinical signs of pneumothorax are **reduced breath sounds** and **hyper-resonance** on the side of the pneumothorax, but these may be difficult to detect.

Respiratory Medicine Lecture Notes, Ninth Edition. Stephen J. Bourke and Graham P. Burns.
© 2015 John Wiley & Sons, Ltd. Published 2015 by John Wiley & Sons, Ltd.
Companion Website: www.lecturenoteseries.com/Respiratory

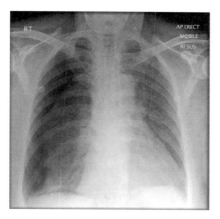

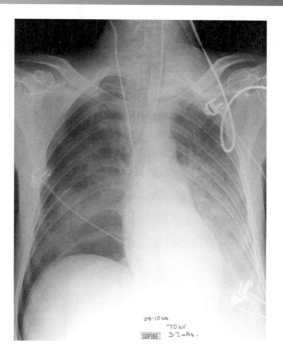

Figure 16.1 This 75-year-old woman presented with sudden onset of breathlessness and right pleuritic pain. Examination showed diminished breath sounds and hyper-resonance over the right lung. The chest X-ray shows a right pneumothorax with a large gas-filled pleural space without lung markings in the right hemithorax, deflation of the right lung and a clear 'pleural line' running parallel to the chest wall at the margin of the collapsed lung. She was given oxygen and analgesia and an intercostal chest tube was inserted into the right pleural space, with successful re-expansion of the lung (see Fig. 16.3a).

Sometimes, a left-sided pneumothorax is associated with a clicking noise, if the cardiac beat produces friction on movement of the layers of the pleura. Signs of **mediastinal shift** such as displacement of the trachea and apex beat to the opposite side may be detectable in a tension pneumothorax.

The **chest X-ray** shows a **black gas space, containing no lung markings**, between the margin of the collapsed lung and the chest wall (Fig. 16.1). Typically, the visceral pleural of the margin of the lung is visible as a laterally convex '**pleural line**' that runs parallel to the chest wall, and the pulmonary vascular markings are absent lateral to this line. Identification of a convex pleural line helps to differentiate a pneumothorax from a large bulla (see Fig. 11.6). A chest X-ray taken after expiration may accentuate the radiological features and help to detect a small pneumothorax, but expiratory X-rays are not needed routinely. It is often difficult to detect a pneumothorax if the chest X-ray is performed with the patient lying supine (e.g. on ventilation in the ITU), because the air in the pleural space, in this position, rises anteriorly, giving an appearance of hyperlucency of the lower chest, such that the mediastinal contours and costophrenic angle are outlined with increased clarity (Fig. 16.2). If the patient cannot be imaged in

Figure 16.2 Chest X-ray of a pneumothorax in a patient lying flat. This patient was in the intensive care unit (ICU) receiving endotracheal ventilation. His condition deteriorated with hypoxia, tachycardia and hypotension. The chest X-ray shows an endotracheal tube in satisfactory position, a cannula in the right internal jugular vein, left lower lobe consolidation and evidence of a right pneumothorax. When a patient with a pneumothorax is lying flat, the air in the pleural space tends to collect anteriorly and inferiorly, giving the appearance of hyperlucency, with unusual clarity of the mediastinal contour and the costophrenic angle, and the typical 'pleural line' at the margin of the lung, which is characteristic of a pneumothorax in an upright patient, is often not present.

an upright position, a lateral decubitus film should be performed. The size of a pneumothorax can be quantified arbitrarily as being 'small' if the rim of air between the margin of the collapsed lung and chest wall is <2 cm or 'large' if it is >2 cm. The volume of a 2 cm rim of air is approximately a 50% pneumothorax.

Treatment

- **No intervention.** A small (rim of air <2 cm) pneumothorax that is not causing respiratory distress may not require any intervention because it will **resolve spontaneously at a rate of about 1–2% per day**. Such patients may be allowed home,

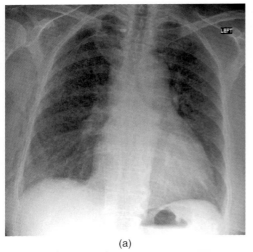

(a)

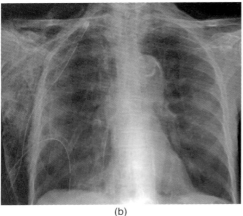

(b)

Figure 16.3 (a) Chest X-ray showing a small-calibre tube inserted using a Seldinger technique (tube passed over a guide wire) into the pleural space of a 75-year-old woman who had presented with a pneumothorax (see Fig. 16.1). (b) Chest X-ray showing two large-calibre tubes inserted by blunt dissection in a patient with COPD who had suffered a secondary pneumothorax with a large air leak. Air has tracked into the tissues of the right chest wall, causing 'subcutaneous emphysema'.

with advice to return to hospital immediately if symptoms deteriorate. They should not undertake an aeroplane flight until 1 week after the chest X-ray shows complete resolution of the pneumothorax, because the reduced barometric pressure at altitude causes expansion of enclosed thoracic air pockets. A follow-up appointment should be arranged for clinical assessment and chest X-ray

to ensure resolution of the pneumothorax and to exclude underlying lung disease. If a patient with a pneumothorax is admitted to hospital for observation, **high-flow oxygen** (e.g. 10 l/min) should be administered – with appropriate caution in patients with COPD, who may be sensitive to higher concentrations of oxygen. Inhalation of oxygen reduces the total pressure of gases in the pleural capillaries by reducing the partial pressure of nitrogen. This increases the pressure gradient between the pleural capillaries and the pleural cavity and increases absorption of air from the pneumothorax.

- **Aspiration.** Air may be aspirated from the pleural space by inserting a French gauge-16 cannula (such as an intravenous cannula) through the second intercostal space in the midclavicular line after injection of local anaesthetic. Once the pleural cavity is entered, the needle is removed and the cannula is connected via a three-way tap to a syringe, and air is aspirated. Aspiration should be abandoned if 2.5 l of air has been aspirated, as this indicates a persistent air leak from the lung. A chest X-ray is performed to assess the success of the procedure. This technique is simple, less distressing to the patient than insertion of a chest tube and very effective for primary pneumothoraces. Even large primary pneumothoraces can be aspirated, but chest tube insertion is needed if aspiration is unsuccessful.

- **Intercostal tube drainage.** Intercostal tube drainage is needed for most secondary pneumothoraces (i.e. in patients with underlying lung disease, such as COPD) or where simple aspiration has failed (Fig. 16.3):

  - **Small-calibre (size 8–14F) tubes** (Fig. 16.3a) can be passed into the pleural space to drain air or fluid using a **Seldinger technique**, whereby, after injection of local anaesthetic (e.g. 10 ml of 1% lidocaine (lignocaine)), a guide wire is inserted via a specially designed cannula and the tube is passed over it into the pleural space. The tube is sutured in place and attached to an underwater seal. These small-calibre tubes are very effective at draining air and fluid from the pleural space and cause less pain and discomfort to the patient than large-calibre tubes. Whenever possible, chest tubes should be inserted in the 'triangle of safety', which is bordered anteriorly by the lateral edge of pectoralis major, laterally by the lateral edge of latissimus dorsi, inferiorly by the line of the fifth intercostal space (level of nipple) and by the base of the axilla. This position minimises the risk of damage to underlying structures (e.g. internal mammary artery) and avoids damage to muscle and breast tissue, which would result in unsightly scarring.

- **Large-calibre (size 24–32F) tubes** (Fig. 16.3b) are required if there is a very large air leak from the lung that exceeds the capacity of the smaller tubes. The insertion of a large-calibre chest tube is a frightening procedure for the patient, who needs adequate **explanation and reassurance**. Premedication with atropine (300–600 mg intravenously) prevents vasovagal reactions, and a small dose of a sedative (e.g. midazolam 1–2 mg intravenously) may be considered for anxious patients. Chest tubes should be inserted in a clean environment using full aseptic technique, including sterile gloves, gowns, drapes and skin cleansing. The skin, subcutaneous tissues, intercostal muscles and parietal pleura are anaesthetised by injection of 10–20 ml of 1% **lidocaine (lignocaine)**. Aspiration of air into the syringe confirms that the pleural space has been entered. The skin is incised and **blunt dissection** with a forceps is used to make a track through the intercostal muscles into the pleural space, taking care to avoid the neurovascular bundle, which is usually situated in the groove on the lower surface of each rib. The chest tube may then be inserted through the track and directed towards the apex. The track made by blunt dissection should be sufficiently wide **to allow the drain to slide in easily without force**, and care must be taken to avoid causing damage to the underlying lung or other structures. The tube is securely **anchored in place** with a suture and connected to an underwater seal. The end of the tube should be 2–3 cm below the level of the water in the bottle. **Oscillation** of the meniscus of the water in the tube indicates that the tube is patent and in the pleural space. **Bubbling** on respiration or coughing indicates continued drainage of air. Breathing with a chest tube in place is painful and **adequate analgesia** should be prescribed. The position of the tube and the degree of re-expansion of the lung should be checked by chest X-ray. Low-pressure (−10 to −20 cmH$_2$O) suction applied to the tube may expedite the removal of air.
- **Surgical intervention.** Surgical treatment is required for persistent or recurrent pneumothoraces. Failure of re-expansion of the lung with profuse bubbling of air through the underwater drain suggests a bronchopleural fistula (i.e. a persistent communication between the lung and pleural space). **Surgical closure of the hole** with

pleurodesis is usually necessary and may be performed via a thoracotomy or via thoracoscopy. The hole is oversewn and blebs on the surface of the lung are excised. **Pleurodesis** involves the obliteration of the pleural space and can be achieved by instilling tetracycline or talc, which provokes adhesions between the visceral and parietal pleura. **Pleurectomy** involves the removal of the parietal pleura. Usually, an apicolateral pleurectomy (leaving the posterobasal pleura intact) prevents recurrence without compromising lung function. There is quite a high risk of recurrence after a first spontaneous primary pneumothorax, with about 50% of patients suffering a second pneumothorax within 4 years. Surgical intervention is usually recommended after a second pneumothorax or when the patient has suffered a pneumothorax on both sides, because of the risk of catastrophic simultaneous bilateral pneumothoraces. Particular thought must be given to the best procedure for patients with complicated pneumothoraces secondary to diseases such as cystic fibrosis, so as not to compromise potential future lung transplantation. A limited apicolateral surgical abrasion pleurodesis may be the best option in these circumstances.

Pleural effusion

A pleural effusion is a collection of fluid in the pleural space.

Pleural fluid dynamics

The parietal and visceral pleural surfaces are normally in close contact and the potential space between them contains only a very thin layer of fluid. Pleural fluid dynamics are complex and incompletely understood, but Fig. 16.4 shows, in a simplified form, some of the main factors governing fluid filtration and absorption. The parietal pleura is perfused by the systemic circulation, and the high systemic capillary pressure, negative intrapleural pressure and pleural oncotic pressure overcome the plasma oncotic pressure, resulting in fluid filtration into the pleural space. The visceral pleura is mainly perfused by the pulmonary circulation with its low pulmonary capillary pressure, so that the balance of forces results in movement of fluid outward from the pleural space to the veins and lymphatics. The balance between **fluid filtration** by the parietal pleura and **fluid absorption** by the visceral pleura is such that fluid does not normally collect in the pleural space. Pleural

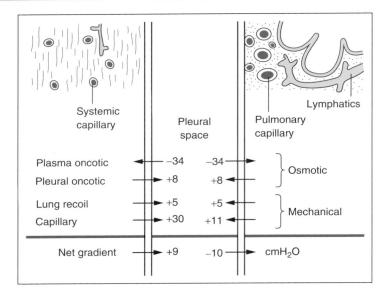

Figure 16.4 Pleural fluid dynamics. In the normal pleural space, the mechanical and oncotic pressures are in equilibrium, such that net filtration of fluid by the parietal pleura is balanced by net absorption of fluid by the visceral pleura. Pleural effusion may arise from changes in the mechanical and oncotic pressures (transudates) or from increased capillary permeability brought about by disease of the pleura (exudates).

effusions may develop from **increased capillary pressure** (e.g. left ventricular failure), **reduced plasma oncotic pressure** (e.g. hypoalbuminaemia), **increased capillary permeability** (e.g. disease of pleura) or **obstruction of lymphatic drainage** (e.g. carcinoma of lymphatics).

Clinical features

Patients with pleural effusions typically present with **dyspnoea**, sometimes with pleuritic pain and often with features of associated diseases (e.g. cardiac failure, carcinoma etc.). The signs of pleural effusion are **decreased expansion** on the side of the effusion, **stony dullness**, **diminished breath sounds** and **reduced tactile vocal fremitus**. Sometimes, **bronchial breathing** is heard at the upper level of the fluid. In taking the patient's history, it is important to enquire about clues to possible causes of pleural effusion, such as asbestos exposure, contact with tuberculosis, smoking, drugs (e.g. dantrolene, bromocriptine) and systemic disease. A full careful physical examination is essential to detect signs of underlying disease (e.g. cardiac failure, breast lump, lymphadenopathy etc.).

Investigations

The causes and investigations of pleural effusions are summarised in Fig. 16.5.

- **Radiology. Chest X-ray** characteristically shows a dense white shadow with a concave upper edge (Fig. 16.6). Small effusions cause no more than blunting of a costophrenic angle, whereas very large effusions cause 'white out' of an entire hemithorax, with shift of the mediastinum to the opposite side. Pleural fluid can be difficult to detect if the chest X-ray is performed with the patient lying supine and may only be suspected by haziness on the affected side. A **lateral decubitus** film may be useful in demonstrating mobility of the fluid, distinguishing the features from pleural thickening. **Ultrasound** imaging is helpful in localising loculated effusions and in positioning chest tubes (Fig. 16.7). **Computed tomography (CT)** may be helpful in detecting pleural tumours (e.g. mesothelioma) and in assessing the underlying lung and mediastinum.
- **Pleural fluid aspiration (thoracocentesis).** This is the key initial investigation. A **protein** level >30 g/l and **lactate dehydrogenase (LDH)** level >200 units/l indicate that the effusion is an exudate and that further investigations for pleural disease are indicated. Both transudates and exudates are typically a yellow, straw colour. **Bloodstained** fluid points towards malignancy, pulmonary infarction or severe inflammation. **Pus** indicates an empyema, **milky** white fluid suggests a chylothorax and frank **blood** suggests a haemothorax (e.g. as a result of trauma). A low **glucose** content points towards infection or a connective tissue disease as a cause of the effusion. A high **amylase** content is characteristic of pleural effusion associated with pancreatitis but also sometimes occurs with adenocarcinoma. **Neutrophils** are the predominant cells in acute inflammation or infection, while **lymphocytes** dominate in chronic effusions particularly caused

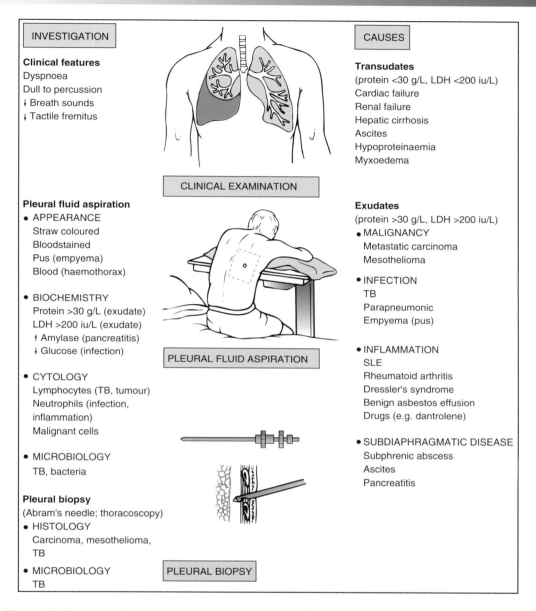

Figure 16.5 Summary of the causes and investigation of pleural effusions. LDH, lactate dehydrogenase; SLE, systemic lupus erythematosus; TB, tuberculosis.

by tuberculosis or malignancy. **Cytology** may show malignant cells (e.g. mesothelioma or metastatic carcinoma). **Microbiology** examination of the fluid may identify tuberculosis or bacterial infection.

- **Pleural biopsy.** This is another key investigation. A 'blind' biopsy can be performed using a specially designed needle such as the **Abram's needle**, but this technique has a low diagnostic yield. **CT-guided biopsy** is particularly useful in diagnosing malignant disease of the pleura when

CT has shown a focal area of pleural thickening. **Video-assisted thoracoscopy** allows direct inspection of the pleural surfaces, with direct biopsy of abnormal tissue. Histology of pleural biopsy samples is particularly useful in diagnosing malignant effusions or tuberculosis (e.g. caseating granuloma). A sample of the biopsy should also be sent for culture for *Mycobacterium tuberculosis*.

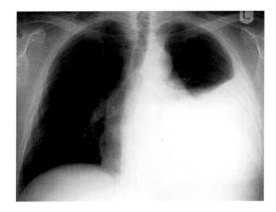

Figure 16.6 This 68-year-old man presented with a 6-week history of progressive breathlessness and left pleuritic pain. On examination, there was stony dullness and diminished breath sounds over the left hemithorax. The chest X-ray shows features of a large pleural effusion, with a dense white shadow with a concave upper border over the left side of the chest. The pleural fluid was bloodstained and showed metastatic adenocarcinoma on cytology. Bronchoscopy showed the primary tumour partly occluding the left lower lobe bronchus. An intercostal drain was inserted to evacuate the fluid and talc was instilled to achieve pleurodesis.

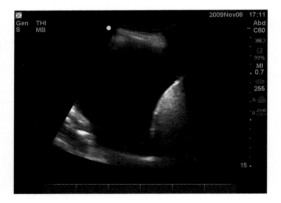

Figure 16.7 Ultrasound is useful in assessing pleural effusions and in guiding the insertion of chest drains. This 40-year-old man had an exudative pleural effusion secondary to a pneumonia. The pleural fluid appears black on ultrasound, with no loculations within it. The curvilinear white line to the right of the image is the diaphragm above the liver.

Further investigations (e.g. bronchoscopy for suspected lung carcinoma or ultrasound of abdomen for suspected subphrenic disease) may be required, depending on the clues to diagnosis elicited on initial assessment.

Causes

Pleural effusions are classified as transudates or exudates. **Transudates** are characterised by a low protein content (<30 g/l) and a low LDH level (<200 units/l). They arise as a result of changes in hydrostatic or osmotic pressures across the pleural membrane rather than from disease of the pleura. **Exudates** are characterised by a high protein (>30 g/l) and LDH (>200 units/l) content, and result from increased permeability associated with disease of the pleura. Sometimes, in patients with borderline protein and LDH levels, there is difficulty in distinguishing between transudates and exudates, and comparison of pleural to serum ratios may be helpful: exudates have a pleural fluid/serum protein ratio >0.5 and an LDH ratio >0.6.

Transudates

The main causes of transudative pleural effusions are **cardiac failure**, **renal failure**, **hepatic cirrhosis** and **hypoproteinaemia** caused by malnutrition or nephrotic syndrome. In most cases, transudative effusions are bilateral, although they may be asymmetrical and initially unilateral. **Ascitic fluid** may pass through pleuroperitoneal communications, which are more common in the right hemidiaphragm. Similarly, **peritoneal dialysis fluid** may give rise to a right pleural effusion. Rare causes of transudates are **myxoedema** and Meigs' syndrome (benign ovarian fibroma, ascites and pleural effusion, which may be a transudate or exudate). Sometimes, treatment of cardiac failure with diuretics results in an increase in fluid protein content, so that the effusion appears to be an exudate. Treatment of transudates involves correction of the underlying hydrostatic or osmotic mechanisms (e.g. treatment of cardiac failure or hypoproteinaemia), and further investigation of the pleura is not usually necessary.

Exudates

A variety of diseases that affect the pleura are associated with increased capillary permeability or reduced lymphatic drainage. Exudates are often unilateral and investigations are directed towards identifying the cause, because this determines treatment.

- **Malignancy. Metastases** to the pleura most commonly arise from **lung**, **breast**, **ovarian** or **gastrointestinal** cancers and from **lymphoma**. **Mesothelioma** is a primary tumour of the pleura related to asbestos exposure (see Chapter 14). In malignant effusions, the fluid is often bloodstained, with a high lymphocyte count, and cytology often shows malignant cells. If cytology of a pleural aspirate is negative, pleural biopsy may be diagnostic. Sometimes, confirmation of the diagnosis is difficult and thoracoscopy with biopsy of lesions under direct vision may be necessary. Malignancy may give rise to pleural effusions by means other than direct involvement of the pleura. **Lymphatic involvement** by tumours may obstruct drainage and cause pleural effusions with negative cytology. **Chylous effusions**, caused by malignancy in the thoracic duct, are characterised by a milky, cloudy appearance of the pleural fluid. **Superior vena caval obstruction** may give rise to pleural effusions as a result of elevation of systemic venous pressure. Treatment of a pleural effusion associated with malignancy is directed against the underlying tumour (e.g. chemotherapy). **Drainage of the fluid** by needle aspiration or intercostal chest tube relieves dyspnoea. It is usually advisable to remove the fluid slowly, at no more than 1.5 l at a time, as too-rapid removal may provoke re-expansion pulmonary oedema, although the risk is small. The risk of recurrence of the effusion may be reduced by the instillation of a sclerosing agent (e.g. tetracycline 1.0–1.5 g, doxycycline 500 mg or sterile talc 2–5 g in 50 ml saline) into the pleural space to provoke chemical **pleurodesis**. Lidocaine (lignocaine) 3 mg/kg (maximum 250 mg) may be instilled intrapleurally before the sclerosing agent to provide local anaesthesia. It is important that the effusion has been drained to dryness before insertion of the sclerosing agent so that the two pleural surfaces can be apposed so as to promote adhesions. If chemical pleurodesis is not successful, surgical pleurodesis or **pleurectomy via thoracoscopy** may be helpful.
- **Infection.** Pneumonia may be complicated by an inflammatory reaction in the pleura resulting in a **parapneumonic effusion**. Secondary infection of this effusion with multiplication of bacteria in the pleural space produces an **empyema**, which is the presence of pus in the pleural cavity. If a parapneumonic effusion has a low pH (<7.2) there is a high risk of an empyema developing and early tube drainage is indicated. Various organisms may give rise to an empyema, including *Streptococcus pneumoniae*, *Staphylococcus aureus*, *Streptococcus anginosus* (*milleri*) and anaerobic organisms (e.g. *Bacteroides*). Empyema is particularly associated with aspiration pneumonia (e.g. related to unconsciousness, alcohol, vomiting, dysphagia etc.). **Actinomycosis** is an unusual infection that spreads from the lung to the pleura and chest wall, with a tendency to form sinus tracts. **Tuberculosis** must always be borne in mind as a cause of pleural effusion or empyema (see Chapter 7). Initial **antibiotic treatment** is often with co-amoxiclav and metronidazole, adjusted in accordance with the results of microbiology tests. The key treatment of empyema, however, is **drainage of the pus**. Placement of the drainage tube is best guided by ultrasound imaging, as the effusion is often loculated as a result of fibrin deposition and adhesions. Instillation of a **fibrinolytic agent** (e.g. streptokinase, urokinase, tissue plasminogen activator), with or without intrapleural DNase (dornase alpha), may improve the outcome in selected patients with loculated empyemas, but the evidence of benefit is uncertain. **Surgical intervention** is necessary if these measures fail. A variety of approaches may be used, including rib resection with open drainage and thoracotomy with removal of infected debris and decortication (stripping of the pleura and empyematous sac).
- **Inflammatory diseases.** Various inflammatory diseases may involve the pleura. Effusions associated with **connective tissue diseases** (e.g. rheumatoid arthritis, systemic lupus erythematosus (SLE)) characteristically have a low glucose content. **Drug reactions** involving the pleura have been described, including with dantrolene, bromocriptine, nitrofurantoin and methysergide. **Asbestos** may give rise to **benign asbestos-related pleural effusions**, which can recur, producing diffuse pleural thickening (see Chapter 14). Small pleural effusions may complicate **pulmonary embolism** and infarction (see Chapter 15). **Dressler's syndrome** consists of inflammatory pericarditis and pleurisy of uncertain aetiology following a myocardial infarction or cardiac surgery.
- **Subdiaphragmatic disease. Pancreatitis** may be associated with pleural effusions, probably as a result of diaphragmatic inflammation. Such effusions are usually left sided and characterised by a high amylase content. **Ascites** may traverse the diaphragm through pleuroperitoneal communications, causing a pleural effusion. Spread of infection or inflammation from a **subphrenic abscess** or **intrahepatic abscess** may also cause a pleural effusion.

Oesophageal rupture

Oesophageal rupture may give rise to a pyopneu-mothorax (air and pus in the pleural cavity). This can result from external **trauma** or may be **iatrogenic** (e.g. perforation during endoscopy). **Spontaneous rupture of the oesophagus** (Boerhaave's syndrome) is a rare but catastrophic condition that typically occurs when the patient attempts to suppress vomiting by closure of the pharyngeal sphincter. Intraoesophageal pressure rises steeply and rupture typically occurs in the lowest third of the oesophagus. It is a more severe form of the Mallory–Weiss syndrome of haematemesis, caused by mucosal tears from protracted vomiting. Characteristically, vomiting is followed by chest pain and subcutaneous emphysema (palpable air in skin) as air and gastric contents leak into the mediastinum. A few hours later, the pleural membrane gives way and air and food debris pass into the pleural cavity, producing pleuritic pain, pleural effusion and empyema. Chest X-ray typically shows an initial pneumomediastinum (a rim of air around mediastinal structures), followed by a hydropneumothorax. The diagnosis is notoriously difficult to make and a radiocontrast oesophagogram is the key investigation. Thoracotomy with repair of the oesophagus is usually required.

- A **chest tube** is needed for a symptomatic secondary pneumothorax (underlying lung disease, e.g. COPD) and for primary pneumothoraces where aspiration has failed. A small-calibre (8–14F) tube is inserted using a Seldinger technique over a guide wire in the 'triangle of safety' and connected to an underwater seal.
- The tube position must be checked on X-ray. The drain should be examined frequently to ensure that it is securely anchored in place and not kinked or blocked. **Oscillation** of the meniscus of water in the tube indicates that the tube is patent. **Bubbling** indicates ongoing drainage of air. Adequate pain control (e.g. ibuprofen and morphine) must be ensured. The drain is removed when bubbling has stopped and X-ray confirms re-expansion of the lung.
- Persistent bubbling indicates an ongoing air leak. **Low-pressure suction** (−10 to −20 cmH$_2$O) may be applied. If the air leak persists, **thoracic surgical assessment** is needed for thoracoscopic closure of the hole and for pleurodesis or pleurectomy.
- At discharge, the patient should be advised **not to smoke** and to avoid air travel for at least 7 days.

Respiratory emergencies Pneumothorax

- Acute **pleuritic pain** and **breathlessness** with diminished breath sounds are the typical features of a pneumothorax. Severe distress with cardiorespiratory compromise suggests a **tension pneumothorax**.
- **Chest X-ray** shows a convex '**pleural line**' at the margin of the collapsed lung, with a black gas space containing **no lung markings** between the collapsed lung and chest wall. If a distinct pleural line in not visible, the appearances may be a result of a **bulla** and CT scan may be needed to clarify. A 2 cm rim of air approximately equates to a 50% pneumothorax.
- A small pneumothorax not causing distress may not require intervention. It is likely to resolve spontaneously at a rate of 1–2% per day.
- **Aspiration** is recommended for a spontaneous primary pneumothorax (no underlying lung disease) using a 16G cannula inserted via the second intercostal space anteriorly.

 KEY POINTS

- Pneumothorax is the presence of air in the pleural space. This usually occurs from rupture of subpleural cysts in the underlying lung.
- A small pneumothorax (<2 cm rim of air) may not require intervention. A larger pneumothorax (>2 cm rim of air) is treated by simple aspiration or insertion of an intercostal tube.
- A pleural effusion is a collection of fluid in the pleural space.
- Transudative effusions result from changes in hydrostatic pressure (e.g. cardiac failure). Exudative effusions result from diseases of the pleura (e.g. malignancy, infection, inflammation).
- Investigation of an exudative effusion involves clinical assessment, imaging (e.g. CT), pleural fluid aspiration (for biochemistry, cytology and microbiology) and pleural biopsy.

📖 FURTHER READING

British Thoracic Society Pleural Disease Guideline Group. British Thoracic Society pleural disease guideline. *Thorax* 2010; **65**(Suppl. II): 1–76.

Cameron RJ, Davies HR. Intra-pleural fibrinolytic therapy versus conservative management in the treatment of adult parapneumonic effusions and empyema. *Cochrane Database Syst Rev* 2008; doi: 10.1002/14651858.CD002312.pub3.

Henry MT. Simple sequential treatment for primary spontaneous pneumothorax: one step closer. *Eur Resp J* 2006; **27**: 448–50.

Light RW. Parapneumonic effusions and empyema. *Proc Am Thorac Soc* 2006; **3**: 75–80.

Rahman NM, Maskell NA, West A, et al. Intrapleural use of tissue plasminogen activator and DNase in pleural infection. *N Engl J Med* 2011; **365**: 518–26.

Multiple choice questions

16.1 The characteristic feature of a pneumothorax is:
  A dullness to percussion
  B bronchial breathing
  C tenderness on palpation of the chest wall
  D decreased breath sounds
  E crackles

16.2 An 18-year-old man who is usually fit and well presents with left pleuritic pain. A chest X-ray shows a small left apical pneumothorax. He is now asymptomatic. The most appropriate management of his pneumothorax is:
  A no intervention
  B aspiration
  C chest drain insertion
  D thoracoscopy with pleurodesis
  E limited apicolateral surgical pleurectomy

16.3 A 50-year-old man is admitted to hospital with a left lower lobe pneumonia. Chest X-ray shows a small left pleural effusion. Pleural aspiration under ultrasound guidance yields straw-coloured fluid with a protein of 40 g/l, LDH of 300 units/l and pH 7.5. These features indicate:
  A an empyema requiring insertion of a chest drain
  B an exudative parapneumonic effusion not requiring insertion of a chest drain
  C a transudative effusion not requiring intervention
  D an exudative parapneumonic effusion requiring insertion of a chest drain
  E probable tuberculosis

16.4 A transudative pleural effusion in a 70-year-old man is most likely to result from:
  A lung carcinoma
  B mesothelioma
  C left ventricular failure
  D pneumonia
  E rheumatoid arthritis

16.5 A 75-year-old man presents acutely unwell with a 16-hour history of left chest pain, breathlessness and fever, following an episode of vomiting the previous night. There is dullness on percussion of the left side of the chest, with diminished breath sounds. Subcutaneous emphysema is palpable in the neck. Chest X-ray shows a left hydropneumothorax. The most likely diagnosis is:
  A oesophageal rupture
  B perforated duodenal ulcer
  C aspiration pneumonia and empyema
  D pneumothorax with bronchopleural fistula
  E aspiration pneumonia and parapneumonic effusion

16.6 The characteristic features of a pneumothorax on chest X-ray are:
  A hyperinflated black lungs
  B a dense white shadow with a concave upper edge
  C a cyst of air within the lungs
  D a black gas space between the margin of the lung and the chest wall, with a convex 'pleural line'
  E an area of consolidation with an associated pleural effusion

16.7 A 70-year-old man who has worked with asbestos as a pipe lagger in shipyards presents with a large right pleural effusion. The pleural fluid is bloodstained but cytology is nondiagnostic. CT scan shows a large pleural effusion with areas of nodular pleural thickening extending on to the mediastinal pleura. The most appropriate investigation is:
  A video-assisted thoracoscopy with pleural biopsy and pleurodesis
  B bronchoscopy and bronchial biopsy
  C PET scan
  D ultrasound
  E mediastinoscopy and lymph node biopsy

16.8 A diagnostic pleural aspirate under ultrasound guidance in a 60-year-old man yields straw-coloured fluid with a protein of 40 g/l and a lactate dehydrogenase of 400 IU/l. This is best classified as:
  A a chlyous effusion
  B an empyema
  C a transudate
  D an exudate
  E a parapneumonic effusion

16.9 A 25-year-old man has had a chest drain inserted for a large left pneumothorax. The next day, inspection of the drain and underwater seal shows that the water in the tube is oscillating with respiration but not bubbling. This is likely to indicate that:

A the pneumothorax has resolved satisfactorily

B the tube is blocked

C the tube is displaced

D he has now developed a pleural effusion

E he has developed a bronchopleural fistula

16.10 Pleural effusions associated with left ventricular dysfunction are usually:

A bloodstained

B left-sided

C exudates

D transudates

E chylous

Multiple choice answers

16.1 D

The typical signs of a pneumothorax are diminished breath sounds, decreased expansion and hyper-resonance on the side of the pneumothorax, although these are often difficult to detect. Shift of the trachea and apex beat to the opposite side with severe distress and cardiorespiratory compromise indicates a tension pneumothorax.

16.2 A

Conservative management of small, asymptomatic primary spontaneous pneumothoraces has been shown to be safe. This man is fit and well, with no known pre-existing lung disease (primary pneumothorax) and is asymptomatic. No intervention is needed. He may be allowed to go home with a follow-up appointment arranged. He should be advised to return to the accident and emergency department in the unlikely event that he deteriorates.

16.3 B

The elevated protein and LDH indicate an exudate. The fluid is straw-coloured, with a normal pH, so that the small pleural effusion is likely to resolve with antibiotics and does not need drainage. A pH <7.2 indicates that a parapneumonic effusion requires drainage.

16.4 C

Transudative pleural effusions have a protein content of <30 g/l and an LDH < 200 units/l. They arise as a result of changes in hydrostatic or osmotic pressures across the pleural membrane, rather than through disease of the pleura. The main causes of transudative effusions are cardiac failure, renal failure, hepatic cirrhosis and hypoproteinaemia.

16.5 A

Spontaneous rupture of the oesophagus (Boerhaave's syndrome) occurs when the patient attempts to suppress vomiting by closure of the pharyngeal sphincter. Air and fluid leak from the ruptured oesophagus into the pleural space, causing a hydropneumothorax. Air can leak into the tissues, giving palpable subcutaneous emphysema.

16.6 D

The chest X-ray in a patient with a pneumothorax typically shows a black gas space, containing no lung markings, between the margin of the collapsed lung and the chest wall. The visceral pleura typically appears as a laterally convex 'pleural line' that runs parallel to the chest wall.

16.7 A

The clinical and radiological features are suspicious for a malignant mesothlioma. Video-assisted thoracoscopy allows biopsy of the pleura under direct vision, and can be combined with pleurodesis.

16.8 D

A pleural fluid protein content >30 g/l and LDH > 200 units/l indicate that the effusion is an exudate, and further investigations are required.

16.9 A

Oscillation of the meniscus of water in the chest tube indicates that the tube is patent and in the pleural space. Bubbling on respiration or on coughing would indicate continued drainage of air.

16.10 D

Left ventricular dysfunction causes elevated left heart pressures and increased hydrostatic pressure in the lungs, resulting in pulmonary oedema and transudative pleural effusions, which are frequently bilateral.

17

Acute respiratory distress syndrome

Introduction

The acute respiratory distress syndrome (ARDS) is a form of **acute respiratory failure** caused by **permeability pulmonary oedema** resulting from **endothelial damage** due to a cascade of **inflammatory events** developing in response to an **initiating injury or illness**.

It has long been recognised that soldiers wounded in battle often die of respiratory failure some days later. During World Wars I and II, it was thought that this was because of lung infection or excessive fluid administration. Further experience of the condition during the Vietnam War showed that despite successful surgical management of wounds and optimal fluid replacement, soldiers were still dying of pulmonary dysfunction some days later and that the lungs showed features such as oedema, atelectasis, haemorrhage and hyaline membrane formation. It was not until 1967 that this condition was recognised as a specific clinical entity separate from the precipitating injury, and that it could also arise from civilian injuries and illnesses. The term 'adult respiratory distress syndrome' was sometimes used, because of the superficial similarity of the pathology of the disease – showing hyaline membranes – to the infant respiratory distress syndrome (caused by surfactant deficiency in premature babies), but the term 'acute respiratory distress syndrome' is more appropriate.

Pathogenesis

In most situations, pulmonary oedema arises as a result of increased pulmonary capillary **pressure** (e.g. left ventricular failure), but in ARDS it arises because of increased alveolar capillary **permeability**.

Pressure pulmonary oedema

In the normal situation, the hydrostatic pressure and the osmotic pressure exerted by the plasma proteins are in a state of equilibrium between the pulmonary capillaries and lung alveoli (Fig. 17.1). An **increase in hydrostatic pressure** is the most common cause of pulmonary oedema, and this typically occurs secondary to elevated left atrial pressure from left ventricular failure (e.g. after myocardial infarction) or from mitral valve disease (e.g. mitral stenosis). **Volume overload** may also increase pulmonary capillary pressure, and this may arise from excessive intravenous fluid administration or fluid retention (e.g. renal failure). **Reduced osmotic pressure** may contribute to pulmonary oedema, and this occurs in hypoproteinaemic states (e.g. severely ill, malnourished patients; nephrotic syndrome with renal protein loss). In the early stages of pulmonary oedema, there is an increase in the fluid content of the interstitial space between the capillaries and alveoli, but as the condition deteriorates, flooding of the alveoli occurs.

Permeability pulmonary oedema

In ARDS, a cascade of inflammatory events arises over a period of hours from a focus of tissue damage. In particular, activated neutrophils aggregate and adhere to endothelial cells, releasing various toxins, oxygen radicals and mediators (e.g. arachidonic acid, histamine, kinins). This **systemic inflammatory response** may be initiated by a variety of injuries or illnesses and gives rise to **acute lung injury** as one

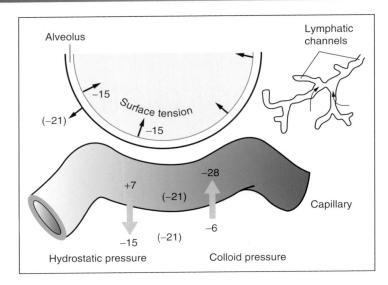

Figure 17.1 Diagram illustrating approximate values for hydrostatic and colloid pressures in millimetres of mercury (mmHg) between the pulmonary capillary and alveolus. Pulmonary oedema may arise from increased hydrostatic pressure (e.g. cardiogenic pulmonary oedema), from reduced colloid pressure (e.g. hypoalbuminaemia) or from increased capillary permeability (e.g. ARDS).

of its earliest manifestations, with the development of **endothelial damage** and **increased alveolar capillary permeability**. The alveoli become filled with a protein-rich exudate containing abundant neutrophils and other inflammatory cells, and the airspaces show a rim of proteinaceous material: the hyaline membrane. The characteristic feature of permeability pulmonary oedema in ARDS is that the pulmonary capillary wedge pressure is not elevated. This may be measured by passing a special balloon-tipped pulmonary artery catheter (e.g. Swan–Ganz catheter) via a central vein through the right side of the heart to the pulmonary artery. The balloon of the catheter is then inflated and is carried forward in the blood flow until it wedges in a pulmonary capillary. The measurement of pulmonary capillary wedge pressure reflects left atrial pressure. In ARDS, it is typically ≤18 mmHg, whereas in cardiogenic pulmonary oedema, it is elevated.

Clinical features

ARDS develops in response to a variety of injuries or illnesses that affect the lungs, either **directly** (e.g. aspiration of gastric contents, severe pneumonia, lung contusion) or **indirectly** (e.g. systemic sepsis, major trauma, pancreatitis). About 12–48 hours after an initiating event, the patient develops respiratory distress, with increasing dyspnoea and tachypnoea. Arterial blood gases show deteriorating hypoxaemia, which responds poorly to oxygen therapy. Diffuse bilateral infiltrates develop on chest X-ray in the absence of evidence of cardiogenic pulmonary oedema. ARDS is the most severe end of the spectrum of acute lung injury and is characterised by the following features:

- A history of an **initiating injury or illness** (Table 17.1).
- **Hypoxaemia** refractory to oxygen therapy (e.g. Po_2, 8.0 kPa (60 mmHg) on 40% oxygen). The degree of hypoxaemia may be expressed as the ratio of arterial oxygen tension (Po_2) to the fractional inspired oxygen concentration (F_iO_2/100% oxygen = F_iO_2 of 1). In ARDS, Po_2/F_iO_2 is <26 kPa (200 mmHg).

Table 17.1 Initiating injuries and illnesses in ARDS

Direct	Indirect
Aspiration of gastric contents	Sepsis
Severe pneumonia	Major trauma
Smoke inhalation	Multiple blood transfusions
Lung contusion	Pancreatitis
Fat embolism	Extensive burns
Amniotic fluid embolism	Anaphylaxis
Chemical inhalation (e.g. silo filler's lung)	Hypotensive shock
Oxygen toxicity/ventilator lung	Disseminated intravascular coagulation

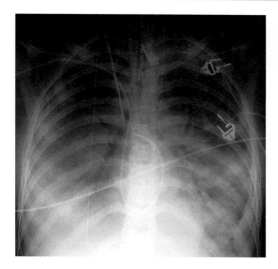

Figure 17.2 This 21-year-old diabetic patient was admitted to the ITU having vomited and inhaled gastric contents while unconscious with severe ketoacidosis. Despite antibiotics and treatment of ketoacidosis, she developed ARDS with progressive respiratory distress and severe hypoxaemia refractory to oxygen therapy. The chest X-ray shows diffuse bilateral shadowing with air bronchograms (black tubes of air against the white background of consolidated lung). An endotracheal tube is in place and the patient is being mechanically ventilated, with a positive end-expiratory pressure (PEEP) of 7.5 cmH$_2$O. Electrocardiogram monitor leads are visible and a central venous line has been inserted via the right internal jugular vein. A Swan–Ganz catheter has been passed from the right subclavian vein and can be seen looped through the right side of the heart into the pulmonary artery. Pulmonary capillary wedge pressure was low at 8 mmHg, indicating that the lung shadowing was not caused by cardiogenic pulmonary oedema but by increased capillary permeability of ARDS. Despite requiring prolonged ventilation and support on ITU, the patient made a full recovery.

- Bilateral **diffuse infiltrates on chest X-ray** (Fig. 17.2).
- No evidence of cardiogenic pulmonary oedema (e.g. **pulmonary capillary wedge pressure < 18 mmHg**).

Recognition of critically ill patients

Patients who subsequently develop ARDS may appear deceptively well in the initial stages of their illness.

Table 17.2 Features indicating a critically ill patient. A patient demonstrating any of these warning signs needs urgent attention and consideration of ITU care

Respiratory rate	<8 or >30/min
Pulse rate	<40 or >130/min
Blood pressure (systolic)	<90 mmHg
Temperature	Hyperthermia (>38 °C, 100.4 °F)
	Hypothermia (<36 °C, 96.8 °F)
Urine output	<30 ml/hour for 3 hours
Level of consciousness	Not responding to commands
Oxygenation	O$_2$ saturation <90% or P$_a$O$_2$< 8 kPa (60 mmHg) despite 60% inspired oxygen
Acidosis	pH <7.2; bicarbonate <20 mmol/l

Early recognition and careful observation of at-risk patients are of crucial importance in detecting the signs of deterioration and identifying the need for intensive therapy unit (ITU) care. Certain warning signs are applicable in a wide variety of clinical circumstances, because there is often a common physiological pathway of deterioration in the severely ill, which can be detected by simple observations of the **pulse rate**, **respiratory rate**, **blood pressure**, **temperature**, **urine output** and **level of consciousness** (Table 17.2). Arterial blood gas measurements provide useful additional information about gas exchange and the metabolic state of the patient.

Treatment

The treatment of ARDS consists of optimal management of the initiating illness or injury, combined with supportive care directed at preserving adequate oxygenation, maintaining optimal haemodynamic function and compensating for multiorgan failure, which often supervenes.

Treatment of initiating illness

Prompt and complete treatment of the initiating injury or illness is essential. This includes rapid resuscitation with correction of hypotension in patients with multiple trauma, for example, as well as eradication of any source of sepsis (e.g. intra-abdominal abscess or ischaemic bowel post-surgery).

Respiratory support

Characteristically, the hypoxaemia of ARDS is refractory to **oxygen therapy** due to shunting of blood through areas of lung that are not being ventilated because the alveoli are filled with a proteinaceous exudate and undergoing atelectasis. **Continuous positive airway pressure (CPAP)** can be applied via a tight-fitting nasal mask to prevent alveolar atelectasis and thereby reduce ventilation/perfusion mismatch and the work of breathing. However, **endotracheal intubation** and **mechanical ventilation** rapidly become necessary and the patient may need to be transferred to a **specialist ITU** with expertise and facilities for treating ARDS. Intermittent positive-pressure ventilation mechanically inflates the lungs, delivering oxygen-enriched air at a set tidal volume and rate. Adjustments in the volume, inflation pressure, rate and percentage oxygen are made to achieve adequate ventilation. A **positive end-expiratory pressure (PEEP)** of $5-15\,cmH_2O$ is usually applied at the end of the expiratory cycle to prevent collapse of the alveoli. High airway pressures may be generated in ventilating the noncompliant stiff lungs in ARDS, and this can reduce cardiac output and carries the risk of barotrauma (e.g. pneumothorax). High ventilation pressures combined with high oxygen concentrations may themselves result in microvascular damage, which perpetuates the problem of permeability pulmonary oedema ('ventilator lung/oxygen toxicity'). A variety of lung-protective ventilatory techniques have been developed to overcome these problems. Ventilation with **lower tidal volumes** can reduce lung damage.

Permissive hypercapnia is a technique that allows the patient to have a high P_aco_2 level (e.g. 10 kPa, 75 mmHg) in order to reduce the alveolar ventilation and avoid excessive airway pressure. **Inverse-ratio ventilation** prolongs the inspiratory phase of ventilation such that it is longer than the expiratory phase, allowing the tidal volume to be delivered over a longer time at a lower pressure. However, this may cause progressive air trapping. **High-frequency jet ventilation** is a technique whereby small volumes are delivered as an injected jet of gas at high frequencies (e.g. 100–300/min). Ventilation of the patient in the **prone posture** may be beneficial, as it reduces gravity-dependent fluid deposition and atelectasis. **Extracorporeal membrane oxygenation** (ECMO) involves the diversion of the patient's circulation through an artificial external membrane to provide oxygen and remove carbon dioxide. None of these ventilatory strategies has yet achieved a major improvement in the overall prognosis of ARDS, but each may be useful in individual circumstances. Nursing patients in a semirecumbent position at 45 degrees reduces the incidence of ventilator-associated pneumonia.

Optimising haemodynamic function

Reducing the pulmonary artery pressure may help to reduce the degree of pulmonary capillary leak. This is achieved by avoidance of excessive fluid administration, by judicious use of **diuretics** and by use of drugs that act as **vasodilators** of the pulmonary arteries. Treatment is sometimes guided by use of a balloon-tipped pulmonary artery catheter (Swan–Ganz) that measures pulmonary artery pressures, pulmonary capillary wedge pressure (reflecting left atrial pressure) and cardiac output (using a thermal dilution technique). Haemodynamic management essentially consists of achieving an **optimal balance** between a **low pulmonary artery pressure** (to reduce fluid leak to the alveoli), an **adequate systemic blood pressure** (to maintain perfusion of tissues and organs, e.g. kidneys), a satisfactory **cardiac output** and an optimal **oxygen delivery** to tissues (oxygen delivery is a function of the haemoglobin level, oxygen saturation of the blood and cardiac output). Most drugs used to vasodilate the pulmonary arteries, such as nitrates and calcium antagonists, also cause systemic vasodilatation with hypotension and impaired organ perfusion. Inotropes and vasopressor agents, such as **dobutamine** and **norepinephrine** (noradrenaline), may be needed to maintain systemic blood pressure and cardiac output, particularly in patients with the sepsis syndrome (caused by septicaemia or peritonitis, for example), in which sepsis is associated with systemic vasodilatation. Inhaled **nitric oxide** (NO) may be used as a selective pulmonary artery vasodilator. Because it is given by inhalation, it is selectively distributed to ventilated regions of the lung, where it produces vasodilatation. This vasodilatation to ventilated alveoli may significantly improve ventilation/perfusion matching, with improved gas exchange. NO is rapidly inactivated by haemoglobin, preventing a systemic action. It is necessary to monitor the level of inspired gas, nitrogen dioxide (NO_2) and methaemoglobin in order to avoid toxicity. Nebulised **prostacyclin** is a vasodilator with similar effects to NO but a reduced risk of toxicity. Unfortunately, these selective pulmonary vasodilator agents have not been shown to reduce mortality.

General management

Correction of anaemia by **blood transfusions** improves oxygen carriage in the blood and oxygen delivery to the tissues. **Nutritional support** (e.g. by enteral feeding via a nasogastric tube) is important in maintaining the patient's overall fitness in the face of critical illness, and correction of hypoalbuminaemia improves the osmotic pressure of the plasma, reducing fluid leak from the circulation. The ventilated patient with ARDS is particularly vulnerable to **hospital-acquired pneumonia**, and bronchoalveolar lavage may be helpful in identifying pathogens. **Multiorgan failure** often complicates ARDS, requiring further specific interventions (e.g. dialysis for renal failure).

Anti-inflammatory therapies

A key target for potential treatment is the cascade of inflammatory events arising from the tissue damage resulting from the initiating illness. Unfortunately, these events are poorly understood and no anti-inflammatory drug has yet achieved an established role in treating ARDS. Corticosteroids have not been beneficial. Ibuprofen has been used in an attempt to reduce neutrophil activation and pentoxifylline has been used because of its action in reducing the production of IL-1. Haemofiltration is a procedure that is primarily used to control fluid balance, but it may have an additional beneficial effect in patients with sepsis via removal of endotoxins.

Prognosis

Advances in the supportive care of patients with ARDS have resulted in improved survival rates, but mortality remains very high, at >40%. Patients who survive ARDS may experience substantial physical impairment, psychiatric morbidity, impaired cognitive function and reduced health-related quality of life, but some patients make a remarkably full recovery despite having been critically ill with gross lung injury requiring prolonged treatment in ITU.

 KEY POINTS

- ARDS is a form of acute pulmonary oedema caused by increased endothelial permeability resulting from an inflammatory response to illness or injury.
- Precipitating factors include systemic sepsis, trauma, burns, pancreatitis and aspiration of gastric contents.
- Patients are severely hypoxic, with diffuse infiltrates on chest X-ray and no evidence of cardiac failure.
- Treatment involves correction of the initiating illness and supportive care using lung-protective ventilation with PEEP.

 FURTHER READING

Adhikari NK, Burns KE, Friedrich JO, et al. Effect of nitric oxide on oxygenation and mortality in acute lung injury: systematic review and meta-analysis. *BMJ* 2007; **334**: 779–82.

Ashbaugh DG, Bigelow DB, Petty TL, Levine BE. Acute respiratory distress in adults. *Lancet* 1967; **ii**: 319–23.

Baudouin S, Evans T. Improving outcomes for severely ill medical patients. *Clin Med* 2002; **2**: 92–4.

Bernard GR, Artigas A, Brigham KL, et al. Report of the American–European Consensus Conference on ARDS. *Intens Care Med* 1994; **20**: 225–32.

Guerin C, Reigner J, Richard JC, et al. Prone positioning in severe acute respiratory distress syndrome. *N Engl J Med* 2013; **368**: 2159–68.

Matthay MA, Zimmerman GA. Acute lung injury and acute respiratory distress syndrome. *Am J Resp Cell Mol Biol* 2005; **33**: 319–27.

Pandharipande PP, Girard TD, Jackson JC, et al. Longterm cognitive impairment after critical illness. *N Engl J Med* 2013; **369**: 1306–16.

Peter JV, John P, Graham PL, et al. Corticosteroids in the prevention and treatment of acute respiratory distress syndrome in adults: meta-analysis. *BMJ* 2008; **336**: 1006–9.

Multiple choice questions

17.1 ARDS was first described in:
A 1918
B 1940
C 1967
D 1980
E 1994

17.2 Pulmonary oedema in ARDS is characterised by:
A an elevated pulmonary artery pressure
B volume overload
C increased hydrostatic pressure
D decreased colloid pressure
E increased alveolar capillary permeability

17.3 A 40-year-old man is admitted to hospital with severe pancreatitis. Three days later, he develops progressive breathlessness, severe hypoxia and diffuse bilateral shadowing on chest X-ray. The most likely diagnosis is:
A pulmonary embolism
B left ventricular failure
C ARDS
D hospital-acquired pneumonia
E fat embolism

17.4 The mortality rate of patients requiring endotracheal ventilation for ARDS is approximately:
A 10%
B 20%
C 30%
D 40%
E 80%

17.5 With regard to ARDS:
A the pulmonary capillary wedge pressure is typically less than 18 mmHg
B pulmonary oedema usually results from excessive fluid administration
C left ventricular failure is usually a major factor in the development of pulmonary oedema
D lung infiltrates on chest X-ray usually indicate pneumonia
E lymphatic obstruction gives rise to pulmonary congestion

17.6 The most common precipitating factor for ARDS is:
A acute pulmonary embolism
B myocardial infarction with cardiogenic shock
C systemic sepsis
D an acute exacerbation of COPD
E multiple blood transfusions

17.7 Acute pulmonary oedema in a patient with a myocardial infarction is usually due to:
A increased alveolar–capillary permeability
B increased hydrostatic pressure
C reduced colloid pressure
D ARDS
E excess fluid administration

17.8 Pulmonary oedema in ARDS is usually treated by:
A mechanical ventilation with positive end-expiratory pressure
B noninvasive ventilation via a tight-fitting mask
C sputum clearance physiotherapy
D renal dialysis to remove excess fluid
E intravenous diuretics

17.9 The most common cause of pneumonia developing in a patient undergoing prolonged ventilation for ARDS is:
A *Legionella pneumophilia*
B *Haemophilus influenzae*
C *Streptococcus pneumoniae*
D *Clostridium difficile*
E Gram-negative bacteria

17.10 The most common cause of death in patients with ARDS is:
A pulmonary embolism
B myocardial infarction
C stroke secondary to brain hypoxia
D multi-organ failure
E brainstem death

Multiple choice answers

17.1 C

ARDS was described in 1967. It had been recognised that soldiers wounded in battle during World Wars I and II often died of respiratory failure some days later, and it was mistakenly thought that this was due to infection or fluid overload. It was only with further experience during the Vietnam War that it was recognised that the respiratory failure was due to permeability pulmonary oedema caused by endothelial damage.

17.2 E

ARDS is characterised by permeability pulmonary oedema. The systemic inflammatory response results in endothelial damage, with leakage of a protein-rich exudate into the alveoli.

17.3 C

Severe pancreatitis is a typical initiating illness. It gives rise to the inflammatory processes and endothelial damage that result in ARDS.

17.4 D

ARDS is a very serious disease, with a high mortality of approximately 40%.

17.5 A

In cardiogenic pulmonary oedema (e.g. caused by left ventricular failure), pulmonary artery pressure is typically elevated, whereas in ARDS the pulmonary oedema results from an increased permeability of the endothelium rather than 'pressure pulmonary oedema', and the pulmonary artery pressure is typically <18 mmHg.

17.6 C

Severe systemic sepsis is the most common cause of ARDS in most circumstances.

17.7 B

Myocardial infarction with left ventricular dysfunction causes elevated left heart pressures, with increased hydrostatic pressure in the lungs and resultant 'pressure pulmonary oedema'.

17.8 A

Patients with ARDS require admission to the ITU with endotracheal intubation and mechanical ventilation. A positive end-expiratory pressure (PEEP) of $5-15$ cmH$_2$O is usually applied at the end of the expiratory cycle to prevent collapse of the alveoli.

17.9 E

Gram-negative bacteria are the most common cause of ventilator-associated pneumonia.

17.10 D

Multiorgan failure often complicates ARDS and is the most common cause of death.

18

Ventilatory failure and sleep-related breathing disorders

Introduction

For the lungs to take up oxygen and expel carbon dioxide, they must be ventilated. Whilst some diseased lungs have an impaired ability to perform 'gas exchange', even a healthy lung is entirely dependent on a constant supply of fresh air in order to do its job. If ventilation fails, oxygen can't be taken up and carbon dioxide can't be expelled. There are a number of conditions that lead to inadequate ventilation; in some, the lungs themselves may be entirely healthy.

People spend almost one-third of their lives asleep, and the relationship between ventilation and sleep is important. Ventilatory drive and ventilation are generally diminished during sleep. In healthy individuals, this causes no deleterious effect, but when ventilation is compromised, problems can be greatly exacerbated during sleep. Some conditions, such as obstructive sleep apnoea (OSA), are only manifest during sleep, although the consequences can impact on the entirety of the patient's life.

Sleep physiology

Although familiar to everyone as a state in which the eyes are closed, postural muscles relaxed and consciousness suspended, sleep is an enigmatic condition that has essential refreshing and restorative effects on the mind and body. Electroencephalogram (EEG) studies show that sleep may be divided into five stages and two major categories. Stages 1–4 are characterised by loss of alpha-wave activity, with a progressive slowing in frequency and increase in amplitude of the EEG waveform. A quite distinct stage is characterized by **rapid eye movements**: **REM sleep**. Typically, a person drifts from an awake, relaxed state through EEG stages 1–4 into a progressively deeper sleep, becoming less responsive to stimuli and less rousable. After about 70 minutes of non-REM sleep, the person usually enters a period associated with rapid eye movements. This usually lasts about 30 minutes and is often followed by a brief awakening and a return to stage 1 sleep. Cycles of REM and non-REM sleep continue throughout the night, with the period spent in REM sleep becoming longer each cycle, such that it occupies about 25% of total sleep time. During REM sleep, the person is difficult to rouse and has reduced muscle tone. This stage of sleep is associated with dreaming and a variety of autonomic changes, including changes in respiration, blood pressure, pulse rate and pupil diameter. Irregularity of respiration and heart rate are common in this stage of sleep and apnoeic episodes lasting 15–20 seconds are common in normal individuals. The exact sleep 'architecture' (depth, character, changes) varies with age and circumstances (e.g. unfamiliar environment, disruption of regular routine), so that it can be difficult to define precisely normal and abnormal patterns by arbitrary cut-off points. Although sleep has major beneficial effects on the mind and body, the physiological changes during sleep may aggravate pre-existing

Respiratory Medicine Lecture Notes, Ninth Edition. Stephen J. Bourke and Graham P. Burns.
© 2015 John Wiley & Sons, Ltd. Published 2015 by John Wiley & Sons, Ltd.
Companion Website: www.lecturenoteseries.com/Respiratory

respiratory disease, and specific breathing disorders may arise during sleep.

Ventilatory failure

Ventilation is the action of pumping air in and out of the lungs (the alveoli, to be precise) (see Chapter 1). Constant mixing of the gas in the alveoli with inspired air replenishes the oxygen and washes out the carbon dioxide. If ventilation is normal, arterial Pco_2 will be normal (in fact, the level of arterial Pco_2 defines the adequacy of ventilation). If ventilation is reduced (**alveolar hypoventilation**), the alveolar O_2 is not replenished properly and alveolar CO_2 is not washed out adequately; arterial Po_2 falls and Pco_2 rises. This is type 2 respiratory failure. The degree to which the Po_2 falls is directly related to the rise in Pco_2 (see the alveolar gas equation in Chapter 1). Note this is a very different mechanism to that which leads to type 1 respiratory failure, in which ventilation/perfusion mismatch within the lungs leads to a failure of gas exchange. In type 1 respiratory failure, Po_2 falls, but, so long as ventilation is adequate, Pco_2 is normal (see Chapter 3).

Not all ventilatory failure (type 2 respiratory failure) is related to lung disease. Alveolar hypoventilation can occur from disorder anywhere along the chain of processes that connect the central drive to breathe

with the movement of air in and out of the alveoli. Depending on the nature of the problem, the severity and the speed of onset, the ventilatory failure can be anything from acute asphyxia to chronic ventilatory failure (see Fig. 18.1).

Ventilation can be significantly impaired by severe obesity. Once a rare condition (known as Pickwickian syndrome, after the Dickens character), **obesity-related hypoventialtion syndrome (OHS)** (high BMI, low Po_2, high Pco_2) is now increasingly common.

Ventilatory failure and sleep

During sleep, the respiratory centre in the medulla receives less stimulation from higher cortical centres and becomes less responsive to chemical (e.g. hypercapnia) and mechanical (e.g. from chest wall and airway receptors) stimuli. Minute ventilation (tidal volume and respiratory rate) falls, Pco_2 rises, functional residual capacity decreases and there is diminished activity of the intercostal and accessory respiratory muscles. These changes are most marked during REM sleep. Although they are not associated with any adverse effects in normal individuals, sleep-related hypoventilation becomes problematic

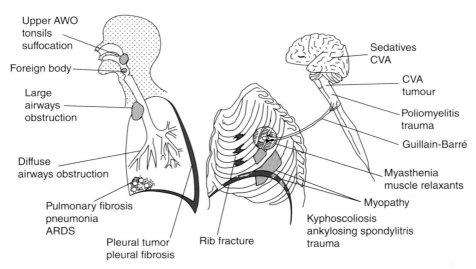

Figure 18.1 Ventilatory failure (type 2 respiratory failure). Examples of processes that can lead to ventilatory failure (often made worse by the physiological changes that occur during sleep), extending (from right to left) from the central nervous system to the upper airway. Severe obesity can additionally have a significant splinting effect on the diaphragm, limiting the ability of the lungs to obtain a full breath. AWO, airway obstruction; ARDS, acute respiratory distress syndrome; CVA, cerebro-vascular accident.

in patients who have pre-existing type 2 respiratory failure. This is most commonly encountered in **chronic obstructive pulmonary disease (COPD)**, **neuromuscular disease** (e.g. muscular dystrophy, motor neurone disease), **thoracic cage disorders** (e.g. kyphoscoliosis) and **OHS**. The nocturnal oxygen desaturation (and hypercapnia) in these disorders results from the deleterious effect of sleep physiology on pre-existing respiratory insufficiency.

Treatment

Optimising the management of any **underlying respiratory disease** (e.g. bronchodilators in COPD) and avoiding **aggravating factors**, such as the use of alcohol or sedative medication, are important. In the case of OHS, **weight loss**, if achieved, can be critical. Supplemental **oxygen** may alleviate oxygen desaturation but may provoke further hypoventilation and carbon dioxide retention, because, in many of these patients, respiratory drive is partly dependent on the stimulant effect of hypoxaemia (see Chapter 1).

If significant nocturnal hypoventilation is present, long-term ventilatory support at night is needed. This is delivered as domiciliary nocturnal **noninvasive positive-pressure ventilation** (NIPPV). A tight-fitting mask is strapped in place over the nose and connected to a specifically designed ventilating machine. The spontaneous inspiratory effort of the patient triggers the ventilator to deliver positive pressure, increasing the volume of air inspired. As the patient begins to breathe out, the machine responds by reducing the pressure and allowing the patient to complete expiration. The expiratory pressure, although substantially lower than the inspiratory pressure, is not usually set at zero. A small amount of positive pressure, against which the patient expires, functions to keep the small airways open for longer, facilitating a more complete expiration. Thus, tidal volume is increased and overall ventilation is improved.

Despite the cumbersome nature of this form of ventilatory support, it is very well tolerated by patients, who can usually manage to sleep while receiving nasal ventilation after a few nights of acclimatisation. Control of nocturnal desaturation by NIPPV improves not only the quality of their sleep and nocturnal symptoms but also their daytime symptoms and gas exchange, via a number of mechanisms. During periods of assisted ventilation, (i) improvements in arterial blood gas levels probably 'reset' the chemoreceptors in the brain stem, (ii) fatigued respiratory muscles are rested, (iii) atelectatic alveoli are opened up and recruited into gas exchange and (iv) sleep deprivation is relieved. These effects result

in general improvement of both gas exchange and ventilation, as well as reduced fatigue during the day. In patients with chronic ventilatory failure, NIPPV can have a worthwhile effect on mortality, and its impact on quality of life can be substantial (see Fig. 18.2).

It is important to understand the difference between this modality of treatment and continuous positive airway pressure (CPAP) in OSA. In CPAP, the pressure delivered is continuous and unchanging; a *difference* between inspiratory and expiratory pressure is required to achieve augmentation of ventilation. NIPPV is a ventilatory treatment, CPAP is not.

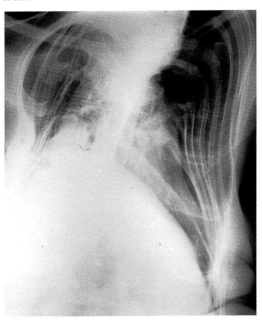

Figure 18.2 This 39-year-old woman with severe kyphoscoliosis developed sleep disturbance, tiredness, headaches and oedema. She was erroneously treated with sedatives for insomnia. Spirometry showed a severe restrictive defect, with a forced expiratory volume in 1 second (FEV$_1$) of 0.4 L and forced vital capacity (FVC) of 0.5 L. Po$_2$ was 5.6 kPa (42 mmHg) and Pco$_2$ 10.2 kPa (76 mmHg). Her sleep was fragmented, with multiple arousals and profound oxygen desaturation. She was unable to tolerate oxygen because of deteriorating hypercapnia. Nocturnal ventilatory support was commenced using NIPPV delivered via a tight nasal mask. After using NIPPV for about 8 hours a night at home for a number of years, she was able to obtain work as a secretary and could work around the house, although she still became breathless on walking 150 m. NIPPV is an effective form of ventilatory support for patients with hypercapnic respiratory failure caused by thoracic cage disorders or neuromuscular disease.

Obstructive sleep apnoea

OSA is a condition of sleep-related pharyngeal collapse in which recurrent episodes of **upper airway occlusion** occur **during sleep**, causing diminution (hypopnoea) or cessation of airflow (**apnoea**) in the pharynx and provoking arousals and **sleep fragmentation**, resulting in daytime **sleepiness** (Fig. 18.3).

With increasing levels of obesity in society, the prevalence of OSA is increasing. There is a much greater awareness of the condition amongst the general public and GPs, although many cases are still thought to be undiagnosed.

Pathogenesis

The **oropharyngeal dilator muscles** play an important part in maintaining patency of the upper airway. During deep sleep, there is reduced muscle tone, so that the pharyngeal airway is most vulnerable to collapse during REM sleep. Use of sedatives or alcohol may cause a further loss of muscle tone. Narrowing of the upper airway predisposes to occlusion; this is usually a result of fat deposition in the neck due to **obesity**, but other factors, such as bone morphology (e.g. micrognathia), soft-tissue deposition (e.g. hypothyroidism, acromegaly) and enlargement of the tonsils or adenoids in children, may also be important. Contraction of the diaphragm and intercostal muscles during inspiration creates a negative pressure in the airways, drawing air into the lungs. This negative pressure also acts to suck in or collapse the upper airway. An increase in upper airway resistance, such as that found in nasal obstruction (e.g. deviated nasal septum, polyps) and in enlargement of the tonsils and adenoids, requires a greater inspiratory effort to overcome it, and thus increases the forces sucking in the pharyngeal airway.

OSA is characterised by recurrent episodes of pharyngeal airway obstruction during sleep, with apnoea, arousal and sleep fragmentation. As the patient with a compromised pharyngeal airway (e.g.

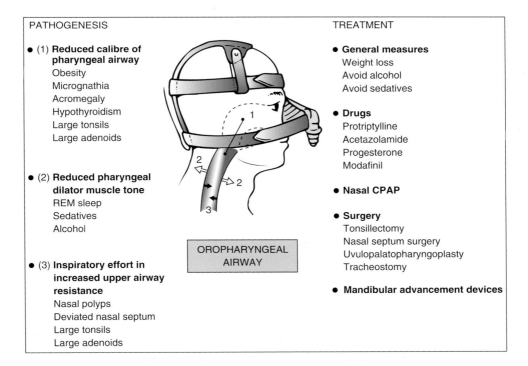

PATHOGENESIS

- (1) **Reduced calibre of pharyngeal airway**
  Obesity
  Micrognathia
  Acromegaly
  Hypothyroidism
  Large tonsils
  Large adenoids

- (2) **Reduced pharyngeal dilator muscle tone**
  REM sleep
  Sedatives
  Alcohol

- (3) **Inspiratory effort in increased upper airway resistance**
  Nasal polyps
  Deviated nasal septum
  Large tonsils
  Large adenoids

OROPHARYNGEAL AIRWAY

TREATMENT

- **General measures**
  Weight loss
  Avoid alcohol
  Avoid sedatives

- **Drugs**
  Protriptylline
  Acetazolamide
  Progesterone
  Modafinil

- **Nasal CPAP**

- **Surgery**
  Tonsillectomy
  Nasal septum surgery
  Uvulopalatopharyngoplasty
  Tracheostomy

- **Mandibular advancement devices**

Figure 18.3 Apnoea results from occlusion of the pharyngeal airway in patients with narrowed airways when there is loss of pharyngeal dilator muscle tone in sleep. Increased inspiratory effort, when there is increased upper airway resistance, 'sucks in' the pharyngeal airway. Nasal CPAP acts as a splint, preventing collapse of the airway, and is the main treatment used for sleep apnoea.

narrowed by obesity) enters deep sleep, the reduction in oropharyngeal dilator muscle tone results in collapse of the airway, causing apnoea (cessation of airflow) or hypopnoea (reduction of airflow), with a fall in oxygen saturation. Inspiratory effort increases as the diaphragm and intercostal muscles try to overcome the closed upper airway. The brain's response is to begin to 'wake up'. As sleep becomes more shallow (often without waking completely), the improved muscle tone relieves the obstruction and terminates the apnoea. This activity is associated with a burst of sympathetic nerve activity, release of catecholamines and fluctuations in pulse rate and blood pressure. Resumption of pharyngeal airflow is usually accompanied by loud snoring, which is an inspiratory noise arising from vibration of the soft tissues of the oropharynx. Once breathing has resumed, the patient drifts back into deep sleep. The cycle then starts again. Hundreds of episodes of apnoea and arousal can occur throughout the night. The patient therefore never experiences any prolonged spell of good-quality, deep sleep. If the episodes of apnoea don't provoke complete wakefulness (and they often don't), by morning the patient can wake believing they've had a solid night's sleep. They will, however, feel entirely unrefreshed.

Clinical features

Patients with OSA may have no detectable respiratory abnormality when awake, but **daytime symptoms** include excessive **sleepiness**, **poor concentration**, **irritability**, **morning headaches** and **loss of libido**. Sleepiness is usually a prominent feature and may result in the patient falling asleep inappropriately, for example when reading, watching television or even driving a car. **The Epworth sleepiness scale** is a useful way of assessing the likelihood of falling asleep in various situations (Table 18.1). Patients with OSA have a high rate of accidents at home, at work and when driving. It is estimated that about 5% of commercial drivers have OSA and that sleep-related **road traffic accidents** make up 15–20% of all crashes, resulting in many serious injuries and deaths. In the UK, patients with OSA must inform the Driver and Vehicle Licensing Agency (DVLA) if they have OSA with symptoms that affect their ability to drive safely. They should be advised to avoid driving until their sleepiness has been controlled by treatment.

The patient might be unaware of **night-time symptoms**, but their bed partner may report loud **snoring**, witnessed **apnoeas** and **restless sleep**. It is important to enquire about use of sedatives or alcohol, which can aggravate OSA.

Table 18.1 The Epworth sleepiness score is useful in screening patients for excessive sleepiness. The patient is asked how likely they are to doze off or fall asleep in the listed situations, according to the following scale: 0, would never doze; 1, slight chance of dozing; 2, moderate chance of dozing; 3, high chance of dozing. A total score of 10 or higher suggests the need for further evaluation for an underlying sleep disorder.

Situation	Score (0–3)
1 Sitting and reading	
2 Watching television	
3 Sitting inactive in a public place (e.g. theatre)	
4 As a passenger in a car for an hour without a break	
5 Lying down to rest in the afternoon	
6 Sitting and talking to someone	
7 Sitting quietly after lunch (when you've had no alcohol)	
8 In a car, while stopped in traffic	

Examination focuses on risk factors for OSA, such as **obesity**, **increased neck circumference**, anatomical abnormalities reducing **pharyngeal calibre** (e.g. micrognathia, enlarged tonsils) and **nasal obstruction** (e.g. polyps, deviated septum).

Cardiovascular complications associated with OSA include hypertension, myocardial infarction, stroke, cardiac arrhythmias, structural cardiac changes and cardiac failure. Although some of these associations may be explained by confounding variables, such as obesity, there is accumulating evidence of an independent direct relationship between OSA and hypertension, stroke and cardiovascular disease, which may result from a combination of factors, including hypoxaemia, changes in blood pressure and sympathetic nervous system activation during apnoeas and arousals. There is an association between OSA and the metabolic syndrome (visceral obesity, insulin resistance, hypertension, dyslipidaemia). Recurrent apnoeas and arousals with deoxygenation and reoxygenation increase the formation of reactive oxygen species (ROS), which are damaging to the vasculature. ROS also provoke inflammatory responses, with activation of cytokines, adhesion molecules, endothelial cells, circulating leucocytes and platelets. It is important to reduce cardiovascular risk factors by checking smoking history, blood pressure and lipid and glucose levels, and intervening as appropriate.

In addition to catecholamine release, OSA is associated with other **hormonal changes**, including reduced testosterone and growth hormone levels. Although hypoxaemia, hypercapnia and elevation of pulmonary artery pressure occur during apnoeas, **cor pulmonale is unusual** unless there is concomitant lung disease (e.g. COPD). Links between **cancer** and OSA have been identified in epidemiological studies; further research is ongoing.

Diagnosis (sleep studies)

A definitive assessment has traditionally involved full polysomnography, including signals relating to **oxymetry**, **airflow** (thermistor at the nose and mouth), **chest wall movement** (magnetometers or impedance), stage of sleep (**electroencephalograph** (EEG) and **electrooculogram** (EOG), to detect rapid eye movement) and heart rate (**electrocardiogram** (ECG)). These tracings are often combined with a video recording of the patient during sleep, which permits observation of the patient's position and movement in relation to apnoeas and arousals. In clinical practice, most sleep studies are now carried out in the patient's home using a portable kit (which doesn't include EEG or EOG).

The number of apnoeas increases with age, and there is a continuum from normality to full-blown OSA, so that it is difficult to define precise diagnostic criteria. However, OSA is usually diagnosed when there are more than 15 apnoeas or hypopnoeas per hour, each lasting 10 seconds (**apnoea/hypopnoea index (AHI) > 15**). These are usually associated with **oxygen desaturation of >4%**. For OSA to be regarded as clinically significant (requiring treatment), the patient should have typical symptoms (e.g. daytime sleepiness) combined with an apnoea/hypopnoea index > 15. Using these criteria, about 4% of middle-aged men and 2% of women have OSA.

Treatment

General measures

Weight loss is an important treatment for patients who are overweight, although it is difficult to achieve. Even a small loss in weight can result in a significant improvement, with a 10% reduction in weight typically resulting in an improvement in the AHI. In very severe cases, bariatric surgery has been employed, which has a proven effect on OSA. Aggravating factors

should be removed by **avoidance of alcohol and sedatives** before sleep. Snoring and OSA are more common when the patient sleeps lying on their back, so measures such as sewing a tennis ball on to the back of the patient's pyjamas have sometimes been employed to **discourage sleeping on the back**. **Tonsillectomy**, excision of nasal polyps or correction of a deviated nasal septum may be appropriate in some cases. Attention should also be directed towards eliminating any **concomitant risk factors** for cardiovascular disease. Any **underlying lung disease** (e.g. COPD) should be treated appropriately.

Nasal CPAP

Nasal CPAP (e.g. 5–15 cmH$_2$O) applied via a tight-fitting **nasal mask** has become the standard first-choice treatment for OSA. It is very effective and acts by splinting the pharyngeal airway open, counteracting the tendency to airway collapse. It can be cumbersome treatment, and some patients have had difficulty in adhering to this treatment in the long term. However, modern CPAP machines are smaller and quieter, with good long-term adherence, especially in those with severe OSA.

When there is coexistent hypoventilation syndrome (e.g. in the very obese), CPAP alone is unlikely to be effective and NIPPV is required.

In addition to the positive benefits on the associated hypersomnolence of OSA, there is evidence of a moderate benefit of CPAP on hypertension. The long-term prognosis of OSA is not fully understood, but some studies have shown a significantly higher mortality in patients who refused treatment than in those whose sleep apnoea was controlled by CPAP.

Other therapies

The lower jaw may be held in an open, slightly advanced position by the use of specifically designed **mandibular advancement devices** that are worn over the teeth. The forward movement of the mandible increases the cross-sectional area of the oropharynx. A recent randomised, controlled trial of dental devices has shown they are effective for mild to moderate OSA.

One unusual study showed that training of the upper airway muscles by didgeridoo playing reduced the collapsibility of the upper airways and improved sleepiness and the AHI. There is ongoing work on **pharyngeal stimulation**.

Uuvulopalatopharyngoplasty (UPPP) involves the surgical excision of redundant tissue of the soft palate, uvula and pharyngeal walls in order to increase the calibre of the pharyngeal airway. It is effective in stopping snoring but its effect on sleep apnoea is unpredictable, and where beneficial, the effect is often short-lived. Side effects include postoperative pain, changes in the quality of the voice and, sometimes, nasal regurgitation during swallowing.

Central sleep apnoea

Central sleep apnoea is a relatively uncommon condition in which cessation of airflow at the nose and mouth is associated with a lack of respiratory muscle activity. It is associated with an **unstable ventilatory control system**, which may arise in a variety of different circumstances. For example, **Cheyne–Stokes respiration** is a pattern of irregular breathing with periods of apnoea followed by hyperventilation seen in patients with cardiac failure when the carotid body is slow in responding to changes in ventilation because of a prolonged circulation time. Periodic breathing develops in most people at high altitude, when hypoxia results in hyperventilation, hypocapnia and ventilatory instability. Sometimes, OSA seems to provoke reflex inhibition of inspiratory drive, so that central apnoeas follow classic obstructive apnoeas. Patients with this reflex central apnoea respond to nasal CPAP. Primary central sleep apnoea is very rare but may result from instability of respiratory drive due to damage to the respiratory centres by brainstem infarcts or syringobulbia. Most of these patients also have hypercapnic respiratory failure when awake, and NIPPV is the main form of treatment used.

> **KEY POINTS**
>
> - Ventilatory failure is often exaggerated during sleep. Treatment involves augmentation of ventilation, such as NIPPV, and not CPAP.
> - OSA is caused by pharyngeal collapse during sleep, resulting in apnoea, arousal, sleep fragmentation and daytime sleepiness.
> - OSA is a serious condition, causing daytime sleepiness, poor quality of life and road accidents.
> - OSA is associated with an increased risk of hypertension, strokes and myocardial infarctions.
> - CPAP is the main treatment for OSA and acts by splinting the pharyngeal airway open during sleep.

FURTHER READING

American Sleep Apnoea Association Web site (www.sleepapnea.org, last accessed 29 December 2014).

Johansson K, Neovius M, Lagerros YT, et al. Effect of a very low energy diet on moderate and severe obstructive sleep apnoea in obese men: a randomised controlled trial. *BMJ* 2009; **339**: 1365.

John MW. A new method for measuring daytime sleepiness: the Epworth sleepiness scale. *Sleep* 1991; **14**: 540–5.

McNicholas WT. Diagnosis of obstructive sleep apnoea in adults. *Proc Am Thorac Soc* 2008; **5**: 154–60.

Ozsancak A, D'Ambrosio C, Hill NS. Nocturnal non-invasive ventilation. *Chest* 2008; **133**: 1275–86.

Peters RW. Obstructive sleep apnoea and cardiovascular disease. *Chest* 2005; **127**: 1–3.

Puhan MA, Suarez A, Cascio CL, et al. Didgeridoo playing as alternative treatment for obstructive sleep apnoea syndrome: a randomised controlled trial. *BMJ* 2006; **332**: 266–8.

Scottish Intercollegiate Guidelines Network. *Management of Obstructive Sleep Apnoea/Hypopnoea Syndrome in Adults*. Edinburgh: Scottish Intercollegiate Guidelines Network, 2003.

Sleep Apnoea Trust Web site (www.sleep-apnoea-trust.org, last accessed 29 December 2014).

Suratt PM, Findley LJ. Serious motor vehicle crashes: the cost of untreated sleep apnoea. *Thorax* 2001; **56**: 505.

Tasali E, Ip MS. Obstructive sleep apnoea and metabolic syndrome: alterations in glucose metabolism and inflammation. *Proc Am Thorac Soc* 2008; **5**: 207–17.

West SD, McBeath HA, Stradling JR. Obstructive sleep apnoea in adults. *BMJ* 2009; **338**: 1165–7.

Multiple choice questions

18.1 The most effective treatment of obstructive sleep apnoea is:
  A oxygen
  B nitrazepam night sedation
  C continuous positive airway pressure (CPAP)
  D uvulopalatopharyngoplasty
  E mandibular advancement devices

18.2 The prevalence of obstructive sleep apnoea in middle-aged men is approximately:
  A 4%
  B 10%
  C 20%
  D 30%
  E 40%

18.3 The main treatment for oxygen desaturation during sleep in patients with neuromuscular disease is:
  A oxygen
  B CPAP
  C weight reduction
  D mandibular advancement devices
  E noninvasive positive pressure ventilation

18.4 Obstructive sleep apnoea:
  A particularly occurs during non-REM sleep
  B is less common in men than women
  C does not occur in children
  D is more common when lying supine
  E only occurs in overweight people

18.5 Obstructive sleep apnoea results from:
  A weakness of the respiratory muscles
  B episodes of upper airway obstruction
  C loss of ventilatory drive from the respiratory centre in the brain stem
  D nocturnal bronchospasm
  E pulmonary oedema and paroxysmal nocturnal dyspnoea

18.6 In ventilatory failure, a typical blood gas finding is:
  A isolated fall in pO_2
  B isolated rise in pCO_2
  C rise in both pCO_2 and pO_2
  D fall in both pCO_2 and pO_2
  E rise in pCO_2 and fall in pO_2

18.7 Recognised causes of chronic respiratory failure include:
  A kyphoscoliosis
  B obesity
  C COPD
  D asthma
  E pneumonia

18.8 In chronic ventilatory failure, ventilation can be improved during sleep using:
  A CPAP
  B bi-level positive airways pressure (BiPAP)
  C supplemental oxygen
  D sedative medication taken at bedtime
  E mandibular advancement splints

18.9 Obstructive sleep apnoea may be associated with:
  A death from road traffic accidents
  B loss of libido
  C daytime hyper-somnolence
  D stroke
  E hypertension

18.10 In chronic ventilatory failure, supplemental oxygen:
  A will prolong life
  B will improve morning headaches if used at night
  C is dangerous and should not be used
  D is purely for symptomatic relief of breathlessness
  E can be used in addition to noninvasive ventilation

Multiple choice answers

18.1 C

CPAP is very effective and has become the standard treatment of obstructive sleep apnoea. Uvulopalatopharyngoplasty is primarily used to reduce snoring but its effect on sleep apnoea is unpredictable.

18.2 A

About 4% of middle-aged men and 2% of middle-aged women have obstructive sleep apnoea.

18.3 E

Patients with neuromuscular weakness who hypoventilate during sleep require non-invasive ventilation rather than CPAP.

18.4 D

Apnoeas are more common when patients are supine, lying on their backs. Sleep apnoea is more common during REM sleep. It is not confined to people who are overweight. It also occurs in children, when it may be related to enlarged tonsils and adenoids.

18.5 B

Obstructive sleep apnoea results from recurrent episodes of upper airway occlusion during sleep. Sleep disturbance from nocturnal wheeze in patients with asthma and from pulmonary oedema in patients with paroxysmal nocturnal dyspnoea due to cardiac failure do not result from obstructive sleep apnoea.

18.6 E

18.7 A,B,C,D

Asthma less commonly so, although it occurs more often in older patients with long-term, fixed airway obstruction

18.8 B

A difference between inspiratory and expiratory pressure is required to augment ventilation. BiPAP does this, CPAP does not.

18.9 All of them

18.10 E

19

Lung transplantation

Introduction

Lung transplantation is an established treatment option for selected patients with end-stage lung disease who have failed to respond to maximum medical treatment. However, the number of donor lungs available is far fewer than the number of patients with advanced lung disease that could potentially benefit from the procedure, and difficult decisions therefore have to be made in order to optimise the use of this scarce resource. Lung transplantation is a major surgical procedure, with substantial mortality and morbidity in patients who are already critically ill, and there is often a short window of opportunity in which patients are sick enough to need transplantation but well enough to undergo the procedure. Unfortunately, deterioration in a patient's condition may happen while they are on the active transplant waiting list, such that about 30% of patients die before donor lungs become available.

The first heart transplantation was performed in 1967 in Groote Schuur Hospital, South Africa, when a man in end-stage cardiac failure received the heart of a young woman killed in a road traffic accident. Initial attempts at lung transplantation were unsuccessful, but surgical advances, better selection of suitable patients and the introduction of ciclosporin immunosuppression allowed the first successful heart–lung transplantation to be performed in 1981 in Stanford, USA in a patient with primary pulmonary hypertension. Today there are about 44 000 patients on the registry of the International Society of Heart Lung Transplantation, which records all those who have undergone lung transplantation worldwide.

Types of operation

Surgical techniques have been developed for the transplant of a single lung, both lungs or the heart and lungs together. Approximately 3700 procedures are now performed every year worldwide.

Heart–lung transplant

The recipient's diseased lungs and heart are removed through a median sternotomy and the donor lungs and heart are implanted as a block. If the recipient's heart is normal, it may be donated to another patient (domino procedure).

Single-lung transplant

A diseased lung is removed through a thoracotomy incision, leaving the heart and contralateral lung intact. The donor lung is then implanted using a bronchial anastomosis. The residual native lung must be free of infection or it will be a source of sepsis in the postoperative period, when the patient is immunosuppressed; this procedure is thus not suitable for patients with cystic fibrosis, for example. The donor's heart and other lung are available to transplant to other patients.

Bilateral lung transplant

- **Double-lung transplant.** The diseased lungs are removed through a median sternotomy, leaving the heart intact. The donor lungs are implanted as a block using a tracheal anastomosis.

Respiratory Medicine Lecture Notes, Ninth Edition. Stephen J. Bourke and Graham P. Burns.
© 2015 John Wiley & Sons, Ltd. Published 2015 by John Wiley & Sons, Ltd.
Companion Website: www.lecturenoteseries.com/Respiratory

- **Bilateral sequential single-lung transplant.** A transverse bilateral thoracotomy is performed, dividing the sternum horizontally (clamshell incision). The diseased lungs are removed and two separated lungs are implanted with separate bronchial anastomoses.

Donor organs are normally procured from patients less than 55 years of age who have suffered a catastrophic spontaneous intracranial haemorrhage or a major head injury, have been ventilated on an intensive therapy unit (ITU) and who have then been diagnosed as having suffered brain stem death. There are strict criteria for the diagnosis of brain stem death and the process of organ donation. The use of lungs from deceased non-heart-beating donors after circulatory death is increasing. The vulnerability of the lungs to injury and infection means that many potential donor lungs are unsuitable for transplantation. Ideally, there should be no history of significant respiratory disease and no major chest trauma. The chest X-ray should be clear and gas exchange should be adequate (Po_2 >12 kPa (90 mmHg) on <35% inspired oxygen). The shortage of donor organs has led to efforts to extend these criteria to allow more transplants without jeopardizing outcomes. A balance must be struck between a patient dying on a transplant waiting list and the use of extended-criteria donor lungs. For example, donor lungs from patients who have smoked are associated with slightly reduced long-term outcomes, but the use of these lungs improves the overall survival of patients registered for lung transplantation. A patient who decides against accepting donor lungs from a smoker is at increased risk of dying on the transplant waiting list.

Techniques have been developed to preserve donor lungs for up to 8 hours, allowing emergency transport of donor organs to the recipient. The donor and recipient are matched for ABO blood group, cytomegalovirus status and chest size.

Living lobar transplantation

This is a less common procedure in which a child or small young adult receives two lower lobes from two living donors, but this technique involves significant risks to the living donors, and the technique is not suitable for the majority of patients on a lung transplant waiting list.

Indications for transplantation

Although, in theory, many types of end-stage lung disease would be amenable to transplantation, in practice the lack of donor organs severely restricts the procedure. The median waiting time to transplantation is about 412 days, and, unfortunately, about 30% of patients identified as suitable candidates to undergo lung transplantation die of their underlying lung disease before an organ becomes available. Lung transplantation has proved a successful treatment for patients with cystic fibrosis, idiopathic pulmonary fibrosis, chronic obstructive pulmonary disease (COPD), emphysema caused by α_1-antitrypsin deficiency and other rare diseases such as idiopathic pulmonary hypertension and lymphangioleiomyomatosis. Overall, about 34% of lung transplants are performed for COPD, 24% for fibrotic lung disease and 17% for cystic fibrosis.

There is usually a window of opportunity in which the patient is **ill enough to need a lung transplant** but **not so ill as to be unable to withstand** the surgery. Furthermore, the patient must be aware of the limitations, risks and benefits of transplantation and must actively **want to undergo** the operation. In patients with cystic fibrosis, for example, a forced expiratory volume in 1 second (FEV_1) of 30% predicted, a Po_2 < 7.5 kPa (55 mmHg) and a Pco_2 > 6.5 kPa (50 mmHg) are associated with a 50% mortality within 2 years, and it is at this stage that lung transplantation may be the best treatment option (Fig. 19.1). The patient needs time to understand the severity of the disease, the predicted prognosis and what is involved in lung transplantation. Addressing these issues is traumatic for the patient and his or her family. Some patients with advanced lung disease want to try all available treatment options, whereas others fear high-intensity unpleasant interventions and would prefer to take a palliative approach to the terminal stages of their disease.

Contraindications to lung transplantation include the presence of other major organ dysfunction, such as **hepatic** or **renal disease, uncontrolled infection, malignancy, inability to adhere** to a complex treatment regimen, the presence of an **aspergilloma** and **poor nutritional** status. Poor outcomes have

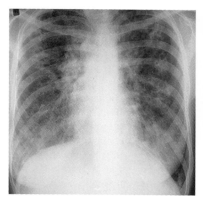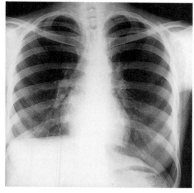

Figure 19.1 This 29-year-old woman developed respiratory failure (Po_2 6 kPa (45 mmHg), Pco_2 8 kPa (60 mmHg)) as a result of advanced cystic fibrosis lung disease (FEV_1 0.5 l). (a) Her chest X-ray shows hyperinflated lungs with diffuse bronchiectasis and peribronchial fibrosis. She was accepted on to a lung transplantation waiting list and supported by oxygen therapy, antibiotics, physiotherapy and nutritional supplements while awaiting donor lungs. Her hypercapnic respiratory failure deteriorated and she was 'bridged' to transplantation by domiciliary intermittent positive-pressure ventilation delivered via a tight-fitting nasal mask. (b) Bilateral sequential single-lung transplantations were performed 14 months after she was accepted on to the waiting list. She subsequently died 5 years post-transplantation of obliterative bronchiolitis.

been reported in patients with cystic fibrosis and coincident *Burkholderia cenocepacia*, such that infection with this organism is now considered a contraindication to transplantation. The success of lung transplantation programmes is based upon careful selection of the small number of patients who can benefit from the procedure and who can be supported long enough to have a realistic chance of getting a donor organ.

Post-transplantation complications and treatment

In the first few days post-transplantation, **reimplantation injury** may occur, with infiltrates developing in the donor lung because of increased capillary permeability as a result of surgical trauma, ischaemia, denervation and lymphatic interruption. Early postoperative **surgical complications** include haemorrhage and dehiscence of the anastomosis.

Prophylactic antibiotics are given to counter **'donor-acquired' infection**, because the donor lungs

are often contaminated by bacteria. Lavage of the donor organ is performed before implantation to identify infection. Intense **immunosuppression**, using a combination of ciclosporin, azathioprine and corticosteroids, is needed to prevent rejection of the donor lungs. Antithymocyte globulin may be given for the first few days to suppress T-cell function.

Patients remain on ciclosporin, prednisolone and azathioprine indefinitely and are at ongoing risk from two particular hazards: **rejection** and **infection**. Both may present with similar clinical features of malaise, pyrexia, infiltrates on chest X-ray, impaired oxygenation and reduced lung function. Bronchoscopy, bronchoalveolar lavage and transbronchial biopsy are the key investigations in identifying rejection of the donor lung and infection. Episodes of **acute rejection** are treated by intensification of immunosuppression (e.g. intravenous methylprednisolone). The treatment of infection is crucially dependent upon identification of the causative organism, because the patient is at risk from both bacterial and **opportunistic infections** (e.g. *Pneumocystis* pneumonia, cytomegalovirus (CMV), fungi; see Chapter 6). *Pneumocystis* pneumonia prophylaxis (e.g. cotrimoxazole) is given routinely. **Lymphoproliferative disorders** such as Epstein–Barr (EB) virus-related B-cell lymphoma may develop as a result of immunosuppression. Treatment consists of aciclovir with a reduction in immunosuppression.

Bronchiolitis obliterans syndrome is the most important complication threatening the long-term survival of patients after lung transplantation. It results from chronic rejection of the donor lungs and is characterised by progressive airway obstruction as a result of obliteration of the bronchioles by organising fibrosis. It may be treated by intensifying or changing the immunosuppressive regimen (e.g. through the use of tacrolimus, sirolimus, mycophenolate mofetil), and azithromycin has a beneficial effect in stabilising lung function. Lung transplant patients are also vulnerable to **gastroesophageal reflux** and gastric aspiration, which is damaging to the lungs.

Drug toxicity is important and levels of drugs such as ciclosporin must be monitored to ensure adequate immunosuppression and to avoid toxicity, such as hypertension, neurotoxicity and renal failure. Care must be taken when prescribing other drugs that might interfere with ciclosporin levels. **Recurrence of the primary disease** in the donor lungs has been documented in recipients with some diseases, such as sarcoidosis, but the outcome has not generally been affected by this in most cases.

Prognosis

Overall, survival rates post-lung transplantation are approximately 80% at 1 year, 55% at 5 years and 30% at 10 years. Patient quality of life is dramatically improved by a successful lung transplantation, but the long-term prognosis is limited, particularly by the occurrence of bronchiolitis obliterans syndrome.

Future prospects

The shortage of donor organs and the occurrence of post-transplant obliterative bronchiolitis are the two main problems to be overcome. Members of the general public are encouraged to volunteer and register for **organ donation** and to discuss their wishes with their families. At present, it is common for families, in the distress of their bereavement, to refuse permission for organ donation, even when the deceased has previously volunteered and registered to donate organs. Fewer than 20% of cadaveric donors have lungs suitable for donation because the lungs of a ventilated patient are very vulnerable to infection,

aspiration and lung injury. Management aimed at **optimising donor lung function** prior to retrieval and better identification of the criteria that make a lung unsuitable for donation might increase the number of useable organs.

Attempts are being made to increase the number of donor organs that can be used through a process of **'reconditioning'**, using a technique of ex vivo lung perfusion, whereby explanted donor lungs are placed in a chamber connected to a heart bypass machine and then treated with nutrient-rich solution to allow damaged cells to repair. This allows some donor organs that initially appear unsuitable to be used. **Xenotransplantation** (the use of animal organs for transplantation in humans) has not been successful because of hyperacute rejection, and there are also concerns about the potential for the spread of animal viruses to humans.

Some new surgical techniques, such as **resizing of lungs**, may also maximise the use of donor lungs. Many women with cystic fibrosis, for example, are of small stature, and many donor lungs may be too large to fit into their thoracic cavity, such that they have a higher death rate because they have to wait longer for suitable lungs. Donor lungs can be 'trimmed' down to size to enable transplantation to proceed.

Some newer techniques can be used to support patients with failing lungs whilst they await transplantation. These include extension of cardiopulmonary bypass technology to add oxygen and remove carbon dioxide, such as **extracorporeal membrane oxygenation** (ECMO) and **Novalung**. However, there may then be a risk of compromising the overall success of transplant surgery, through inclusion of patients who have deteriorated to the extent that they are beyond the transplant window and are at an unacceptably high risk of not surviving transplant surgery. Careful judgement is needed in deciding which patients might benefit from such respiratory support and which may be better served by palliative care. Some patients (e.g. those with COPD) can remain reasonably stable whilst awaiting transplantation, whereas others (e.g. those with cystic fibrosis or idiopathic pulmonary fibrosis) are at particularly high risk of dying. **Lung allocation systems** based on medical urgency might reduce death rates.

It is hoped that the occurrence of bronchiolitis obliterans syndrome can be reduced by measures that reduce gastroesophageal reflux, developments in immunosuppressive therapies (e.g. total lymphoid irradiation) and the use of drugs (e.g. tacrolimus, sirolimus, mycophenolate mofetil and ciclosporin microemulsion formulations).

KEY POINTS

- Lung transplantation is now an established option for some patients with end-stage lung disease.
- There is a critical shortage of donor organs.
- The transplanted lungs are very vulnerable to infection and rejection.
- Bronchiolitis obliterans syndrome is a form of chronic rejection that limits long-term survival.
- Survival rates post-lung transplantation are 80% at 1 year and 55% at 5 years.

 FURTHER READING

Bonser RS, Taylor R, Collett D, et al. Effect of donor smoking on survival after lung transplantation: a cohort study of a prospective registry. *Lancet* 2012; **380**: 747–55.

Cystic Fibrosis Trust. Hope for more: improving access to lung transplantation and care for people with cystic fibrosis 2014 (http://www.cysticfibrosis.org.uk/hopeformore, last accessed 29 December 2014).

Fuehner T, Kuehn C, Hadem J, et al. Extracorporeal membrane oxygenation in awake patients as a bridge to lung transplantation. *Am J Respir Crit Care Med* 2012; **185**: 763–8.

Iversen M, Corris PA. Lung transplantation: immuno-suppression. *Eur Respir Monog* 2009; **45**: 147–68.

Meachery G, DeSoyza A, Nicholson A, et al. Outcome of lung transplantation for cystic fibrosis in a large UK cohort. *Thorax* 2008; **63**: 725–31.

National Institute for Health and Clinical Excellence. *Living-Donor Lung Transplantation for End-Stage Lung Disease. Interventional Procedure Guidance 170.* London: NICE, 2006 (http://www.nice.org.uk/guidance/ipg170/resources/ipg170-living-donor-lung-transplantation-for-endstage-lung-disease-information-for-the-public2, last accessed 29 December 2014).

Verleden GM, Fisher AJ. Indication, patient selection and timing of referral for lung transplantation. *Eur Respir Mon* 2009; **45**: 1–5.

Yusen RD, Christie JD, Edwards LB, et al. The registry of the international society for heart and lung transplantation: transplant report 2013. *J Heart Lung Transplant* 2013; **329**: 65–78.

Multiple choice questions

19.1 Patients with cystic fibrosis are not suitable for:
A single-lung transplantation
B bilateral lung transplantation
C living lobar transplantation
D heart–lung transplantation
E double-lung transplantation

19.2 Patients with cystic fibrosis are not suitable for lung transplantation if they have:
A *Pseudomonas aeruginosa* infection
B respiratory failure
C *Burkholderia cenocepacia* infection
D diabetes
E previous pneumothorax

19.3 The 5-year survival post-lung transplantation is approximately:
A 80%
B 70%
C 55%
D 30%
E 10%

19.4 A major late complication, occurring 5–10 years post-transplantation, is:
A reimplantation injury
B lung cancer
C donor-acquired infection
D dehiscence of the anastomosis
E bronchiolitis obliterans syndrome

19.5 Lung transplantation is not a suitable option for patients with:
A idiopathic pulmonary fibrosis
B lung cancer
C idiopathic pulmonary hypertension
D emphysema
E cystic fibrosis

19.6 The number of lung transplants performed each year worldwide is about:
A 1000
B 1400
C 2200
D 3700
E 5200

19.7 Lungs from donors who have smoked:
A are never used for transplantation
B are associated with a slightly reduced longterm survival rate post-lung transplant
C have the same long-term outcome as donor lungs from nonsmokers
D are not used for young adults with advanced cystic fibrosis
E are not used for patients with emphysema

19.8 The death rate for patients on a lung transplant waiting list is approximately:
A 5%
B 10%
C 20%
D 25%
E 30%

19.9 The most common disease treated by lung transplantation is:
A cystic fibrosis
B idiopathic pulmonary fibrosis
C primary pulmonary hypertension
D COPD
E bronchiolitis obliterans syndrome

19.10 The first successful heart–lung transplantation was performed in:
A 1968
B 1981
C 1991
D 2001
E 2005

Multiple choice answers

19.1 A

Patients with cystic fibrosis are not suitable for single-lung transplantation, as the residual native lung contains infection, which would act as a source of sepsis in the postoperative period.

19.2 C

Unfortunately, the results of the transplantation of patients with cystic fibrosis who had *Burkhoderia cenocepacia* infection were so poor that transplant centres now regard this infection as a major contraindication to transplantation. Previous pneumothorax is not a contraindication to transplantation.

19.3 C

Survival rates post-lung transplantation are approximately 80% at 1 year, 55% at 5 years and 30% at 10 years.

19.4 E

Reimplantation injury, dehiscence of the anastomosis and donor-acquired infection are risks early after transplantation. Bronchiolitis obliterans syndrome is the most important complication threatening the long-term survival of patients with transplanted lungs.

19.5 B

Lung transplantation is a potential treatment for many forms of advanced lung disease, but is not suitable for patients with lung cancer.

19.6 D

Worldwide, about 3700 lung transplants are currently performed each year.

19.7 B

Because of the significant prevalence of smoking in the general population, many potential donor lungs come from patients who have smoked. Research studies show that the results of transplantation are slightly less good with lungs from patients who have smoked than with those from patients who have not. However, using appropriate lungs from donors who have smoked reduces the overall death rate in those on the waiting list. Patients have difficult decisions to make in balancing the immediate high risk of dying while awaiting donor lungs from the slightly less favourable long-term outcome of accepting organs from a donor who has smoked.

19.8 E

Unfortunately, about 30% of patients on an active lung-transplant waiting list die before donor lungs become available

19.9 D

The Registry of the International Society for Heart and Lung Transplantation shows that 34% of lung transplants are performed for COPD, 24% for fibrotic lung disease and 17% for cystic fibrosis.

19.10 B

The first successful combined heart–lung transplant was performed in 1981. This marked the start of the modern era of lung transplantation.

Index

Respiratory Medicine Lecture Notes, Ninth Edition. Stephen J. Bourke and Graham P. Burns.
© 2015 John Wiley & Sons, Ltd. Published 2015 by John Wiley & Sons, Ltd.
Companion Website: www.lecturenoteseries.com/Respiratory